Sports Neurology

Editor

TAD SEIFERT

NEUROLOGIC CLINICS

www.neurologic.theclinics.com

Consulting Editor
RANDOLPH W. EVANS

August 2017 • Volume 35 • Number 3

ELSEVIER

1600 John F. Kennedy Boulevard • Suite 1800 • Philadelphia, Pennsylvania, 19103-2899

http://www.theclinics.com

NEUROLOGIC CLINICS Volume 35, Number 3
August 2017 ISSN 0733-8619, ISBN-13: 978-0-323-53245-7

Editor: Stacy Eastman
Developmental editor: Donald Mumford

Neurologic Clinics (ISSN 0733-8619) is published quarterly by Elsevier Inc., 360 Park Avenue South, New York, NY 10010–1710. Months of issue are February, May, August, and November. Periodicals postage paid at New York, NY, and additional mailing offices. Subscription prices are $306.00 per year for US individuals, $607.00 per year for US institutions, $100.00 per year for US students, $383.00 per year for Canadian individuals, $736.00 per year for Canadian institutions, $423.00 per year for international individuals, $736.00 per year for international institutions, and $210.00 for Canadian and foreign students/residents. To receive student/ resident rate, orders must be accompanied by name of affiliated institution, date of term, and the *signature* of program/residency coordinator on institution letterhead. Orders will be billed at individual rate until proof of status is received. Foreign air speed delivery is included in all *Clinics* subscription prices. All prices are subject to change without notice. **POSTMASTER:** Send address changes to *Neurologic Clinics*, Elsevier Health Sciences Division, Subscription Customer Service, 3251 Riverport Lane, Maryland Heights, MO 63043. **Customer Service: Telephone: 1-800-654-2452 (U.S. and Canada); 314-447-8871 (outside U.S. and Canada). Fax: 314-447-8029. E-mail: journalscustomerservice-usa@elsevier.com (for print support); journalsonlinesupport-usa@elsevier.com (for online support).**

Reprints. For copies of 100 or more of articles in this publication, please contact the Commercial Reprints Department, Elsevier Inc., 360 Park Avenue South, New York, New York, 10010-1710; Tel.: +1-212-633-3874; Fax: +1-212-633-3820, and E-mail: reprints@elsevier.com.

Neurologic Clinics is also published in Spanish by Nueva Editorial Interamericana S.A., Mexico City, Mexico.

Neurologic Clinics is covered in *Current Contents/Clinical Medicine*, *MEDLINE/PubMed (Index Medicus)*, *EMBASE/Excerpta Medica*, and *PsycINFO*, and *ISI/BIOMED*.

Contributors

CONSULTING EDITOR

RANDOLPH W. EVANS, MD
Clinical Professor, Department of Neurology, Baylor College of Medicine, Houston, Texas

EDITOR

TAD SEIFERT, MD
Director, Sports Concussion Program, Norton Healthcare, Neurologist, Norton Neuroscience Institute, Team Neurologist, Western Kentucky University, Department of Athletics, Chairman, Kentucky Boxing and Wrestling Commission, Medical Advisory Panel, Association of Boxing Commissions, Medical Committee, Head, NCAA Headache Task Force, Norton Healthcare, Norton Neurology Services–St. Matthews, Louisville, Kentucky

AUTHORS

MARTINA ANTO-OCRAH, MPH
Departments of Emergency Medicine and Public Health Sciences, University of Rochester, School of Medicine and Dentistry, Rochester, New York

BRETON ASKEN, MS, ATC
Graduate Student, Department of Clinical and Health Psychology, University of Florida, Gainesville, Florida

JULIAN E. BAILES, MD
Department of Neurosurgery, NorthShore University HealthSystem, Evanston, Illinois

JEFFREY J. BAZARIAN, MD, MPH
Departments of Emergency Medicine, Public Health Sciences, Neurology, Neurosurgery, and Physical Medicine and Rehabilitation, University of Rochester, School of Medicine and Dentistry, Rochester, New York

HEIDI K. BLUME, MD, MPH
Associate Professor, Division of Child Neurology, Seattle Children's Hospital and Research Institute, University of Washington, Seattle, Washington

ANDREW BLAKE BULETKO, MD
Fellow, Department of Neurology, Cleveland Clinic, Cleveland, Ohio

R. DAWN COMSTOCK, PhD
Professor, Department of Epidemiology, Colorado School of Public Health, University of Colorado Denver, Aurora, Colorado

HOWARD DERMAN, MD
Associate Professor, Department of Neurology, Weill-Cornell Medical College, Houston Methodist Hospital, Houston Methodist Concussion Center, Houston, Texas

DANIELLE DIACOVO, BA
Department of Emergency Medicine, University of Rochester, School of Medicine and Dentistry, Rochester, New York

THOMAS P. DOMPIER, PhD, ATC
President and Lead Epidemiologist, Datalys Center for Sports Injury Research and Prevention, Indianapolis, Indiana

COURTNEY MARIE CORA JONES, PhD, MPH
Departments of Emergency Medicine and Public Health Sciences, University of Rochester, School of Medicine and Dentistry, Rochester, New York

MELISSA C. KAY, MS, LAT, ATC
Matthew Gfeller Sport-Related Traumatic Brain Injury Research Center, Department of Exercise and Sport Science, Curriculum in Human Movement Science, The University of North Carolina at Chapel Hill, Chapel Hill, North Carolina

ZACHARY Y. KERR, PhD, MPH
Assistant Professor, Department of Exercise and Sport Science, Research Scientist, Injury Prevention Research Center, University of North Carolina, Chapel Hill, North Carolina

SYLVIA LUCAS, MD, PhD, FAHS
Clinical Professor of Neurology and Neurological Surgery, Adjunct Clinical Professor of Rehabilitation Medicine, Department of Neurological Surgery, University of Washington Medical Center, Seattle Sports Concussion Program, Harborview Medical Center, Seattle, Washington

RAMAN K. MALHOTRA, MD
Director, Sleep Medicine Fellowship, Co-Director, Sleep Disorders Center, Associate Professor of Neurology, Saint Louis University School of Medicine, St Louis, Missouri

ROBERT J. MARQUARDT, DO
Resident, Department of Neurology, Cleveland Clinic, Cleveland, Ohio

STEPHEN W. MARSHALL, PhD
Professor, Department of Epidemiology, Director, Injury Prevention Research Center, University of North Carolina, Chapel Hill, North Carolina

MICHAEL A. McCREA, PhD
Professor and Eminent Scholar, Director of Brain Injury Research, Department of Neurosurgery, Medical College of Wisconsin, Milwaukee, Wisconsin

LINDSAY D. NELSON, PhD
Assistant Professor, Department of Neurosurgery, Medical College of Wisconsin, Milwaukee, Wisconsin

RICARDO OLIVO, MD
Assistant Professor of Neurology, Loma Linda University School of Medicine, Loma Linda, California

KENNETH PODELL, PhD
Associate Professor, Department of Neurology, Weill-Cornell Medical College, Houston Methodist Hospital, Houston Methodist Concussion Center, Houston, Texas

CHASE PRESLEY, MS
Department of Neurology, Houston Methodist Hospital, Houston Methodist Concussion Center, Houston, Texas

CLAUDIA L. REARDON, MD
Associate Professor, Department of Psychiatry, University of Wisconsin School of Medicine and Public Health, Counseling and Consultation Services, University Health Services, Madison, Wisconsin

JOHNA K. REGISTER-MIHALIK, PhD, LAT, ATC
Assistant Professor, Department of Exercise and Sport Science, Research Scientist, Injury Prevention Research Center, Matthew Gfeller Sport-Related Traumatic Brain Injury Research Center, The University of North Carolina at Chapel Hill, Chapel Hill, North Carolina

ANDREW NEIL RUSSMAN, DO
Staff Physician, Department of Neurology, Cleveland Clinic, Cleveland, Ohio

TAD SEIFERT, MD
Director, Sports Concussion Program, Norton Healthcare, Neurologist, Norton Neuroscience Institute, Team Neurologist, Western Kentucky University, Department of Athletics, Chairman, Kentucky Boxing and Wrestling Commission, Medical Advisory Panel, Association of Boxing Commissions, Medical Committee, Head, NCAA Headache Task Force, Norton Healthcare, Norton Neurology Services–St. Matthews, Norton Medical Plaza 2–St. Matthews, Louisville, Kentucky

BRIAN SINDELAR, MD
Department of Neurosurgery, NorthShore University HealthSystem, Evanston, Illinois; Department of Neurosurgery, University of Florida, Gainesville, Florida

AMAAL JILANI STARLING, MD
Assistant Professor, Neurology, Mayo Clinic, Phoenix, Arizona

KRISTEN STEENERSON, MD
Neuro-Otology Fellow, Neurology, Barrow Neurological Institute, Phoenix, Arizona

BRYAN TSAO, MD
Chair, Associate Professor, Department of Neurology, Loma Linda University School of Medicine, Loma Linda, California

TAMARA C. VALOVICH MCLEOD, PhD, ATC, FNATA
Professor, Athletic Training Programs, School of Osteopathic Medicine, A.T. Still University, Mesa, Arizona

ERIN B. WASSERMAN, PhD
Sports Injury Epidemiologist, Director of the NCAA Injury Prevention Program, Datalys Center for Sports Injury Research and Prevention, Indianapolis, Indiana

SCOTT L. ZUCKERMAN, MD
Resident Fellow, Department of Neurological Surgery, Vanderbilt University Medical Center, Vanderbilt University School of Medicine, Nashville, Tennessee

Contents

Concussion is a complex injury that requires a multimodal assessment to identify and manage the resulting dysfunction. To appropriately manage concussion, clinicians must be aware of the accompanying pathophysiology and dysfunction that occurs following the injury. The current best practice model of care includes symptom, motor, and neurocognitive assessment and management. Furthermore, clinicians should be aware that lifetime accumulation of head impacts may also play a role in neurologic presentation and response to concussion. This article reviews recent evidence concerning terminology, pathophysiology, epidemiology, and best practices in concussion management and potential long-term and cumulative implications of concussion.

Concussion pathophysiology is complicated and involves numerous mechanisms, including excessive neurotransmitter release, metabolic derangements, neuroinflammation, cerebral blood flow changes, and axonal disruption. The initial biomechanical impact in a concussion results in abnormal function at the cellular level, which initiates a cascade of events that leads to microstructural changes and, in the minority of cases, more persistent, permanent damage.

Numerous sports injury surveillance systems exist with the capability of tracking concussion incidence data. It is important for the consumers of sport-related concussion data, be they researchers or the public, to have a comprehensive understanding of the strengths and limitations of sports injury surveillance systems. This article discusses issues of system design and analysis that affect the interpretation and understanding of sport-related concussion incidence data from sports injury surveillance systems. Such understanding will help inform the design of sports injury surveillance systems and research studies that aim to identify risk factors, develop prevention strategies, and evaluate prevention mechanisms.

provide a brief, high-level overview of current approaches to best practice in neuropsychological assessment of SRC.

Sylvia Lucas and Heidi K. Blume

Headache occurring in a sports setting may be primary or secondary headache. Headache is the primary symptom reported after concussion. Cumulative incidence and prevalence of posttraumatic headache (PTH) are higher following mild traumatic brain injury (TBI) compared with moderate to severe TBI. Frequency is higher in those with more severe PTH. Migraine or probable migraine is the most common headache type after any severity TBI using primary headache disorder criteria. Management is empiric. Expert opinion recommends treating PTH according to clinical characteristics of primary headache. The most important factor in this approach is the recognition of the severity of headache.

Tad Seifert

Neurologic injuries of both an acute and chronic nature have been reported in the literature for various combat sport styles; however, reports of the incidence and prevalence of these injury types vary greatly. Combat sports clinicians must continue to strive for the development, implementation, and enforcement of uniform minimum requirements for brain safety. These health care providers must also seize on the honor to provide this oft-underserved population with the health care advocacy they very much deserve, but often do not receive.

Claudia L. Reardon

Athletes are not immune to mental illness, despite outward appearances of strength and wellness. Depression and anxiety disorders may occur in athletes at least as commonly as in the general population. Eating disorders, attention-deficit/hyperactivity disorder, and substance use disorders may occur even more frequently in athletes than in the general population. Thus, it is imperative that medical professionals across all specialties are aware of these psychiatric comorbidities, and how to initiate evaluation for and treatment of them.

Raman K. Malhotra

Poor sleep can lead to decreases in performance and recovery for athletes. Sleep disorders and symptoms are commonly seen in athletes, and may be unrecognized. It is important to educate athletes on adequate duration, quality, and timing of sleep. Interventions may include changes to practice times or careful planning for travel to games in different time zones. It is important to screen and treat sleep disorders such as sleep apnea and insomnia that are seen in some athletes. In patients who suffer concussion, it is important to address sleep issues, as poor sleep can prolong or exacerbate other concussion symptoms.

Sport-related peripheral nerve injuries (SRNIs) can occur in virtually any sport whether or not enjoyed by an amateur or in the career of a professional athlete. The diagnosis of SRNIs can be difficult, especially when trying to differentiate nerve injury from musculoskeletal pain. Clinicians should be able to recognize when a significant SRNI occurs and how to initiate a diagnostic and treatment pathway and referral to a specialist. This article reviews SRNIs and their specific sports, how to diagnose SRNIs, and how to select conservative or surgical management of these injuries.

Noncontact sports are associated with a variety of neurologic injuries. Concussion, vascular injury (arterial dissection), and spinal cord trauma may be less common in noncontact sports, but require special attention from the sports neurologist. Complex regional pain disorders, muscle injury from repetitive use, dystonia, heat exposure, and vascular disorders (patent foramen ovale), occur with similar frequency in noncontact and contact sports. Management of athletes with these conditions requires an understanding of the neurologic consequences of these disorders, the risk of injury with return to play, and consideration for the benefits of exercise in health restoration and disease prevention.

NEUROLOGIC CLINICS

RELATED INTEREST

Physical Medicine and Rehabilitation Clinics of North America
May 2017 (Vol. 28, Issue 2)
Traumatic Brain Injury Rehabilitation
Blessen C. Eapen and David X. Cifu, *Editors*

THE CLINICS ARE AVAILABLE ONLINE!
Access your subscription at:
www.theclinics.com

Preface

Sports Neurology

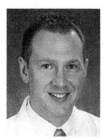

Tad Seifert, MD
Editor

Sports neurology is an evolving field with wide-reaching implications for multiple medical providers. Countless disciplines encounter active individuals, from both a competitive and a layperson standpoint. These expert providers include general neurologists, neurosurgeons, orthopedists, pediatricians, internists, physiatrists, certified athletic trainers, neuropsychologists, physical therapists, chiropractors, sports psychologists, and many others. Despite recent strides made within the field of sports neurology, much remains unknown. The spectrum of sports concussion pathophysiology provides an ideal example, as the management of this injury at times requires as much art of medicine as do approaches grounded in evidence-based science. There is also no other medical discipline where knowing the patient is so imperative to the ensuing recovery. Such preexisting conditions and comorbidities often are amplified in the context of neurologic-related injury; subsequently, providing "whole patient" care is often necessary to ensure optimal recovery.

Despite these inherent challenges, the frontline of sports neurology is not a place for doubt to prevail. Unmitigated confidence among all practitioners is necessary for the consummate protection of the central and peripheral nervous systems in sport. This issue of *Neurologic Clinics* provides 13 articles specific to the practice of sports neurology. The content extends far beyond sports concussion, although this remains the most prominent injury within our field; however, as the popularity of other sports continues to grow, so does our role as sideline, training room, and traditional outpatient clinic providers. Despite headache being the most common symptom of competitive athletes presenting for formal neurologic input, other clinical states exist. These include peripheral nerve injuries, sleep disruption, psychiatric comorbidities, and the overall process of an athlete returning to sport participation safely after injury.

This issue nicely merges the knowledge gained from prior studies with new data from ongoing projects, such as the National Collegiate Athletic Association (NCAA) and the US Department of Defense's (DoD) landmark $30 million initiative known as

http://dx.doi.org/10.1016/j.ncl.2017.05.001
0733-8619/17/© 2017 Published by Elsevier Inc.
neurologic.theclinics.com

the NCAA-DoD Grand Alliance. Within this framework, the *Concussion Assessment, Research, and Education Consortium* serves as the scientific and operational framework for the Concussion Research Initiative of the Grand Alliance. Within this issue, you will learn more about this project as well as its ongoing data collection. I am extremely grateful to each outstanding contributor within concussion as well as other subtopics. They are truly the expert researchers, physicians, clinicians, and leaders within this unique field of medicine.

It is an exciting time to practice within the context of sports neurology. Each day I'm allowed to unite my two key clinical interests: sports medicine and neurology. I've been blessed to have a number of incredible mentors within the field, such as Jeff Kutcher, MD, Barry Jordan, MD, MPH, Chris Giza, MD, Vern Williams, MD, Ninan Mathew, MD, Randy Evans, MD, Merle Diamond, MD, Timothy Smith, MD, Rph, Dawn Buse, PhD, Anthony Alessi, MD, Sylvia Lucas, MD, Brian Hainline, MD, Allen Sills, MD, James Couch, MD, Mya Schiess, MD, Margaret Goodman, MD, James Ferrendelli, MD, Grant Iverson, PhD, James Andrews, MD, Brad Bluestone, ATC, Bill Edwards, ATC, and Scott Anderson, ATC. Through this issue, each reader is afforded that same opportunity of attaining knowledge, but also establishing a fellowship of like-minded clinicians within our field. Feel free to reach out to me or any of my coauthors at any time via the e-mail address provided below. I hope you enjoy this special issue of *Neurologic Clinics*, and continued success to each of you.

Tad Seifert, MD
Norton Neurology Services
3991 Dutchmans Lane, Suite 310
Louisville, KY 40207, USA

E-mail address:
tad.seifert@nortonhealthcare.org

The Current State of Sports Concussion

Johna K. Register-Mihalik, PhD, LAT, ATC[a,b,*], Melissa C. Kay, MS, LAT, ATC[a,c]

KEYWORDS

- Brain injury • Head injury • Sport-related concussion • Return to play • Management
- Assessment • Concussion • Head trauma

KEY POINTS

- Concussion is a complex injury that requires a multimodal assessment and treatment process.
- The varying terminology and lack of consensus on treatment make it key for clinicians to educate and discuss expectations with patients and their families.
- The approach to concussion management should address all aspects of patients' lives, including daily activities and return to school, work, and sport.
- This multimodal approach should include a strong clinical evaluation with symptom, motor/balance, and neurocognitive considerations.
- Using these best practices, clinicians will have a more complete picture of the concussion puzzle initially and throughout the recovery process to guide decision-making and management.

CONCUSSION OVERVIEW AND DEFINITION

Sport-related concussion is one of the most complex sport-related injuries clinicians manage. In addition, there is increased societal interest and a growing body of evidence in the medical literature concerning the sequelae following concussion that is evolving at a rapid pace. Therefore, there are several concussion definitions and guidelines in which clinicians and the lay community turn for information and guidance. Because of the complexity of concussion (**Fig. 1**), these multiple definitions and guidelines often lead to variation in how an individual concussion is managed. Athletes may experience an injury that is managed in a conservative nature by a clinician, whereas

[a] Matthew Gfeller Sport-Related Traumatic Brain Injury Research Center, Department of Exercise and Sport Science, The University of North Carolina at Chapel Hill, Chapel Hill, NC, USA; [b] Injury Prevention Research Center, The University of North Carolina at Chapel Hill, Chapel Hill, NC, USA; [c] Curriculum in Human Movement Science, The University of North Carolina at Chapel Hill, Chapel Hill, NC, USA
* Corresponding author. Injury Prevention Research Center, The University of North Carolina at Chapel Hill, Chapel Hill, NC.
E-mail address: johnakay@email.unc.edu

Neurol Clin 35 (2017) 387–402
http://dx.doi.org/10.1016/j.ncl.2017.03.009   **neurologic.theclinics.com**
0733-8619/17/© 2017 Elsevier Inc. All rights reserved.

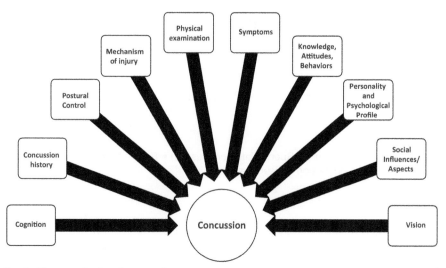

Fig. 1. The complexity of concussion.

other individuals who have similar presentations are minimized. Previously, it was common practice for an individual to only be diagnosed with a concussion if they experienced a loss of consciousness (LOC) and/or amnesia.[1] However, literature suggests that only 9% of concussed individuals also experience a LOC, whereas only 23% experience posttraumatic amnesia.[2] Despite literature suggesting that LOC has no bearing on severity of injury, including symptomology, neurocognition, and recovery,[3–5] many of the available resources for concussion diagnosis imply the opposite. In addition, many individuals, especially in the sport community, still think that LOC always accompanies a concussion.[6]

Concussions are often distinguished as a subset of mild traumatic brain injury (TBI).[7] Even though this subset is agreed on by experts in the field, the true definition of concussion is evolving and suffers from frequent disagreement in the use of descriptive terminology.[8] In fact, in 2012, experts discussed not including *mild* when discussing a concussion but simply labeling concussion a brain injury to be sure the effects were not minimized.[7] In recent years, experts continue to rely on a consensus process to determine appropriate components of a concussion definition, which include an injury that results from a blow to the head or body that causes an alteration in mental status and one or more of the following symptoms: headache, nausea, vomiting, dizziness/balance problems, fatigue, difficulty sleeping, drowsiness, sensitivity to light or noise, blurred vision, memory deficits, and difficulty concentrating.[2,9] Other definitions include "a complex pathophysiological process affecting the brain, induced by traumatic biomechanical forces,"[7] and "a clinical syndrome of biomechanically induced alteration of brain function, typically affecting memory and orientation, which may involve loss of consciousness."[10] Despite the varying definitions that exist, each contains the same basic components: a biomechanical mechanism, altered mental status, and some type of resulting, typically transient, symptomology. The International Concussion in Sport Group's definition also highlights key clinical features of concussion such as the following: typically results in rapid onset of neurologic impairments, concussion is a functional, not structural, injury, may or may not include LOC, and is not identifiable on standard imaging (computed tomography [CT], MRI).[7]

EPIDEMIOLOGY

There are more than 1,224,000 emergency department visits, 290,000 hospitalizations, and 51,000 deaths each year resulting from TBIs, making it one of the most disabling and burdensome injuries in the United States.[11] The Centers for Disease Control and Prevention estimates that between 1.6 and 3.8 million sports-related brain injuries occur each year and concussions account for approximately 10% to 15% of all sport-related injuries.[1,12] Problems and disabilities following TBI, such as concussion, may lead to emotional, physical, academic, cognitive, and social dysfunction, all of which may result in overall decreased quality of life and burden to families as well as the general health care system.[13–15]

As expected, collision sports, such as football and ice hockey, continue to have the highest incidence of concussion[16–20]; but sports such as soccer, lacrosse, and basketball also have high concussion rates. However, it should be noted that concussion occurs in all sports and activities.[21] Concussion rates in football range from 3.52 per 1000 athlete exposures in college to 1.61 in high school and 2.13 at youth levels during competition.[22] Concussion rates in soccer range from 1.08 per 1000 athlete exposures in college[23] to 2.78 per 10,000 athlete exposures in high school[24] and 0.19 per 1000 athletic exposure at youth levels.[25] As stated, recent reports suggest concussion itself accounts for up to 14% of all injuries occurring in sport.[26] In the high school population, it is estimated that more than 700,000 concussions occurred from 2005 to 2010, with 13% of these injuries being recurrent or subsequent concussions.[27]

In matched women's sports, such as soccer and basketball, female athletes have nearly 2.0 times the risk of concussion compared with their male counterparts in the high school age group[28] and around 1.4 times higher in college.[29] There are no confirmations as to why this difference exists. However, anthropometrics,[30] such as neck muscle strength, and preparation have been posited as potential explanations. There are also medical reports that indicate females are more likely to seek medical care and report symptoms of many various conditions than males.[31–33] Overall, the literature has become consistent that in male and female matched sports, females have a higher incidence of concussion, especially at the high school level. The summary of recent publications indicates that in these similar sports, females' risk of concussions is almost twice that of males.[28]

The population of youth sport athletes presents unique characteristics that make the epidemiologic study of concussion and other injuries particularly difficult. One characteristic is the varying levels of coverage at youth sporting events that is often much less in comparison with high school and collegiate events. Unlike the high school and collegiate populations, there are no surveillance systems in place at the youth level nationally, regionally, or even statewide in which epidemiologic data can be gathered. Because of the lack of medical presence, few studies to date exist that examine the epidemiologic concerns of injury. Among the literature that exists, similar patterns are shown when compared with high school and collegiate concussive injury rates. For example, a study of American youth football found a concussion incidence rate to be 1.76 per 1000 athlete exposures that is higher in competition (6.16) and lower in practice (0.24).[34]

Unlike the youth population, there are more available data highlighting the presence of concussion at the high school level of play. When examining the data, it shows that concussion rates have increased in the past few years, up through 2014.[28] Part of this may be attributed to greater awareness and understanding of concussion and the passage of state concussion legislation, which may have influenced the reporting of concussionlike symptoms and improved identification. In high school sports, the concussion incidence rates are relatively consistent across recent studies but variable among sports. Overall incidence has been suggested to be 0.23 to 0.24 per 1000 athlete exposures, with sport-specific values of the following: football 0.47 to 0.60, boys lacrosse 0.28 to 0.30, girls lacrosse 0.21,[35] boys soccer 0.17 to 0.22, girls soccer 0.35 to 0.36, girls volleyball 0.05, boys basketball 0.07 to 0.10, girls basketball 0.16 to 0.21, wrestling 0.17 to 0.18, baseball 0.05 to 0.06, softball 0.07 to 0.11, cheerleading 0.06 to 0.09,[36] and field hockey 0.10.[21,28]

In collegiate athletics, some studies suggest concussions occur at a higher incidence and that there is a more even distribution between sexes in comparison with high school athletes.[21] Within specific collegiate sports, the incidence rates of concussions have been shown to be the following per 1000 athlete exposures: football 0.37 to 0.61, men's lacrosse 0.26, women's lacrosse 0.25, men's soccer 0.28 to 0.49, women's soccer 0.41 to 0.63, men's basketball 0.07 to 0.09, women's basketball 0.22 to 0.43, wrestling 0.25 to 0.42, softball 0.14 to 0.19, and field hockey 0.18.[21,37] Despite heavy public focus on the realm of professional sports, there are little data to support epidemiologic findings related to concussions. Two of the primary sports in which this has been studied is in ice hockey (National Hockey League [NHL]) and football (National Football League [NFL]). In the NHL, the concussion incidence rate is 1.8 per 1000 athlete exposures, whereas the NFL has a rate of 6.43 per 1000 athlete exposures.

Because of the ever-evolving definition of concussion as previously highlighted, it can be difficult to acquire epidemiologic data that are reliable and of high quality. Studies range from requiring a LOC to constitute a concussion[38] to extremely broad definitions in which reported injuries may or may not be a concussion.[21] These varying definitions can cause the clinicians who are reporting these injury data to provide variable results due to the symptoms of a concussion also overlapping with and being influenced by other conditions, such as hydration level, fatigue, and time in season.[39–41] Furthermore, because concussion may not be identified if the athlete does not disclose the injury, epidemiologic studies likely underestimate the incidence of concussion in sport.

MECHANISM/PATHOPHYSIOLOGY OF CONCUSSION
Mechanism of Injury

Concussion is often described as a diffuse injury that involves an acceleration-deceleration mechanism[42] leading to more functional, not structural damage. This damage causes transient neurologic deficits.[43] The brain accelerates, which causes a lag and maximizes shearing forces on impact.[42,44] Forces can be compressive, tensile, or rotational and result in a coup (same side) and/or countercoup (opposite side) injury. Coup injuries typically occur when there is a blow to a moving head or body, whereas countercoup injuries more commonly occur when a moving head or body hits a stationary object.[42,44] The countercoup injury is speculated to produce most deficits in concussive injury.[45] Recent real-time collection of head impacts have identified a few areas of important clinical relevance, including the following: (1) There is no known specific threshold for concussive injury, as concussive injuries occur across various magnitudes. (2) There is no support from these recent studies to suggest a relationship between a specific magnitude or location of impact and the result being a concussive injury.[46–48] Although these data have provided important context to the impacts around concussion, there are still many questions that research is attempting to answer.

Overview of Pathophysiology

The previously described forces produce a variety of signs and symptoms due to a complex neuro-metabolic cascade of events. In the acute phase of injury, there is an abrupt release of neurotransmitters and unchecked ionic influxes. As the cascade continues, further neuronal depolarization occurs via an efflux of potassium and influx of calcium affecting cellular physiology. This process causes an energy crisis because the sodium-potassium pump must work overtime to rebalance the ionic shift, which in turn requires more energy. This increased energy need causes glucose metabolism to increase dramatically, resulting in the following presentation: decreased cerebral blood flow, depleted glucose supply, and high glucose (energy) demand. The energy crisis mechanism is speculated to be the cause of postconcussive vulnerability to repeat injury.[43] Following the acute phase of injury, the injured brain goes through a period of depressed metabolic activity. At this time, there are increases in the calcium level potentially impairing cellular function and creating an even larger energy crisis. This continued influx in calcium that is not attenuated may also lead to cell death.[43] Although the acute phase is thought to be the initial cause of symptoms following concussion, the brain is still in a vulnerable state when the metabolic activity remains depressed.

The lack of obvious structural damage with a concussion, coupled with no current ability to measure the metabolic dysfunction in real time, makes it difficult to create a diagnostic gold standard. Therefore, concussions do not show abnormal results on standard imaging measures, such as MRI and CT scans.[49,50] Because of the inability to diagnose via imaging, clinicians primarily focus on the presentation of signs and symptoms warranting management as a potential concussive injury, making the multimodal assessment of concussion essential.

ASSESSMENT

Following a potential concussive injury, it is imperative to diagnose and manage the injury appropriately to avoid unnecessary sequelae and complications. Concussion is often considered a silent epidemic, as several of the symptoms are invisible to the physical eye and require clinical judgment and a battery of assessments to identify. Because of these less visible signs and symptoms, along with variability in presentation, the lack of a gold standard for diagnosis, and the general lack of awareness from those in the community, many concussions go unidentified or unreported.[51–53] When these injuries are not identified or reported appropriately, an individual may be placed at greater risk for future injury or more complicated recovery processes.[9,54,55]

Given these complexities, the assessment and management of concussion should be a multimodal process (**Fig. 2**) that assesses the interaction of the many systems that may be affected following a concussive injury. At a minimum, this process should include a detailed clinical interview and neurologic examination, symptom assessment, cognitive assessment, and motor assessment.[7,10,56] However, recent data have suggested additional metrics should also be used to understand deficits and potential opportunities for treatment, including vestibular and visual screenings.[57]

The clinical interview and examination are the cornerstone of the evaluation and provide the demographic and historical context to understand a patient's concussive injury. Key factors to consider in this process are previous history of head trauma, psychological disorders, neurologic disorders, family history, headache disorders, and additional trauma.

The symptom assessment should be completed using a clinical interview but should also include a checklist whereby individuals rate presence and severity. There are

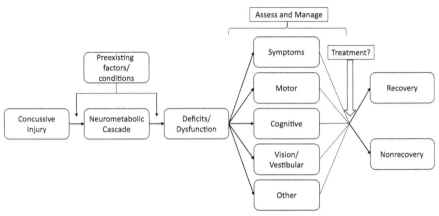

Fig. 2. Progression of concussion management.

various reliable and valid tools from the graded symptoms checklist to the postconcussion symptom scale, which are freely available to clinicians.[58] This type of approach allows clinicians to track symptom trajectory and recovery, including changes in the presence of various symptoms and the severity of those symptoms over time. Recent data suggest the checklist approach is more conservative and allows to better understand what symptoms patients are experiencing.[59] Clusters of symptoms that present together are also important clinical considerations.[7,8] Recent data suggest that the presence of certain clusters of symptoms may be related to recovery time.[9–11] For instance, recent studies highlight that on-field dizziness[10] and potentially the migraine-fatigue cluster[12] may be associated with prolonged recovery. Total symptom severity burden has also been shown to be predictive of prolonged recovery.[13] An additional key advantage to using a symptom checklist is that tracking of symptoms over time or serial assessment guides clinical decision-making concerning both management and treatment options. Assessing symptoms over time also allows for a more informed decision on when to introduce various physical and cognitive activities along the recovery path. These assessments may also aid in knowing when activity should be further limited.

The cognitive assessment may have many levels. There are brief mental status examinations, such as the Standardized Assessment of Concussion (SAC), that may be used. However, the SAC is most sensitive in the first 48 to 72 hours after injury.[2,60] There are other simple screens, such as immediate word memory, delayed word memory, and serial 7s, that can also be included. Traditionally, in the assessment of concussion, computerized neurocognitive testing is used. This assessment includes a computerized assessment of memory, reaction time, processing, attention, and other cognitive domains. These tests often take between 25 and 40 minutes to complete and are offered in a variety of batteries or assessments. For concussion assessments, these computerized programs (ImPACT [ImPACT Applications Inc., San Diego, CA], Automated Neuropsychological Assessment Metrics [ANAM], Concussion Vital Signs, and so forth) consist of a battery including the aforementioned domains in a single tool. Paper and pencil metrics are also available and provide more direct patient interaction. These metrics take a longer amount of time to administer and require additional training in administration and interpretation. One key note when using such measures is that clinicians should be trained in the use of and familiar with the tools being used. Clinicians should also use appropriate expertise of individuals who can interpret and recommend the most appropriate treatment options around the results of neurocognitive measures.[6]

The motor assessment should include an assessment of balance as well as overall co-ordination. There are tools/tests, such as the Balance Error Scoring System (BESS),[61–64] that are not costly and can provide a more objective assessment than a traditional Romberg test as there are varying conditions and associated scores. There are also additional measures, although more costly, that can provide more specific information, such as the Sensory Organization Test (SOT) (NeuroCom, Nautus, Clackamas, OR). These tools may aid in understanding sensory integration in addition to overall balance deficits.[65,66] The American Academy of Neurology's "Summary of Evidence-Based Guideline Update" states deficits on measures such as the BESS and SOT are "likely to be associated with more severe or prolonged concussive impairments."[10]

More recent literature has also suggested that gait metrics should also be considered in the assessment of postural control and coordination,[67–71] as deficits on these metrics may outlast those on more static measures of balance that have been more traditionally used. In addition, recent literature also highlights the potential inclusion of both motor and cognitive tasks concurrently performed to elicit deficits of divided attention, as few to no activities of daily living or sport are completed without attention division. There are various paradigms[72–79] in the literature, including balance or gait tasks, inclusive of cognitive tasks and virtual-reality environments. Examples of these activities include a simple walking task while performing a word memory or digit span task as well as balance tests, such as the BESS, while performing cognitive tasks.

Recently, studies suggest additional measures that may be of great value to the concussion assessment process. These measures include visual and vestibular screenings,[57,80–82] which have been shown to predict prolonged recovery and to delineate concussed patients from controls. However, more studies are needed to fully understand the role of these tools in the concussion assessment process. Another visual screening task of recent interest is the King-Devick Test (R) (King-Devick Test, Inc, Oakbrook Terrace, IL),[83–85] which is a test of visual tracking. Although recent studies show utility,[83,84,86] others question the specificity and its use in various settings, such as the emergency department.[87] Furthermore, there are more advanced diagnostic and prognostic metrics that are currently only used in a research capacity. These metrics include neuroimaging and blood biomarkers. These tools have shown ambiguous results in their abilities to diagnose and understand concussion[88–90]; however, research continues to move the mark toward a more definitive gold standard diagnostic tool for concussion.

MANAGEMENT AND TREATMENT

Management of concussion has typically been characterized by cognitive and physical rest until symptoms resolve. However, recent literature suggest that complete or strict rest may not be most beneficial[91] and that some level of controlled, symptom-guided level of activity may be the best course of action. Following symptom resolution, the recommended steps in the management of concussion are to follow a gradual return-to-play progression for sport. A graduated return protocol is the accepted paradigm for returning an athlete to sport; however, there is varied evidence on the most effective approach. In addition, implementation of the progression varies across settings and health care professionals.

The current recommended graduated return to play (GRTP) protocol seems relatively safe in a college age group. Therefore, clinicians should use, at a minimum, the GRTP protocol guidelines outlined in the CIS group consensus statement[7] in developing and implementing physical return-to-play progressions for concussed athletes. There is limited information on the true efficacy of the protocol in younger age groups. In addition, for school-aged individuals, academic adjustments, such as shortened days, changes in work load, and rest breaks, are likely necessary during the recovery period; before return to activity, a gradual and progressive approach should be used.[56]

Furthermore, there is currently no treatment paradigm for concussion. There are pharmacologic interventions that may be used to treat symptoms, such as headache or sleep disturbances, but none for the concussion itself.[92] In addition, no rehabilitation paradigm has been developed for concussion. Recent evidence suggests that various levels of exercise and types of rehabilitation may be beneficial for individuals with prolonged concussion symptoms. Recent studies, including the Buffalo Concussion Treadmill Test (BCTT), illustrate that the use of symptoms and heart rate to guide intensity of exercise for patients with prolonged concussion symptoms may lead to improvements in symptoms and recovery time.[93–96] The current data suggest that individuals participating in the BCTT and aerobic activity at the threshold heart rate for symptoms have improvements in symptoms.[93–96] In addition, vestibular/cervicogenic programs among individuals with prolonged symptom presentation in these domains have shown success,[97] with individuals having symptoms in those domains and completing a rehabilitation protocol decreasing time for medical clearance to sport. To date, few to no studies have addressed acute intervention and its effect on outcomes.

RECOVERY PATTERNS AND LONG-TERM EFFECTS
Recovery

The definition of recovery in the concussion literature is often vague. Following concussion, one of the primary indicators of recovery among athletes is time to return to play. Studies over the past 15 years have varied in the timing of return to play, with older studies indicating shorter return times[2] and more recent studies highlighting longer return times.[22] Other studies use recovery on a specific metric, such as symptoms. Delayed recovery may be defined as symptoms lasting longer than 10, 14, 21, or 30 days. Many of the current studies use the 3- or 4-week mark as a protracted recovery time. These studies report that approximately 10% to 20% of patients have prolonged symptoms.[57,98,99] There are mixed results on what the key prognostic indicators of symptoms presence may be; however, initial total symptom burden is one of the factors that continues to be present in many studies.[100,101] An additional area of recovery for consideration is cognitive and academic recovery for individuals who are to return to work or school. Few studies have examined return-to-learn times and recovery for school-based activities in combination with return to sport and physical activity.

One study during the 2005 to 2008 school years observed that 15% percent of concussed high school football athletes, who sustained a LOC, returned to play in less than 1 day.[102] In this same study, boys were more likely than girls to return 1 to 2 days after sustaining more severe injuries, 12.0% versus 5.9%.[102] Approximately 40% of concussed athletes returned to play prematurely under the American Academy of Neurology's guidelines and 15% according to the international consensus return-to-play guidelines.[102] A more recent study[22] comparing recovery and symptoms across age groups (youth, high school, college) observed that 15.3% were returned at least 30 days after concussion and 3.8% were returned within the first 24 hours, a much smaller percentage than the earlier study. In this same study, a lengthier return-to-play time period (beyond 30 days) was more likely among youth athletes compared with high school or college.

Literature suggests that adolescent-aged individuals may experience a greater symptom burden, changes in academic performance, and protracted recoveries from subsequent injuries compared with older athletes.[54,55] High school athletes also report more symptoms after concussion.[22] These recovery differences following TBI may also result from the varied cognitive maturity in pediatric individuals.[2,103,104] The younger brain may be particularly vulnerable to injury during this stage of rapid neural development. All current consensus documents recommend no athlete return to participation while symptomatic; this line of best practice, coupled with increased awareness, has likely been the key driver behind extended return-to-play times.

Cumulative and Long-term Effects

Cumulative and potential long-term effects are one of the most discussed topics of concussion. These issues range from suffering multiple concussions (recurrent concussion) to damage that may result from suffering multiple head impacts over the course of a lifetime, even in the absence of a clinically diagnosed concussion. Although no causal studies have been conducted, evidence to date highlights associations between recurrent concussion (specifically 3 or more) and increased initial severity of subsequent concussions; memory issues; concentration deficits; regular headache presence; psychological issues, such as depression and anxiety; or more complicated, later-life issues, such as dementia.[9,54,105,106] More complicated injuries may include more severe signs and symptoms and longer or protracted recovery times. In addition, catastrophic injury, such as second impact syndrome, may result if an individual is returned to activity too soon after an initial concussion.[104] The age at which accumulation of head impacts becomes problematic is unknown. Furthermore, the effects of concussion on neural plasticity and development are unknown.

Despite concussions being defined as an acute injury, sustaining subconcussive impacts is a chronic problem that has received increased discussion over the past 5 years. These subconcussive impacts do not meet the threshold causing an individual to be symptomatic. However, they may still cause an alteration in the neurometabolic cascade, just not to the same extent of initial clinical manifestation. When experienced in a cumulative manner, these additive subconcussive impacts have been associated with potential neurodegeneration and even chronic traumatic encephalopathy (CTE), but more research is needed to deem causality.[107,108] Therefore, current policies and rules have been aimed at reducing the frequency of head impacts in sport to reduce not only concussions but also cumulative exposure to head impacts in sport.

Much of this exposure discussion has largely focused on CTE, a neurodegenerative disease that has been found in former boxing, football, wrestling, and ice hockey athletes and has hallmark signs of diffuse tauopathy with tau-immunoreactive neurofibrillary tangles and threads.[109] The clinical manifestation of the disease is associated with judgment impairments, memory loss, confusion, issues with impulse control, aggression, and depression, which overtime progresses to dementia. It is essential to note that currently, CTE can only be diagnosed postmortem,[109] through an autopsy and corresponding pathologic study, despite many individuals and providers claiming to identify cases of CTE. There are more recent studies that suggest various forms of imaging may be able to pick up the tau protein deposits, characteristic of CTE. However, these are yet to be fully clinically validated and the sample sizes are too small to make conclusions.[110]

The earliest studies of such a condition were in boxers.[37,38] Early estimates suggest that approximately 10% of individuals who receive multiple impacts as a result of sport will develop the disease.[111–113] However, no true epidemiologic studies have confirmed these estimates. Recommendations around these early findings have been centered on limiting exposure to head impacts over a person's lifetime. In addition, no casual studies have been conducted in this area; more research is needed to determine the cause/effect relationship between head impacts and this disease as well as other neurodegenerative conditions.

Much of the data concerning neurodegenerative conditions have been attained from former professional and elite-level athletes. These data suggest associations between concussion and previous history of concussion and depression, mild cognitive impairment, and other psychological and memory-related issues in former American football players.[105,113,114] In ice hockey, similar findings have also been observed.[115] The data concerning former soccer players are more ambiguous. Some data suggest that, when returned, former elite soccer athletes have a prevalence of neurodegenerative conditions in line with the general population.[116] On the contrary, other studies have suggested that exposure to soccer, specifically heading, may be a precursor to such conditions.[117,118] In many instances, the messaging has outpaced the science in our understanding of the link between head impacts and neurodegenerative conditions and the subset of the population that may be most affected by these head impacts. There are numerous studies currently underway to better understand these complex issues and the preventative efforts that should be used.

SUMMARY

Concussion is a complex injury that requires a multimodal assessment and treatment process. The varying terminology and lack of consensus on treatment make it key for clinicians to educate and discuss expectations with patients and their families. The approach to concussion management should address all aspects of patients' lives, including daily activities and return to school, work, and sport. This multimodal approach should include a strong clinical evaluation with symptom, motor/balance, and neurocognitive considerations. Using these best practices, clinicians will have a more complete picture of the concussion puzzle initially and throughout the recovery process to guide decision-making and management. Clinicians should address the key domains of dysfunction following concussion and should ensure that they and their team have the expertise to use and interpret the tools of choice. Current discussions around the treatment and management of concussion include more active approaches that will allow clinicians to provide better patient-centered care for concussive injury.

REFERENCES

1. Powell JW, Barber-Foss KD. Traumatic brain injury in high school athletes. JAMA 1999;282(10):958–63.
2. McCrea M, Guskiewicz KM, Marshall SW, et al. Acute effects and recovery time following concussion in collegiate football players: the NCAA Concussion Study. JAMA 2003;290(19):2556–63.
3. Collins MW, Iverson GL, Lovell MR, et al. On-field predictors of neuropsychological and symptom deficit following sports-related concussion. Clin J Sport Med 2003;13:222–9.
4. Guskiewicz KM, Ross SE, Marshall SW. Postural stability and neuropsychological deficits after concussion in collegiate athletes. J Athl Train 2001;36:263–73.
5. Lovell MR, Iverson GL, Collins MW, et al. Does loss of consciousness predict neuropsychological decrements after concussion. Clin J Sport Med 1999;9: 193–8.

6. Register-Mihalik JK, Guskiewicz KM, McLeod TC, et al. Knowledge, attitude, and concussion-reporting behaviors among high school athletes: a preliminary study. J Athl Train 2013;48(5):645–53.

7. McCrory P, Meeuwisse WH, Aubry M, et al. Consensus statement on concussion in sport: the 4th International Conference on Concussion in Sport held in Zurich, November 2012. Br J Sports Med 2013;47(5):250–8.

8. Gioia GA, Isquith PK, Schneider JC, et al. New approaches to assessment and monitoring of concussion in children. Top Lang Disord 2009;29(3):266–81.

9. Guskiewicz KM, McCrea M, Marshall SW, et al. Cumulative effects associated with recurrent concussion in collegiate football players: the NCAA Concussion Study. JAMA 2003;290(19):2549–55.

10. Giza CC, Kutcher JS, Ashwal S, et al. Summary of evidence-based guideline update: evaluation and management of concussion in sports: report of the Guideline Development Subcommittee of the American Academy of Neurology. Neurology 2013;80(24):2250–7.

11. Rutland-Brown W, Langlois JA, Thomas KE, et al. Incidence of traumatic brain injury in the United States, 2003. J Head Trauma Rehabil 2006;21(6):544–8.

12. Guskiewicz KM, Weaver NL, Padua DA, et al. Epidemiology of concussion in collegiate and high school football players. Am J Sports Med 2000;28(5): 643–50.

13. Mainwaring LM, Hutchison M, Bisschop SM, et al. Emotional response to sport concussion compared to ACL injury. Brain Inj 2010;24(4):589–97.

14. Kontos AP, Covassin T, Elbin RJ, et al. Depression and neurocognitive performance after concussion among male and female high school and collegiate athletes. Arch Phys Med Rehabil 2012;93(10):1751–6.

15. Soberg HL, Røe C, Anke A, et al. Health-related quality of life 12 months after severe traumatic brain injury: a prospective nationwide cohort study. J Rehabil Med 2013;45(8):785–91.

16. Buckley WE. Concussions in college football. A multivariate analysis. Am J Sports Med 1988;16(1):51–6.

17. Bruce DA, Schut L, Sutton LN. Brain and cervical spine injuries occurring during organized sports activities in children and adolescents. Clin Sports Med 1982; 1(3):495–514.

18. Cantu RC. Minor head injuries in sports. Adolesc Med 1991;2(1):141–54.

19. Gerberich SG, Finke R, Madden M, et al. An epidemiological study of high school ice hockey injuries. Childs Nerv Syst 1987;3(2):59–64.

20. Gerberich SG, Priest JD, Boen JR, et al. Concussion incidences and severity in secondary school varsity football players. Am J Public Health 1983;73(12): 1370–5.

21. Gessel LM, Fields SK, Collins CL, et al. Concussions among United States high school and collegiate athletes. J Athl Train 2007;42(4):495–503.

22. Kerr ZY, Zuckerman SL, Wasserman EB, et al. Concussion symptoms and return to play time in youth, high school, and college American Football Athletes. JAMA Pediatr 2016;170(7):647–53.

23. Agel J, Evans TA, Dick R, et al. Descriptive epidemiology of collegiate men's soccer injuries: National Collegiate Athletic Association Injury Surveillance System, 1988-1989 through 2002-2003. J Athl Train 2007;42(2):270–7.

24. Comstock RD, Currie DW, Pierpoint LA, et al. An evidence-based discussion of heading the ball and concussions in high school soccer. JAMA Pediatr 2015; 169(9):830–7.

25. Pfister T, Pfister K, Hagel B, et al. The incidence of concussion in youth sports: a systematic review and meta-analysis. Br J Sports Med 2016;50(5):292–7.
26. Meehan WP 3rd, d'Hemecourt P, Collins CL, et al. Assessment and management of sport-related concussions in United States high schools. Am J Sports Med 2011;39(11):2304–10.
27. Castile L, Collins CL, McIlvain NM, et al. The epidemiology of new versus recurrent sports concussions among high school athletes, 2005-2010. Br J Sports Med 2012;46(8):603–10.
28. Lincoln AE, Caswell SV, Almquist JL, et al. Trends in concussion incidence in high school sports: a prospective 11-year study. Am J Sports Med 2011; 39(5):958–63.
29. Covassin T, Moran R, Elbin RJ. Sex differences in reported concussion injury rates and time loss from participation: an update of the National Collegiate Athletic Association Injury Surveillance Program from 2004-2005 through 2008-2009. J Athl Train 2016;51(3):189–94.
30. Tierney RT, Sitler MR, Swanik CB, et al. Gender differences in head-neck segment dynamic stabilization during head acceleration. Med Sci Sports Exerc 2005;37(2):272–9.
31. Verbrugge LM. Sex differentials in health. Public Health Rep 1982;97(5):417–37.
32. Verbrugge LM, Wingard DL. Sex differentials in health and mortality. Women Health 1987;12(2):103–45.
33. Dick RW. Is there a gender difference in concussion incidence and outcomes? Br J Sports Med 2009;43(Suppl 1):i46–50.
34. Kontos AP, Elbin RJ, Fazio-Sumrock VC, et al. Incidence of sports-related concussion among youth football players aged 8-12 years. J Pediatr 2013; 163(3):717–20.
35. Lincoln AE, Hinton RY, Almquist JL, et al. Head, face, and eye injuries in scholastic and collegiate lacrosse: a 4-year prospective study. Am J Sports Med 2007;35(2):207–15.
36. Schulz MR, Marshall SW, Yang J, et al. A prospective cohort study of injury incidence and risk factors in North Carolina high school competitive cheerleaders. Am J Sports Med 2004;32(2):396–405.
37. Hootman JM, Dick R, Agel J. Epidemiology of collegiate injuries for 15 sports: summary and recommendations for injury prevention initiatives. J Athl Train 2007;42(2):311–9.
38. Thurman DJ, Branche CM, Sniezek JE. The epidemiology of sports-related traumatic brain injuries in the United States: recent developments. J Head Trauma Rehabil 1998;13(2):1–8.
39. Wang Y, Chan RC, Deng Y. Examination of postconcussion-like symptoms in healthy university students: relationships to subjective and objective neuropsychological function performance. Arch Clin Neuropsychol 2006;21(4):339–47.
40. Patel AV, Mihalik JP, Notebaert AJ, et al. Neuropsychological function performance, postural stability, and symptoms after dehydration. J Athl Train 2007; 42(1):66–75.
41. Iverson GL. Misdiagnosis of the persistent postconcussion syndrome in patients with depression. Arch Clin Neuropsychol 2006;21(4):303–10.
42. Guskiewicz K, Bruce SL, Cantu RC, et al. National Athletic Trainers' Association position statement: management of sport-related concussion. J Athl Train 2004; 39(3):280–97.
43. Giza CC, Hovda DA. The neurometabolic cascade of concussion. J Athl Train 2001;36:228–35.

44. Field M, Collins M, Lovell M, et al. Does age play a role in recovery of sports related concussion. J Pediatr 2003;142(5):546–53.
45. Drew LB, Drew WE. The contrecoup-coup phenomenon: a new understanding of the mechanism of closed head injury. Neurocrit Care 2004;1:385–90.
46. Guskiewicz KM, Mihalik JP, Shankar V, et al. Measurement of head impacts in collegiate football players: relationship between head impact biomechanics and acute clinical outcome after concussion. Neurosurgery 2007;61:1244–52.
47. McCaffrey MA, Mihalik JP, Crowell DH, et al. Measurement of head impacts in collegiate football players: clinical measures of concussion after high- and low-magnitude impacts. Neurosurgery 2007;61:1236–43.
48. Mihalik JP, Bell DR, Marshall SW, et al. Measurement of head impacts in collegiate football players: an investigation of positional and event-type differences. Neurosurgery 2007;61:1229–35.
49. Mendez MF, Paholpak P, Lin A, et al. Prevalence of traumatic brain injury in early versus late-onset Alzheimer's disease. J Alzheimers Dis 2015;47(4):985–93.
50. Schnadower D, Vazquez H, Lee J, et al. Controversies in the evaluation and management of minor blunt head trauma in children. Curr Opin Pediatr 2007; 19:258–64.
51. Kaut KP, DePompei R, Kerr J, et al. Reports of head injury and symptom knowledge among college athletes: implications for assessment and educational intervention. Clin J Sport Med 2003;2003(13):213–21.
52. Valovich McLeod TC, Bay RC, Heil J, et al. Identification of sport and recreational activity concussion history through the preparticipation screening and a symptom survey in young athletes. Clin J Sport Med 2008;18:235–40.
53. Valovich McLeod TC, Schwartz C, Bay RC. Sport-related concussion misunderstandings among youth coaches. Clin J Sport Med 2007;17:140–2.
54. Collins MW, Lovell MR, Iverson GL, et al. Cumulative effects of concussion in high school athletes. Neurosurgery 2002;51(5):1175–9 [discussion: 1180–1].
55. Moser RS, Schatz P, Jordan BD. Prolonged effects of concussion in high school athletes. Neurosurgery 2005;57(2):300–6 [discussion: 300–6].
56. Broglio SP, Cantu RC, Gioia GA, et al. National Athletic Trainers' Association position statement: management of sport concussion. J Athl Train 2014;49(2): 245–65.
57. Henry LC, Elbin RJ, Collins MW, et al. Examining recovery trajectories after sport-related concussion with a multimodal clinical assessment approach. Neurosurgery 2016;78(2):232–41.
58. McLeod TC, Leach C. Psychometric properties of self-report concussion scales and checklists. J Athl Train 2012;47(2):221–3.
59. Elbin RJ, Knox J, Kegel N, et al. Assessing symptoms in adolescents following sport-related concussion: a comparison of four different approaches. Appl Neuropsychol Child 2016;5(4):294–302.
60. Barr WB, McCrea M. Sensitivity and specificity of standardized neurocognitive testing immediately following sports concussion. J Int Neuropsychol Soc 2001;7(6):693–702.
61. Valovich TC, Perrin DH, Gansneder BM. Repeat administration elicits a practice effect with the balance error scoring system but not with the standardized assessment of concussion in high school athletes. J Athl Train 2003;38(1):51–6.
62. Finnoff JT, Peterson VJ, Hollman JH, et al. Intrarater and interrater reliability of the Balance Error Scoring System (BESS). PM R 2009;1(1):50–4.
63. Riemann BL, Guskiewicz K, Shields EW. Relationship between clinical forceplate measures of postural stability. J Sport Rehabil 1999;8:71–82.

64. Riemann BL, Guskiewicz KM. Effects of mild head injury on postural stability as measured through clinical balance testing. J Athl Train 2000;35(1):19–25.

65. Broglio SP, Ferrara MS, Sopiarz K, et al. Reliable change of the sensory organization test. Clin J Sport Med 2008;18(2):148–54.

66. Cavanaugh JT, Guskiewicz KM, Giuliani C, et al. Detecting altered postural control after cerebral concussion in athletes with normal postural stability. Br J Sports Med 2005;39(11):805–11.

67. Howell DR, Osternig LR, Christie AD, et al. Return to physical activity timing and dual-task gait stability are associated 2 months following concussion. J Head Trauma Rehabil 2016;31(4):262–8.

68. Howell DR, Osternig LR, Koester MC, et al. The effect of cognitive task complexity on gait stability in adolescents following concussion. Exp Brain Res 2014;232(6):1773–82.

69. Register-Mihalik JK, Littleton AC, Guskiewicz KM. Are divided attention tasks useful in the assessment and management of sport-related concussion? Neuropsychol Rev 2013;23(4):300–13.

70. Lee H, Sullivan SJ, Schneiders AG. The use of the dual-task paradigm in detecting gait performance deficits following a sports-related concussion: a systematic review and meta-analysis. J Sci Med Sport 2013;16(1):2–7.

71. Catena RD, van Donkelaar P, Chou LS. Different gait tasks distinguish immediate vs. long-term effects of concussion on balance control. J Neuroeng Rehabil 2009;6:25.

72. Teel EF, Register-Mihalik JK, Troy Blackburn J, et al. Balance and cognitive performance during a dual-task: preliminary implications for use in concussion assessment. J Sci Med Sport 2013;16(3):190–4.

73. Ross LM, Register-Mihalik JK, Mihalik JP, et al. Effects of a single-task versus a dual-task paradigm on cognition and balance in healthy subjects. J Sport Rehabil 2011;20(3):296–310.

74. Resch JE, May B, Tomporowski PD, et al. Balance performance with a cognitive task: a continuation of the dual-task testing paradigm. J Athl Train 2011;46(2):170–5.

75. Catena RD, van Donkelaar P, Chou LS. Cognitive task effects on gait stability following concussion. Exp Brain Res 2007;176(1):23–31.

76. Catena RD, van Donkelaar P, Halterman CI, et al. Spatial orientation of attention and obstacle avoidance following concussion. Exp Brain Res 2009;194(1):67–77.

77. Cavanaugh JT, Mercer VS, Stergiou N. Approximate entropy detects the effect of a secondary cognitive task on postural control in healthy young adults: a methodological report. J Neuroeng Rehabil 2007;4:42.

78. Howell DR, Osternig LR, Chou LS. Dual-task effect on gait balance control in adolescents with concussion. Arch Phys Med Rehabil 2013;94(8):1513–20.

79. Okumura MS, Cooper SL, Ferrara MS, et al. Global switch cost as an index for concussion assessment: reliability and stability. Med Sci Sports Exerc 2013;45(6):1038–42.

80. Matuszak JM, McVige J, McPherson J, et al. A practical concussion physical examination toolbox: evidence-based physical examination for concussion. Sports Health 2016;8(3):260–9.

81. Ventura RE, Jancuska JM, Balcer LJ, et al. Diagnostic tests for concussion: is vision part of the puzzle? J Neuroophthalmol 2015;35(1):73–81.

82. Ellis MJ, Cordingley D, Vis S, et al. Vestibulo-ocular dysfunction in pediatric sports-related concussion. J Neurosurg Pediatr 2015;16(3):248–55.

83. Leong DF, Balcer LJ, Galetta SL, et al. The King-Devick test for sideline concussion screening in collegiate football. J Optom 2015;8(2):131–9.

84. King D, Hume P, Gissane C, et al. Use of the King-Devick test for sideline concussion screening in junior rugby league. J Neurol Sci 2015;357(1–2):75–9.

85. Galetta KM, Brandes LE, Maki K, et al. The King-Devick test and sports-related concussion: study of a rapid visual screening tool in a collegiate cohort. J Neurol Sci 2011;309(1–2):34–9.

86. King D, Gissane C, Hume PA, et al. The King-Devick test was useful in management of concussion in amateur rugby union and rugby league in New Zealand. J Neurol Sci 2015;351(1–2):58–64.

87. Silverberg ND, Luoto TM, Öhman J, et al. Assessment of mild traumatic brain injury with the King-Devick test in an emergency department sample. Brain Inj 2014;28(12):1590–3.

88. Cubon VA, Putukian M, Boyer C, et al. A diffusion tensor imaging study on the white matter skeleton in individuals with sports-related concussion. J Neurotrauma 2011;28(2):189–201.

89. Shan R, Szmydynger-Chodobska J, Warren OU, et al. A new panel of blood biomarkers for the diagnosis of mild traumatic brain injury/concussion in adults. J Neurotrauma 2016;33(1):49–57.

90. Schulte S, Podlog LW, Hamson-Utley JJ, et al. A systematic review of the biomarker S100B: implications for sport-related concussion management. J Athl Train 2014;49(6):830–50.

91. Thomas DG, Apps JN, Hoffmann RG, et al. Benefits of strict rest after acute concussion: a randomized controlled trial. Pediatrics 2015;135(2):213–23.

92. Reddy CC, Collins M, Lovell M, et al. Efficacy of amantadine treatment on symptoms and neurocognitive performance among adolescents following sports-related concussion. J Head Trauma Rehabil 2013;28(4):260–5.

93. Leddy J, Hinds A, Sirica D, et al. The role of controlled exercise in concussion management. PM R 2016;8(3 Suppl):S91–100.

94. Clausen M, Pendergast DR, Willer B, et al. Cerebral blood flow during treadmill exercise is a marker of physiological postconcussion syndrome in female athletes. J Head Trauma Rehabil 2016;31(3):215–24.

95. Leddy JJ, Willer B. Use of graded exercise testing in concussion and return-to-activity management. Curr Sports Med Rep 2013;12(6):370–6.

96. Kozlowski KF, Graham J, Leddy JJ, et al. Exercise intolerance in individuals with postconcussion syndrome. J Athl Train 2013;48(5):627–35.

97. Schneider KJ, Meeuwisse WH, Nettel-Aguirre A, et al. Cervicovestibular rehabilitation in sport-related concussion: a randomised controlled trial. Br J Sports Med 2014;48(17):1294–8.

98. McCrea M, Guskiewicz K, Randolph C, et al. Incidence, clinical course, and predictors of prolonged recovery time following sport-related concussion in high school and college athletes. J Int Neuropsychol Soc 2013;19(1):22–33.

99. Sandel NK, Lovell MR, Kegel NE, et al. The relationship of symptoms and neurocognitive performance to perceived recovery from sports-related concussion among adolescent athletes. Appl Neuropsychol Child 2013;2(1):64–9.

100. Meehan WP 3rd, O'Brien MJ, Geminiani E, et al. Initial symptom burden predicts duration of symptoms after concussion. J Sci Med Sport 2016;19(9):722–5.

101. Meehan WP 3rd, Mannix R, Monuteaux MC, et al. Early symptom burden predicts recovery after sport-related concussion. Neurology 2014;83(24):2204–10.

102. Yard EE, Comstock RD. Compliance with return to play guidelines following concussion in US high school athletes, 2005-2008. Brain Inj 2009;23(11): 888–98.
103. Bleiberg J, Cernich AN, Cameron K, et al. Duration of cognitive impairment after sports concussion. Neurosurgery 2004;54(5):1073–8 [discussion: 1078–80].
104. Buzzini SR, Guskiewicz KM. Sport-related concussion in the young athlete. Curr Opin Pediatr 2006;18(4):376–82.
105. Guskiewicz KM, Marshall SW, Bailes J, et al. Association between recurrent concussion and late-life cognitive impairment in retired professional football players. Neurosurgery 2005;57(4):719–26.
106. Cantu RC. Chronic traumatic encephalopathy in the National Football League. Neurosurgery 2007;61(2):223–5.
107. Belanger HG, Vanderploeg RD, McAllister T. Subconcussive blows to the head: a formative review of short-term clinical outcomes. J Head Trauma Rehabil 2015; 31(3):159–66.
108. Montenigro PH, Bernick C, Cantu RC. Clinical features of repetitive traumatic brain injury and chronic traumatic encephalopathy. Brain Pathol 2015;25(3): 304–17.
109. Brandenburg W, Hallervorden J. Dementia pugilistica with anatomical findings. Virchows Arch 1954;325(6):680–709 [in German].
110. Small GW, Kepe V, Siddarth P, et al. PET scanning of brain tau in retired National Football League players: preliminary findings. Am J Geriatr Psychiatry 2013; 21(2):138–44.
111. McKee AC, Cantu RC, Nowinski CJ, et al. Chronic traumatic encephalopathy in athletes: progressive tauopathy after repetitive head injury. J Neuropathol Exp Neurol 2009;68(7):709–35.
112. Gavett BE, Stern RA, Cantu RC, et al. Mild traumatic brain injury: a risk factor for neurodegeneration. Alzheimers Res Ther 2010;2(3):18.
113. Gavett BE, Stern RA, McKee AC. Chronic traumatic encephalopathy: a potential late effect of sport-related concussive and subconcussive head trauma. Clin Sports Med 2011;30(1):179–88, xi.
114. Guskiewicz KM, Marshall SW, Bailes J, et al. Recurrent concussion and risk of depression in retired professional football players. Med Sci Sports Exerc 2007;39(6):903–9.
115. Caron JG, Bloom GA, Johnston KM, et al. Effects of multiple concussions on retired National Hockey League players. J Sport Exerc Psychol 2013;35(2): 168–79.
116. Vann Jones SA, Breakey RW, Evans PJ. Heading in football, long-term cognitive decline and dementia: evidence from screening retired professional footballers. Br J Sports Med 2014;48(2):159–61.
117. Webbe FM, Ochs SR. Recency and frequency of soccer heading interact to decrease neurocognitive performance. Appl Neuropsychol 2003;10(1):31–41.
118. Stalnacke BM, Tegner Y, Sojka P. Playing soccer increases serum concentrations of the biochemical markers of brain damage S-100B and neuron-specific enolase in elite players: a pilot study. Brain Inj 2004;18(9): 899–909.

Pathophysiology of Sports-Related Concussion

Kristen Steenerson, MD[a], Amaal Jilani Starling, MD[b],*

KEYWORDS

- Concussion • Traumatic brain injury • TBI • Trauma

KEY POINTS

- Concussion pathophysiology is complex and still under investigation.
- Concussion pathophysiology involves excessive neurotransmitter release, excitotoxicity, neuroinflammation, and axonal disruption.
- It remains unclear how these mechanisms are affected by genetics, premorbid conditions, and environmental factors.

INTRODUCTION

Sports concussion is a public health epidemic with 1.6 to 3.8 million sports-related concussions occurring annually.[1] Our current recommendations for treatment include rest, symptomatic treatment, and a gradual return to mental and physical activity. At this time, we do not have specific treatment options for the treatment of an acute concussion or to prevent prolonged or permanent symptoms. To develop more targeted management and treatment options, the underlying pathophysiology needs to be better defined.

In addition, a concussion is not the same as a moderate or severe traumatic brain injury. There is currently a large body of evidence demonstrating the mechanisms underlying moderate to severe traumatic brain injury; however, the pathophysiology underlying concussion and mild traumatic brain injury remains under investigation. Sports concussion is complicated and its pathophysiology will likely vary depending on the mechanism and characteristics of the impact, susceptibility of the individual including genetics and premorbid risk factors, and environmental factors. Thus, it is not surprising that numerous mechanisms have been demonstrated in both animal models and in vivo advanced neuroimaging studies. These mechanisms are likely

Dr K. Steenerson has nothing to disclose. Dr A.J. Starling has received consulting fees from Eneura, Amgen, and Lilly.
[a] Neurology, Barrow Neurological Institute, 350 West Thomas Road, Phoenix, Arizona 85013, USA; [b] Neurology, Mayo Clinic, 5777 East Mayo Boulevard, Phoenix, Arizona 85054, USA
* Corresponding author.
E-mail address: starling.amaal@mayo.edu

Neurol Clin 35 (2017) 403–408
http://dx.doi.org/10.1016/j.ncl.2017.03.011
0733-8619/17/© 2017 Elsevier Inc. All rights reserved.

neurologic.theclinics.com

not mutually exclusive and are most likely occurring concurrently in varying degrees in different individuals affected by a sports concussion. This evidence-based article reviews the current understanding in the diverse pathophysiology of sports concussion in efforts to educate and inspire additional research.

DEFINITION OF CONCUSSION

The definition of concussion is widely debated, but the most accepted definition by McCrory et al[2] states that a concussion is a complex pathophysiological process affecting the brain, induced by biomechanical forces with alteration in mental status with or without loss of consciousness.[3] A concussion is a subset of mild traumatic brain injury and is commonly used interchangeably. More recently, it has been recommended to use the diagnosis of concussion for injuries with more complete recovery and the diagnosis of mild traumatic brain injury for the injuries that are associated with more persistent symptoms.[2] Several prognostic risk factors have been identified for prolonged recovery after concussion, including younger age, female gender, premorbid migraine history and psychiatric history, prior concussion, and history of migraine, higher symptom severity score acutely, and duration of posttraumatic amnesia.[4–6]

Concussion symptomatology can be divided into 4 domains: physical (headache and dizziness), cognitive (concentration and memory), emotional (depression, anxiety, and mood lability), and sleep (hypersomnia and insomnia). Although the most commonly reported symptoms are typically headache, dizziness, and difficulties with concentration and memory, oftentimes the most bothersome symptoms fall within the emotional and sleep domains.

Despite the presence of significant symptomatology and acute disability, routine neuroimaging is typically unhelpful at demonstrating evidence of neuropathologic changes. These symptoms are likely caused by functional, metabolic, and microstructural abnormalities as opposed to gross macrostructural damage. A better understanding of concussion pathophysiology and its associated functional and microstructural abnormalities will improve the management and treatment of concussion. It may also be helpful to determine preventive or at least protective measures.

Pathophysiology in Sports Concussion

It is a common misconception that a mechanical injury to the brain results in direct structural damage; however, these biomechanical forces result in abnormal function at the level of the individual cell. Abnormal cellular function is what results in functional impairment and may lead to microstructural and even eventually macrostructural damage.

NEUROTRANSMITTER DYSREGULATION

Massive unregulated, unchecked excitatory neurotransmitter release results in functional impairment, excitotoxicity, and possibly permanent damage. Mechanical injury disrupts cellular membranes causing an efflux of intracellular potassium through voltage-gated channels, resulting in neuronal depolarization.[7] With open voltage-gated channels, a feedback loop is created resulting in increased extracellular potassium, depolarization, and further neurotransmitter release. One excitatory neurotransmitter clearly implicated is glutamate.[8] Glutamate has been identified as not only promoting potassium efflux, stimulating receptors, and inducing ligand-gated potassium channels, but also in binding N-methyl-D-aspartate receptors allowing for unrestricted cortical depolarization and increased hyperexcitability.[9] In addition, the increased release of excitatory neurotransmitters results in the accumulation of intracellular calcium, which activates further cell damage by signaling proteases, reactive oxygen species, and mitochondrial impairment.[10] Neurotransmitters seem to be implicated in not only increased cortical activation and hyperexcitability, but also in initiating cascades that can lead to cell damage and even death.

METABOLIC MISMATCH

In the acute period, the massive depolarization described above due to neurotransmitter dysregulation and excitotoxcity results in a metabolic mismatch. During this time, the mitochondria struggles to meet the cellular demands of ATP production.[11,12] Without ATP, the ATP-dependent Na^+–K^+ pump will fail to maintain ionic homeostasis. The metabolic mismatch and specifically the increased energy demands activate glycolysis, which produces lactic acid. Accumulation of lactic acid will break down the blood–brain barrier and can result in massive cerebral edema.[13]

NEUROINFLAMMATORY RESPONSE

Abnormal metabolism will trigger a local neuroinflammatory response, mediated by microglial infiltration, within hours of injury to the brain.[14] Although the initial neuroinflammatory response is local, the response itself stimulates the release of cytokine mediators, proteases, and reactive oxygen species, which promotes a more global inflammatory response and can result in increased blood–brain barrier permeability and cerebral blood flow changes.[15,16] Ongoing debate exist as to the actual impact of such an inflammatory response: protective and ultimately therapeutic versus overcompensation and damaging. It is unclear, based on currently available evidence, the necessary and sufficient neuroinflammatory response for optimal recovery. Once this parameter is better defined, activation or inhibition of inflammatory pathways could serve as novel target sites for therapeutic intervention and drug discovery.

CEREBRAL BLOOD FLOW CHANGES

Alterations in cerebral blood flow occur in acute sports concussion. Carbon dioxide levels seem to alter acute and chronic vasoreactivity, resulting in changes in cerebral blood flow. There is a transient increase in carbon dioxide production related to metabolic derangements in the acute period, which reduces overall central nervous system vasoreactivity, resulting in relative hypoventilation and dampening of normal vasoconstrictive and vasodilatory properties.[17] Changes in vasoreactivity as a result of increased nitric oxide production may be the underlying mechanism of acute symptom worsening with exertion.[18] Acute symptom worsening with exertion is a hallmark feature of concussion symptomatology.

Functional MRI has demonstrated that cerebral blood flow changes correlate with initial symptom severity, but may return to baseline or normative ranges slower than subjective symptom reporting and neurocognitive testing.[19,20] This suggests that cerebral blood flow changes likely persists even after symptoms and signs have resolved. It is unclear how this information should or should not impact return to play. As discussed elsewhere in this article, persistent cerebral blood flow alterations likely contribute to long-term symptoms and risk for recurrent injury.

DIFFUSE AXONAL INJURY

In addition to the cellular changes discussed, there is disruption of the neuronal pathways that occurs acutely in sports concussion. It entails the disruption of neuronal pathways integral to cortical function. From a gross perspective, cortical coup–contrecoup injuries were implicated as part of the acute disruption of pathways in concussion.[21] This macrostructural model, however, has been refined to detail the microscopic pathway disruption from shear forces and injury that occurs in sports concussion resulting in diffuse axonal injury. Diffuse axonal injury from shearing forces either owing to direct blows to the head or from neck acceleration–deceleration injuries has been implicated in many different aspects of altered central nervous system function and microstructural damage. The acceleration and deceleration of the central nervous system results in shear stress and tension resulting in cytoskeletal injury, which in turn leads to disrupted transport and accumulation of products to injured regions.[22,23] Disrupted axonal transport and accumulation of products results in impaired metabolism, as well as activation of calpain and calcineurin, potentiating further cytoskeletal damage.[24,25] In addition, axonal rupture from shear and tensile forces can result in Wallerian degeneration, transection, and even cell death, compromising cortical and subcortical pathways, and deleteriously impacting overall functional ability.[26]

Advanced neuroimaging techniques including susceptibility-weighted imaging and gradient echo imaging can demonstrate hemosiderin deposition consistent with microhemorrhages as a result of diffuse axonal injury. Susceptibility-weighted imaging lesions have been demonstrated in mild, moderate, and severe traumatic brain injury. These lesions correlate with the severity of injury.[27] In addition, the volume of lesions has a direct relationship with the presence of long-term neurocognitive and psychiatric symptoms.[28]

CHRONIC PATHOPHYSIOLOGY

The majority of patients will recover completely after a concussion; however, a minority will suffer persistent symptoms. Acute mechanisms for pathophysiology in sports concussion also contribute to the mechanisms underlying persistent changes after a concussion. As the acute process alters function and disrupts microstructural networks, there is a greater vulnerability for more persistent and possibly neurodegenerative changes especially in the setting of repetitive traumatic brain injuries or even possibly subconcussive hits. Neuroinflammation is present in the underlying pathophysiology of known neurodegenerative disease processes, including Alzheimer's disease and amyotrophic lateral sclerosis.[29,30] Thus, a persistent and sustained neuroinflammatory response may lead to the development of more permanent neurocognitive symptoms and possibly neurodegenerative changes after traumatic brain injury. Disrupted neuronal pathways and axonal pathology are present in the underlying pathophysiology of known neurodegenerative disease processes. Thus, the diffuse axonal injury present in concussion may play a role in the development of a possible neurodegenerative condition associated with traumatic brain injury. Studies have demonstrated that white matter tract disruption and persistent microglial activation after repetitive mild traumatic brain injury may result in permanent changes.[31]

SYMPTOMS AND PATHOPHYSIOLOGY

Beyond the need for basic understanding, pathophysiology of sports concussion also sheds light on the vast array of symptoms and timing of symptoms experienced by athletes. Giza and Hovda[7] described some of these mechanisms:

a. Ionic flux resulting in acute and chronic migrainelike symptoms;
b. Energy crisis and vulnerability for second hit syndrome;

c. Axonal dysfunction and neurocognitive slowing; and

d. Altered neurotransmission, slowed cognition, and reaction time.

SUMMARY

Sports concussion pathophysiology is a complex and multifactorial process. Although many mechanisms have been identified, there is much more to be learned. It is clear that biomechanical forces cause changes that start at the level of the individual cell, affecting metabolism and neuronal vitality. Changes in cerebral blood flow and neuro-inflammation result in changes in both the acute and possibly chronic phase of brain injury. Pathway disruption, microstructural damage, and specifically diffuse axonal injury also plays a role in both stages of injury. However, it is still unclear if and how genetics, age, gender, premorbid conditions, and environmental factors alter the underlying pathophysiology. These nuances are key to the individualized management and treatment of patients who have suffered from an acute concussion. By continuously seeking to understand these pathophysiologic mechanisms, management and treatment options for sports concussion can continue to improve.

REFERENCES

1. Langlois JA, Rutland-Brown W, Wald MM. The epidemiology and impact of traumatic brain injury: a brief overview. J Head Trauma Rehabil 2006;21:375–8.

2. McCrory P, Meeuwisse WH, Aubry M, et al. Consensus statement on concussion in sport: the 4th International Conference on Concussion in Sport held in Zurich, November 2012. Br J Sports Med 2013;47:250–8.

3. Giza CC, Kutcher JS, Ashwal S, et al. Summary of evidence-based guideline update: evaluation and management of concussion in sports: report of the Guideline Development Subcommittee of the American Academy of Neurology. Neurology 2013;80:2250–7.

4. Ponsford J, Willmott C, Rothwell A, et al. Factors influencing outcome following mild traumatic brain injury in adults. J Int Neuropsychol Soc 2000;6:568–79.

5. Gould KR, Ponsford JL, Johnston L, et al. Predictive and associated factors of psychiatric disorders after traumatic brain injury: a prospective study. J Neurotrauma 2011;28:1155–63.

6. McCrea M, Guskiewicz K, Randolph C, et al. Incidence, clinical course, and predictors of prolonged recovery time following sport-related concussion in high school and college athletes. J Int Neuropsychol Soc 2013;19:22–33.

7. Giza CC, Hovda DA. The new neurometabolic cascade of concussion. Neurosurgery 2014;75:S24–33.

8. Yi JH, Hazell AS. Excitotoxic mechanisms and the role of astrocytic glutamate transporters in traumatic brain injury. Neurochem Int 2006;48:394–403.

9. Katayama Y, Becker DP, Tamura T, et al. Massive increases in extracellular potassium and the indiscriminate release of glutamate following concussive brain injury. J Neurosurg 1990;73:889–900.

10. Cheng G, Kong RH, Zhang LM, et al. Mitochondria in traumatic brain injury and mitochondrial-targeted multipotential therapeutic strategies. Br J Pharmacol 2012;167:699–719.

11. Hovda DA, Yoshino A, Kawamata T, et al. The increase in local cerebral glucose utilization following fluid percussion brain injury is prevented with kynurenic acid and is associated with an increase in calcium. Acta Neurochir Suppl 1990;51:331–3.

12. Kawamata T, Katayama Y, Hovda DA, et al. Administration of excitatory amino acid antagonists via microdialysis attenuates the increase in glucose utilization seen following concussive brain injury. J Cereb Blood Flow Metab 1992;12:12–24.

13. Verweij BH, Amelink GJ, Muizelaar JP. Current concepts of cerebral oxygen transport and energy metabolism after severe traumatic brain injury. Prog Brain Res 2007;161:111–24.

14. Loane DJ, Byrnes KR. Role of microglia in neurotrauma. Neurotherapeutics 2010; 7:366–77.

15. Khuman J, Meehan WP 3rd, Zhu X, et al. Tumor necrosis factor alpha and Fas receptor contribute to cognitive deficits independent of cell death after concussive traumatic brain injury in mice. J Cereb Blood Flow Metab 2011;31:778–89.

16. Habgood MD, Bye N, Dziegielewska KM, et al. Changes in blood-brain barrier permeability to large and small molecules following traumatic brain injury in mice. Eur J Neurosci 2007;25:231–8.

17. Clausen M, Pendergast DR, Willer B, et al. Cerebral blood flow during treadmill exercise is a marker of physiological postconcussion syndrome in female athletes. J Head Trauma Rehabil 2016;31:215–24.

18. DeWitt DS, Prough DS. Traumatic cerebral vascular injury: the effects of concussive brain injury on the cerebral vasculature. J Neurotrauma 2003;20:795–825.

19. Meier TB, Bellgowan PS, Singh R, et al. Recovery of cerebral blood flow following sports-related concussion. JAMA Neurol 2015;72:530–8.

20. Wang Y, Nelson LD, LaRoche AA, et al. Cerebral blood flow alterations in acute sport-related concussion. J Neurotrauma 2016;33:1227–36.

21. Goodman JC. Pathologic changes in mild head injury. Semin Neurol 1994;14: 19–24.

22. Smith DH, Wolf JA, Lusardi TA, et al. High tolerance and delayed elastic response of cultured axons to dynamic stretch injury. J Neurosci 1999;19:4263–9.

23. Dixon CE, Lyeth BG, Povlishock JT, et al. A fluid percussion model of experimental brain injury in the rat. J Neurosurg 1987;67:110–9.

24. Buki A, Farkas O, Doczi T, et al. Preinjury administration of the calpain inhibitor MDL-28170 attenuates traumatically induced axonal injury. J Neurotrauma 2003;20:261–8.

25. von Reyn CR, Spaethling JM, Mesfin MN, et al. Calpain mediates proteolysis of the voltage-gated sodium channel alpha-subunit. J Neurosci 2009;29:10350–6.

26. Povlishock JT, Erb DE, Astruc J. Axonal response to traumatic brain injury: reactive axonal change, deafferentation, and neuroplasticity. J Neurotrauma 1992; 9(Suppl 1):S189–200.

27. Beauchamp MH, Anderson V. Cognitive and psychopathological sequelae of pediatric traumatic brain injury. Handb Clin Neurol 2013;112:913–20.

28. Wang X, Wei XE, Li MH, et al. Microbleeds on susceptibility-weighted MRI in depressive and non-depressive patients after mild traumatic brain injury. Neurol Sci 2014;35:1533–9.

29. Eikelenboom P, van Exel E, Hoozemans JJ, et al. Neuroinflammation - an early event in both the history and pathogenesis of Alzheimer's disease. Neurodegener Dis 2010;7:38–41.

30. Brettschneider J, Libon DJ, Toledo JB, et al. Microglial activation and TDP-43 pathology correlate with executive dysfunction in amyotrophic lateral sclerosis. Acta Neuropathol 2012;123:395–407.

31. Shitaka Y, Tran HT, Bennett RE, et al. Repetitive closed-skull traumatic brain injury in mice causes persistent multifocal axonal injury and microglial reactivity. J Neuropathol Exp Neurol 2011;70:551–67.

Estimating Concussion Incidence Using Sports Injury Surveillance Systems
Complexities and Potential Pitfalls

Zachary Y. Kerr, PhD, MPH[a],*, Scott L. Zuckerman, MD[b],
Johna K. Register-Mihalik, PhD, LAT, ATC[c], Erin B. Wasserman, PhD[d],
Tamara C. Valovich McLeod, PhD, ATC, FNATA[e],
Thomas P. Dompier, PhD, ATC[d], R. Dawn Comstock, PhD[f],
Stephen W. Marshall, PhD[g]

KEYWORDS

- Concussion • Surveillance • Sports injury • National Collegiate Athletic Association
- High School Reporting Information Online • Traumatic brain injury

KEY POINTS

- Numerous sports injury surveillance systems exist with the capability of tracking concussion incidence data, but it is important to understand their strengths and limitations.
- Current sports injury surveillance lacks access to sports with lower visibility and settings that lack medical staff.

Continued

Disclosure Statement: The National Collegiate Athletic Association Injury Surveillance Program, National Athletic Treatment, Injury and Outcomes Network, and Youth Football Surveillance System are run by the Datalys Center for Sports Injury Research and Prevention, at which E.B. Wasserman and T.P. Dompier are employed. Dr. R.D. Comstock is the director of the National High School Sports-Related Injury Surveillance System, High School Reporting Information Online. All remaining authors have nothing to disclose.
[a] Department of Exercise and Sport Science, Injury Prevention Research Center, University of North Carolina, Woollen 313, CB#8700, Chapel Hill, NC 27599-8700, USA; [b] Department of Neurological Surgery, Vanderbilt University Medical Center, Vanderbilt University School of Medicine, Medical Center North T-4224, Nashville, TN 37212, USA; [c] Department of Exercise and Sport Science, Injury Prevention Research Center, University of North Carolina, Fetzer 125, CB#8700, Chapel Hill, NC 27599-8700, USA; [d] Datalys Center for Sports Injury Research and Prevention, 401 West Michigan Street, Suite 500, Indianapolis, IN 46202, USA; [e] Athletic Training Programs, School of Osteopathic Medicine, A.T. Still University, 5850 East Still Circle, Mesa, AZ 85206, USA; [f] Department of Epidemiology, Colorado School of Public Health, University of Colorado Denver, Anschutz, Mail Stop B119, 13001 East 17th Place, Aurora, CO 80045, USA; [g] Department of Epidemiology, Injury Prevention Research Center, University of North Carolina, Suite 500, Bank of America Building, CB#7505, Chapel Hill, NC 27599-7505, USA
* Corresponding author.
E-mail address: zkerr@email.unc.edu

Neurol Clin 35 (2017) 409–434
http://dx.doi.org/10.1016/j.ncl.2017.03.001
0733-8619/17/© 2017 Elsevier Inc. All rights reserved.

neurologic.theclinics.com

Continued

- Potential variations in the definitions of injury and at-risk exposure may affect comparability across findings.
- Sports injury surveillance is able to assess both the immediate and longitudinal effects of rule/policy changes.

INTRODUCTION

Concussions remain a high-profile topic given the research that has elucidated both potential short- and long-term effects.[1–4] Because of this burgeoning research, it is imperative to obtain valid and reliable estimates of concussion incidence.[5] Although estimates related to those individuals presenting at emergency departments or other traditional health care system touchpoints are important,[6–10] they do not fully capture the breadth of concussions that occur as a result of participation in sport and recreational activities.[10–14] Partially because of this known limitation, numerous studies have utilized sports injury surveillance systems to estimate the incidence of sport-related concussion across multiple levels of competition, including youth,[10,15–17] high school,[14–16,18–24] collegiate,[15,16,25–28] and professional[29–35] (**Table 1**). These estimates can be used to monitor trends over time, help identify individuals most at risk, examine the settings and characteristics that exacerbate risk, inform the development of interventions/prevention strategies to reduce the incidence and severity of concussion, and help improve management and care. In addition to research and clinical uses, surveillance findings can be informative to the numerous stakeholders within a sports setting, including parents, players, coaches, policy makers, and industry.[36]

Like all public health surveillance systems, sports injury surveillance systems are focused on capturing and distributing timely information that monitors a clearly defined problem. Given these time pressures, the data captured by surveillance systems are not guaranteed to be high-quality research data. Thus, it is important for all consumers of the sports injury surveillance data to understand the strengths and limitations of estimating sport-related concussion incidence using data captured by sports injury surveillance systems.

Previous research examining general methodologies and data quality of sports injury surveillance systems[37,38] was broad and did not examine specific injuries such as concussion. This article describes some issues pertinent to system design and data analysis that can affect the interpretation and understanding of concussion incidence data captured by sports injury surveillance systems. Such understanding will help improve decision making based on these data and could inform the design of future sports injury surveillance systems and research studies aiming to identify risk factors and develop and evaluate prevention strategies.

WHO COLLECTS THE DATA?

To date, most sports injury surveillance systems have relied upon sports medicine clinicians to collect and report data. In some parts of the world (eg, Europe, Australia, New Zealand), sports injury surveillance systems have traditionally been established in settings where athletic teams are covered by trained sports medicine clinical teams including physiotherapists and physicians.[33,34] In those settings, the team medical staff is capable of collecting and reporting high quality data to sports injury surveillance systems. In the United States, such extensive clinical coverage is usually

Table 1
Sampling of sports injury surveillance systems capturing published concussion data

Sports Injury Surveillance System[a]	Athletes	Type of Sample	Data Collectors	Concussion Definition Provided	Concussion Rates Sports Included in Estimate	Study Period	Estimate[b]
Youth							
Youth Football Safety Study (YFSS)	Youth football players aged 5–15 y	Convenience	Athletic trainers	No definition provided, but after its publication, ATs were encouraged to follow Zurich Consensus Statement on Concussion in Sport[67]	Football	2012/13–2013/14 seasons	0.99 concussions per 1000 AEs[17]
High school							
National High School Sports-Related Injury Surveillance System, High School Reporting Information Online (HS RIO)	High school student-athletes from a large national sample of schools	Stratified random sample and concurrent convenience sample	ATs	No definition provided	Boys' football, wrestling, soccer, basketball, baseball; Girls' volleyball, soccer, basketball, softball	2011/12 academic year	0.51 concussions per 1000 AEs[20]

(continued on next page)

Table 1
(continued)

National Athletic Treatment, Injury and Outcomes Network (NATION)	High school student-athletes	Convenience	ATs	No definition provided, but after its publication, ATs were encouraged to follow Zurich Consensus Statement on Concussion in Sport[67]	Boys' football	2012/13–2014/15 academic years	Game: 1.16 concussions per 1000 AEs; Practice: 0.47 concussions per 1000 AEs[16]
North Carolina High School Athletic Injury Study (NCHSAIS)	High school student-athletes within the North Carolina High School Athletic Association (NCHSAA)	Stratified random	AT or athletic director	Congress of Neurological Surgeons Committee on Head Injury Nomenclature definition	Boys' football, wrestling, soccer, basketball, baseball, track; Girls' soccer, basketball, softball, track; Cheerleading	1996/97–1998/99 academic years	0.17 concussions per 1000 AEs[22]
National Athletic Trainer Association (NATA) injury surveillance program	High school student-athletes from a large national sample of schools	Stratified cluster sample	ATs	No definition provided	Boys' football, wrestling, baseball, soccer, basketball; Girls' volleyball, field hockey, softball, soccer, basketball	1995/96–1997/1998 academic years	Reported separately per sport[24]

Fairfax County Public School System Injury Surveillance Database	All high school student-athletes from a large public school system	Census	ATs	Based upon examination of the athletic trainer	Boys' football, wrestling, soccer, basketball, lacrosse, baseball; Girls' field hockey, soccer, basketball, lacrosse, softball, cheerleading	1997/98–2007/08 academic years	0.24 concussions per 1000 AEs[21]
College							
NCAA Injury Surveillance Program (ISP)	NCAA student-athletes	Convenience	ATs	No definition provided, but after its publication, ATs were encouraged to follow Zurich Consensus Statement on Concussion in Sport.[67]	Men's football, wrestling, ice hockey, soccer, basketball, lacrosse, baseball; Women's volleyball, ice hockey, soccer, basketball, lacrosse, baseball	2011/12–2014/15 academic years	0.55 concussions per 1000 AEs[25]
Professional							
MLB Health and Injury Tracking System (HITS)	All major and minor league baseball players within the MLB	Census	ATs and team physicians	Zurich Consensus Statement on Concussion in Sport definition[67]	Baseball	2011–2012 seasons	0.42 concussions per 1000 AEs[32]

(continued on next page)

Table 1
(continued)

	Population	Sampling	Data collector	Definition	Sport	Seasons	Concussion rate
NHL- NHL Players Association (NHLPA) Concussion Program	All professional ice hockey players within the NHL	Census	Team physicians	Internal definition, followed by 2001 Consensus Statement on Concussion in Sport definition[92]	Ice hockey	1997/98–2003/04 seasons	1.8 concussions per 1000 game player-hours[31]
NFL Injury Surveillance System (ISS)	All professional football players within the NFL (game only)	Census	Team physicians and athletic trainers	Internal definition provided by the NFL Mild Traumatic Brain Injury (MTBI) committee[93]	Football	2002/03–2007/08 seasons	0.19 concussions per team-game[29]
Australian Football League (AFL) annual injury survey	All professional Australian Football Players	Census	Team medical staff	No definition provided, only injuries requiring the player to miss a match recorded	Australian Rules Football	2003–2012 seasons	0.5 concussions per club-season[33]
England Professional Rugby Injury Surveillance Project	13 English Premiership Rugby Union clubs	Convenience	Team Medical Staff	2001 Consensus Statement on Concussion in Sport definition[92] and Maddocks questions[94]	Rugby	2002/03, 2003/04, and 2005/06 seasons	4.1 concussions per 1000 player-hours[34]
Qatar Stars League (QSL) Injury Surveillance	7–10 QSL Clubs per season	Census (study used subsample)	Team medical staff	Based upon examination of the team medical staff	Soccer	2008/09–2011/12 seasons	0.016 concussions per 1000 player-hours[35]

[a] Only sports injury surveillance systems with publications specific to concussion were included; when multiple publications regarding concussion were available, only those publications with the most recent data were included.

[b] If sports injury surveillance systems include multiple sports, only the concussion rate reported across all sports is shown in this table.

available only to athletes competing in the professional or upper level collegiate settings.[29,31,32] Youth and high school sports are usually covered by only a shared athletic trainer (AT), if they have any on-site medical coverage at all.[39] Thus, several existing surveillance systems covering youth and high school sports have utilized ATs as data reporters (see **Table 1**). When compared with physicians, ATs provided comparable injury reports, particularly for concussions.[40]

Research at the high school level found that ATs were more likely to report more injury and exposure data than coaches.[41] Using coaches to report injury data can be challenging, because they are not as educated as ATs regarding the identification of concussion. They are first and foremost focused on coaching duties, and may not regularly keep detailed injury logs. They may also feel pressures to win, which could influence their decision making regarding pulling athletes with suspected concussions from play and reporting those injuries.

As an alternative, parents have been used as data collectors or as assistants to clinical data collectors.[42,43] In 1 youth soccer study, each team designated an assistant coach or parent to record exposure data. When an injury occurred, this designee initiated the injury tracking form, which was then completed by an onsite AT.[42] In another study, both ATs and parents reported injuries via Web-based surveys with good agreement noted.[43] With the lack of AT resources in many youth and high school settings,[39,44] coupled with the influx of injury tracking devices on handheld mobile devices, it may be feasible for parents to report concussion data. However, future research is needed to establish the validity and reliability of parent reports of concussion. As demonstrated previously, while it is not always feasible, when available, trained sports medicine clinicians should be utilized to collect and report injury data to sports injury surveillance systems.

WHAT SPORTS ARE INCLUDED?

Sports such as football and soccer have typically been included in large numbers in previous sports injury surveillance systems (see **Table 1**). In fact, football comprises a large proportion of participation in organized high school and collegiate sports[45,46] and is estimated to comprise the largest proportion of all concussions within high school and collegiate sports.[23,25] Yet, it is imperative to generate estimates of concussion incidence among under-represented sports to help identify sport-specific risk factors and prevention strategies. Other sports, such as golf, beach volleyball, and sailing, are seldom examined, which may be due to lower participation numbers in those sports or these sports being perceived as low risk. A recent study examined a small sample of crew injuries in high school,[47] but numbers for concussions were limited. What may be of the utmost concern is that sports not traditionally included in prior sports injury surveillance systems may have higher concussion incidence. For example, surveillance on rugby concussions is limited in the United States; however, 1 study examining injuries in football and rugby across 3 seasons at 1 National Collegiate Athletic Association (NCAA) member institution found that concussion rates were higher in rugby than football.[48] Potentially high concussion rates may also be present in low-visibility sports, such as water polo, equestrian, and figure skating.

In addition, the sports included in prior sports injury surveillance systems have varied widely. Thus, readers should compare all-sport concussion rates from various surveillance systems with caution. Including sports with lower concussion incidence will naturally reduce the resulting all-sport concussion rate. For example, when examining data from the National High School Sports-Related Injury Surveillance System, High School Reporting Information Online (HS RIO) during the 2008/09 to 2009/10 academic years,[18] the all-sport concussion rate was 2.5 concussions per 10,000 athlete exposures (AEs) ; however, when excluding the sports with concussion rates under 1.0 concussions per 10,000 AEs (boys' baseball, track/field, swim/dive, and girls' gymnastics, volleyball, swim/dive, and track/field), the resulting all-sport concussion rate was 3.5 concussions per 10,000 AEs.

At the same time, there is debate given what activities are even eligible to be considered sport and thus, included in sports injury surveillance. **Table 2** presents the definitions of sport provided by: the NCAA, the US Department of Education's Office for Civil Rights (OCR), and the Women's Sports Foundation (WSF). All 3 organizations utilize criteria that specify: athletic physical activity, whether explicitly or implicitly stated, competition, and administration of the sport by staff and/or rules. However, such criteria hinder some organized physical activities from being considered a sport. For example, competitive cheerleading requires great gymnastic ability from its participants,[49] is considered a sport under Title IX in many states,[50] and has oversight from The National Federation of State High School Associations (NFHS).[51] But within the NCAA, cheerleading is not considered a sport, and thus does not need to abide by NCAA by-laws restricting practice durations and frequencies, requiring coach certification and concussion education, and ensuring safe practice facilities and equipment, as done with sanctioned sports.[52] Cheerleading has been included in HS RIO but historically not been included in the NCAA-ISP, a direct reflection of the difference in NFHS and NCAA categorization of cheerleading. In the context of OCR or WSF definitions, cheerleading is also not considered a sport, as cheerleading's primary purpose is to cheer for a competitive team on the sidelines, not compete against other teams, although many cheer squads compete in regional and national competitions.[53] In addition, a US judge in Connecticut ruled that cheerleading is too undeveloped and unorganized to be suitably labeled a competitive sport.[54] Yet, the need to examine such an activity is essential given recent high school sports injury surveillance data on concussion reported that practice concussion rates in cheerleading are higher than many sanctioned sports.[55] Other examples of the blurred lines of what is and is not a sport include nonschool-sanctioned sporting activities, such as pick-up basketball, or nontraditional sports such as snowboarding, skateboarding, or rock climbing. Because of the inevitable financial and personnel limitations, all sports injury

Table 2
Criteria for organizations' definition of sport

Organization	Criteria
National Collegiate Athletic Association[95]	• An institutional activity involving physical exertion with the purpose of competition within a collegiate competition structure • At least 5 regularly scheduled competitions within a season • Standardized rules with official rating/scoring systems
US Department of Education's Office for Civil Rights[96]	• Athletic ability • Athletic competition • Preparation similar to other athletic teams • Multilevel championship competitions • Administration by an athletics department
Women's Sports Foundation[96]	• Physical activity involving mass resistance • Against/with an opponent • Governing rules • Skill-based competition

surveillance studies are faced with difficult decisions regarding which sports should be covered, and little consensus exists.[56]

DEFINING AT-RISK EXPOSURE TIME

In many epidemiologic studies, calculating at-risk person time is straightforward. At-risk person time is continuous (ie, the populations of concern are always at risk for the disease outcome by simply being alive). In sports injury epidemiology, at-risk person time is staggered, comprised of times at which athletes compete, practice, and/or train. Accurately defining at-risk exposure time is of the utmost importance if valid between-sport comparisons are to be made. An objective time measure (ie, hours and minutes) would seem the most logical method of tracking at-risk person time, and this has been proposed by previous researchers as the preferred method of capturing athlete exposure.[57,58] However, sports settings vary widely across geographic locations, competitive levels, and age groups; thus, it may simply be unrealistic for data collectors in some surveillance systems to be able to capture such detailed exposure data. For example, in the US high school setting, where 1 AT covers all sports, it is impossible for that single AT to be present at every school-sanctioned competition and practice for every sport simultaneously to track every athlete's participation to the exact minute. Furthermore, one must consider the true concept of being at risk. For example, even those surveillance systems capable of capturing exposure as athlete minutes still fail to accurately capture the exact amount of time an athlete is at risk at practice (ie, actually active rather than listening to coaches or watching as other athletes take their turn in drills). Even in competition, accurately capturing minutes at risk can be difficult. For example, in football, should one include all the time in which the game clock is running, or only the time when athletes are actually directly involved in sport-specific physical activity? A *Wall Street Journal* article[59] estimated that each 60 minute football game is comprised of only approximately 11 minutes of time that the ball is in play. For other sports, such as baseball, there can be even more disparity between the length of a game and the number of minutes any individual athlete is actual at risk of injury from sport-specific physical activity.[60]

AEs are a common alternative to tracking at-risk time and have been recommended.[38] The AE is a measure of activity (eg, practices attended, games played in) rather than time (eg, athlete minutes, person years), and is thus an abstract estimate of at-risk person time. Prior surveillance systems have defined AE as "one athlete's participation in a practice or competition."[61] The quantification of AEs is more feasible for most surveillance systems than measuring minutes played/practiced by each athlete, because it only requires the knowledge of an athlete's attendance at practice or competition, not their specific activities within each. Yet, the AE presents a paradox in which it may be simultaneously a superior and inferior measure of at-risk time compared with minute-based measures. Consider the following scenario. During a high school football game, a kicker and quarterback are both injured in the last minutes of the first quarter, and leave the game. The at-risk time for both players would be 1 AE. With a minute-based exposure, the at-risk time for the kicker, who is on the field for only a few plays a game, is far less than that of the quarterback. Is it accurate then to state the quarterback has the same at-risk time? In this scenario, the AE may overestimate injury risk among athletes who play sparingly. Considering another scenario, the quarterbacks from 2 opposing teams both sustain similar injuries with similar severities from a clinical perspective, but one is injured in the first minute of the game while the other is injured in the last minute of the game. The at-risk time for both quarterbacks would be 1 AE, but using a minute-based exposure, one quarterback's at-risk time would be far less than the others, due to leaving the game earlier. However, both will likely face similar rehabilitation needs and similar time loss from play. Additionally, both attended practices and trained with the team, and were on the roster for the entire season consuming the same team resources (uniforms, travel, food, coaching, medical care). Use of a minute-based exposure, if scenarios like this occur over the course of seasons in large population samples, will introduce a healthy player bias similar to the previously reported healthy worker bias.[62] Therefore, it may make sense to treat their at-risk exposure as comparable.

Another complex decision is which athletes on a team contribute exposure. Athletes listed on the game roster for each competition may be counted as having a competition AE, regardless of whether they played in the game, if they participated in precompetition warm-ups. One method, known as the athlete-participation model, includes all athletes on the roster, regardless of playing time. This method has the potential to underestimate injury rates.[57,63] In this scenario, the magnitude of the underestimation will depend on the ratio of athletes on the roster to the number of athletes who played in that game.[63] In addition, if an injury took place during pre-game warm-ups, this is counted as a competition-related injury, when in reality it did not occur during competitive play. These scenarios, as well as those provided previously, demonstrate the difficulty in declaring 1 measure of exposure preferred over others. Researchers must be diligent in documenting how data were collected, and readers must be aware of these nuances. These considerations are especially important when comparing information across multiple studies using different estimates of time at risk. **Table 1** highlights the use of a variety of at-risk exposure time measures in prior sports injury surveillance systems.

Alongside the specific measurement of at-risk exposure time, defining the parameters of when injuries occur is essential. Many sports injury surveillance systems will track concussions that occur in competitions and practices sanctioned by the overarching organization (eg, league,[15,16] high school,[15,16,18] NCAA[64,65]). However, publications using the National Football League (NFL) Injury Surveillance System (ISS) and National Hockey League (NHL)-NHL Players Association (NHLPA) Concussion Program only included competition concussion data.[29,31] This is a limitation as it fails to provide data on the frequency of practice-related concussions. Although concussion rates are higher in competitions for most sports, many have large absolute numbers of practice-related concussions.[18,25] Also, most players on a squad participate in practice while not all play in competitions, which means more individual athletes are at risk during practices, particularly during game-speed, full-contact drills and scrimmages.[66]

There are additional settings and scenarios outside competition and practice that may be underexamined. For example, many surveillance systems do not collect data from individual training or weightlifting sessions that occur outside of formal practice sessions.[18,65] Also, surveillance systems often exclude nonsport-related concussions (eg, falls, motor vehicle crashes), even when such injuries occurred during team-related activities (eg, fall in locker room or team travel). Capturing such concussions that occur outside team-sanctioned sport-specific physical activities is arduous and likely not possible for many sports injury surveillance systems. Thus, this will likely remain another area of variation across surveillance systems that researchers must clearly define, and readers must understand.

DEFINING INJURY/CONCUSSION

Rather than providing a specific definition of concussion, most prior sports injury surveillance systems have instead relied upon the professional judgment of the sports medicine clinicians serving as data collectors and reporters (see **Table 1**). This is both, because sports medical professionals such as ATs and team physicians typically maintain a good, up-to-date, knowledge base regarding concussions and because currently numerous professionally accepted definitions of concussion exist.[67] In some surveillance systems, a working clinical definition is endorsed. For example, ATs participating in sports injury surveillance programs, such as NCAA Injury Surveillance Program (NCAA-ISP), the National Athletic Treatment, Injury and Outcomes Network (NATION), and Youth Football Surveillance System (YFSS),[15,16] have, in recent years, been encouraged to follow the definition provided by the Consensus Statement on Concussion in Sport.[67] The NFL ISS and NHL-NHLPA Concussion Programs instead provide internally created frameworks for concussion reporting.[27,29]

Defining concussion consistently across studies is complex given that concussion injuries have varying effects among athletes, and diagnosis and management of such injuries varies by clinician.[68] Whereas orthopedic injuries can be defined using standardized structural imaging techniques, a diagnosis of concussion may depend on the disclosure of symptoms by the athlete to a clinician. Athletes' willingness to make such disclosure may depend on gender, age, and many other factors.[16] At the same time, concussions that remain unreported because of athlete nondisclosure[69–76] are not identified by medical professionals and thus cannot be captured by surveillance systems using clinicians as data reporters. Although acquiring a consensus on the definition of concussion in sports may never be reached, researchers should specify their definition of concussion utilized, report whether data collectors were trained in the definition, and, if so, describe how they were trained.

DETERMINING WHICH MEASURES OF INCIDENCE TO USE

Most published concussion data from sports injury surveillance systems present concussion incidence as rates (see **Table 1**). Although injury rates may be typically preferred because they account for all cases of injury in the numerator and for variation in the amount of exposure time via the denominator, they may not be intuitive for all of the various sports stakeholders (eg, policy makers, parents, or coaches). Few studies have utilized risk, which may be a more intuitive measure, as it simply measures the probability that an injury will occur during sports participation within a specific timeframe (eg, 1 season). This metric merits strong consideration in outreach and communication settings, as it is frequently requested, and most people who understand probability have an intuitive concept of risk.

As the number of epidemiologic studies of concussions over the past decade has increased,[77] Kerr and colleagues[36] argued that it was necessary to broaden the range of metrics utilized to measure concussion incidence. Using concussion data from the NCAA-ISP, Kerr and colleagues[36] computed 4 measures of concussion incidence: rates, risk, the average number of concussions per team season, and the proportion of team seasons with at least 1 concussion. Despite some variation in the rank order of included sports, full-contact sports such as wrestling, football, and ice hockey consistently generated the highest incidence of concussion. However, squad size may serve as a confounder, particularly in football.[45] Furthermore, such measures can be biased when comparing incidence across teams (or sports) that vary greatly by the number of athletic sessions per season. Thus, it is important for readers to understand the strengths and limitations of measures of concussion incidence utilized by various researchers.

SAMPLING CHALLENGES AND GENERALIZABILITY

Many sports injury surveillance programs at the professional level, such as those for the NFL, Major League Baseball (MLB), National Basketball Association, and NHL, are census data (ie, they obtain data from all teams) (see **Table 1**). However, in many cases, sports injury surveillance relies upon a sample of participating programs. Thus, findings may not be generalizable to nonparticipating programs. This is especially true for programs in which data are collected using a convenience or volunteer sample; programs that choose to participate may differ from those that do not. However, in general, such concerns are outweighed by the merits of obtaining some surveillance information, even from a nonrandom sample.

Findings may also not be generalizable to other organizations and programs within the same level of competition. For example, data from 1 NCAA conference or division may not apply to the entire NCAA due to different rules, officiating, school resources, or personnel. Furthermore, although the NCAA-ISP obtains data from all 3 divisions, data from programs within the National Association of Intercollegiate Athletics (NAIA) and the Junior National Collegiate Athletics Association (JNCAA) are seldom examined. Only 1 study utilizing data from the NAIA and JNCAA exists to the authors' knowledge,[78] and it reported differences in injury rates among the 3 NCAA divisions, NAIA, and JNCAA. Because resources such as staffing may not be equitable across settings within the same level of competition and may confound observed injury estimates, researchers should fully describe their sample characteristics to help readers determine comparability across studies. It is also recommended that, when feasible, sports injury surveillance systems should attempt to recruit across diverse populations (eg, institutions, geographic regions, levels of competitiveness) in order to best account for the broadest spectrum of athletes within the population. Such a breadth of findings can also help to determine whether the incidence of concussion varies within population subgroups.

MONITORING TRENDS ACROSS TIME

Given the long durations in which many have existed, 1 strength of sports injury surveillance is the potential to ascertain secular trends. In a recent examination of concussion data from the NCAA-ISP, Zuckerman and colleagues[25] found that a linear trend did not exist in the national estimates across 5 years (2009/10–2013/14 academic years); however, increases were reported for specific sports, including men's football, women's ice hockey, and men's lacrosse. Similar trends were observed in high school level data.[20] Furthermore, Zuckerman and colleagues[25] found that annual national estimates were the lowest in 2009/10 and the highest in 2011/12. This may be partially attributable to the introduction of concussion policy in April 2010 by the NCAA Executive Committee that mandated each school adopt a concussion management plan; observed increase in incidence may be due to heightened awareness and reporting due to such policies. Using the same timeframe, Wasserman and colleagues[27] found that the proportion of sport-related concussions that required at least a week before return to participation increased from 42.7% in 2009/10% to 70.2% in 2013/14. The authors noted that these findings likely do not indicate increased injury severity, but rather reflect improved symptom monitoring and management protocols. However, it is also essential for future research to directly examine the implementation of, and compliance with, such concussion-related policy. In addition, given that continued surveillance efforts occur across multiple settings, it is imperative to utilize such data to generate a better understanding of the trends over time in concussion incidence and management.

Despite the ability to monitor trends, variation in annual participation may potentially influence estimates of incidence. Zuckerman and colleagues[25] found that men's wrestling has a concussion rate higher than any other NCAA sport. In response to the need to further analyze data from men's wrestling given this finding, Kerr[79] noted two important aspects related to data collection. First, during the 2009/10 to 2013/14 academic years, NCAA-ISP participation in men's wrestling was lower than that of many other sports, which consequently yielded less precise concussion rate estimates (**Fig. 1**).[25] In contrast, football had a larger number of programs participating, and thus, concussion rates were more precise (**Fig. 2**). Part of this increased precision is due to the larger squad size in football.[45] Second, when annual injury rates fluctuate, resulting aggregated rates may vary based upon the time periods examined. For example, the men's wrestling concussion rate was 10.9 concussions per 10,000 AEs in 2009/10 to 2013/14, but 8.2 concussions per 10,000 AEs in 2012/13 to 2014/15 (see **Fig. 1**). When comparing concussions rates from 2012/13 to 2014/15 in wrestling and football, both estimates were more similar than comparisons from 2009/10 to 2013/14 (see **Fig. 2**). Providing precision metrics such as confidence intervals can help readers gauge the quality of findings presented.

EVALUATION OF RISK FACTORS AND INTERVENTIONS

An additional benefit of sports injury surveillance is the ability to identify risk factors and evaluate interventions aimed to reduce concussion incidence and severity across large, population-based groups. For example, to measure neck strength, Collins and colleagues[80] developed a hand-held tension scale, which served as a cost-effective alternative to the commonly used hand-held dynamometer. This hand-held tension scale was then used with 6704 high school athletes in boys' and girls' soccer,

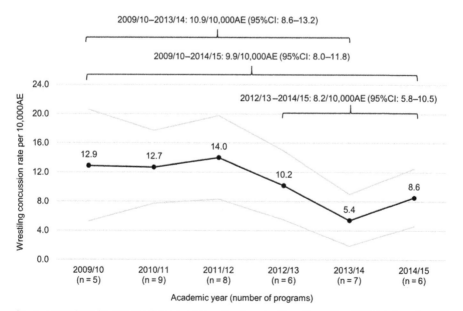

Fig. 1. Variations in reported concussion rates in wrestling from the NCAA Injury Surveillance Program, based upon academic years included. AE, athlete-exposure; CI, confidence interval. Note: gray lines represent 95% CI.

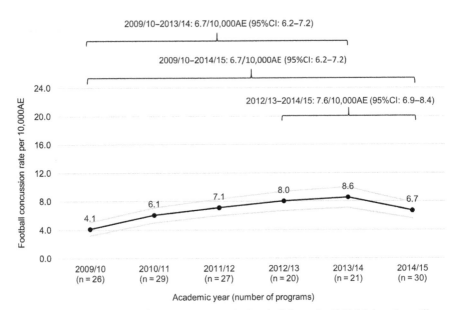

Fig. 2. Variations in reported concussion rates in football from the NCAA Injury Surveillance Program, based upon academic years included. AE, athlete-exposure; CI, confidence interval. Note: gray lines represent 95% CI.

basketball, and lacrosse from 51 high schools in 25 states. Concussion and exposure data were captured via HS RIO. The study found that, after adjusting for gender and sport, for every 1-pound increase in neck strength, the odds of concussion decreased 5%.

Another study examined youth football leagues implementing the Heads Up Football (HUF) educational program and Pop Warner practice contact restriction guidelines.[44] In the HUF educational program, each league had a player safety coach who was responsible for providing other coaches with educational resources on concussion, heat illness, and recognition and immediate management of cardiac events, and hands-on training of proper equipment fitting, proper tackling technique, and strategies for reducing player-to-player contact. The Pop Warner practice contact restriction guidelines forbade full-speed head-on blocking or tackling drills in which the players lined up more than 3 yards apart, and reduced the amount of contact at each practice to a maximum of one-third of practice time. Concussions and all other injuries were tracked using the YFSS. Overall injury rates were lowest among leagues utilizing both the HUF educational program and Pop Warner practice contact restriction guidelines. Concussion rates did not differ significantly, with the exception of leagues of 11- to 15-year-olds using both the HUF educational program and Pop Warner practice contact restriction guidelines, which had a lower concussion rate than leagues using neither. Nevertheless, in an additional study comprised of 6 Indiana high school football programs, all of which were required to have coaches undergo concussion education, those utilizing the HUF educational program with a player safety coach had a lower concussion rate in practices.[81]

Despite the promising surveillance-based findings regarding interventions and programming intending to reduce the incidence of concussion, it is important to continue examining the efficacy of such prevention strategies with additional samples, settings, and study designs. Several survey studies have highlighted organized concussion education plans, only to show a lack of meaningful change in knowledge. Kroshus and colleagues[82] evaluated the effectiveness of mandated, institutional concussion education among male collegiate hockey players, but found no improvements in knowledge and a minimal decrease in intention to continue playing through a concussion. Another study[83] cluster-randomized 256 adolescent boys from 12 ice hockey teams into 3 groups that were provided either one of two concussion education videos, or an informational handout. No changes in concussion knowledge were seen in posteducation surveys, and 1 video actually led to an increase in under-reporting of concussions at 1-month after the survey. These studies emphasize an important point regarding public health mandates; implementation alone may not lead to meaningful change. The use of mixed methods to assess implementation and effectiveness of concussion interventions could help pinpoint areas of focus for future research efforts.

COMPARABILITY ACROSS SPORTS INJURY SURVEILLANCE SYSTEMS

One challenge in comparing surveillance data is that the data elements collected vary across systems. For example, whereas the NCAA-ISP, NATION, and YFSS collect similar data on concussion symptoms (17 symptoms ranging from headache to sensitivity to light),[16,27] HS RIO collects data on 13 symptoms, excluding symptoms such as insomnia and excess excitability. Thus, caution must be taken when comparing findings across systems, particularly related to the average number of symptoms reported (ie, a smaller number reported in HS RIO compared to NATION may simply be due to a smaller number of options available). Previous research has examined concussion incidence across levels of competition from sports injury surveillance systems that utilize the same data collection methods.[16,23,27] However, even these studies note the inability to account for varying level-specific factors that may confound concussion reporting, such as team medical staff coverage and variation in individual clinicians' diagnostic practices.

Readers must also be aware of different dynamics of data collection among varying levels of competition. For a professional or division I collegiate athletic team, there is often at least 1 AT or team physician per team, with abundant resources and constant contact with athletes. In contrast, there may be at best a single AT for multiple sports at the high school level with significantly decreased resources and limited contact with some athletes. Some high school and youth sports settings may have very limited or no access to ATs and data collection infrastructures.[39,44] Thus, many high school sports injury surveillance programs only collect data from schools with AT coverage.[16,18,21,27] Moreover, changes in data collection measures, such as shifts from paper-and-pencil forms to an electronic system, may lead to changes in school participation and subsequent data quality.[65] Readers should be aware of such inherent limitations of sports injury surveillance systems, particularly when attempting to compare data from multiple systems, and critically evaluate how reported findings may be affected.

ACCESS TO DATA

Both orthopedic injury studies[84] and concussion studies have used public records of injuries among professional athletes rather than actual medical records.[85–88] However, because data based on media reports have not been validated, use of an organization's internal sports injury surveillance system data would likely be more valid. Unfortunately, access to existing sports injury surveillance data currently varies widely. Some systems such as HS RIO, NATION, and NCAA-ISP provide data to external researchers through an application process. However, many professional level datasets are not as accessible. Currently, the MLB Health and Injury Tracking System (HITS) allows researchers to apply for access, but assigns priority to particular areas of research. Papers on concussions using MLB HITS data have been published only by the researchers managing the system.[32] Accessing data from NFL ISS is even more limited. The primary purpose of many sports injury surveillance systems is to allow organizations to internally examine injury trends and patterns so they can make evidence-based policy and guideline decisions. Yet, publications reporting data captured by sports injury surveillance systems help external researchers, clinicians, and the general public understand the most up-to-date sports injury patterns. Furthermore, surveillance systems providing access to external researchers not involved with the organizations overseeing the surveillance systems reduce concern regarding lack of objectivity. Just as readers are more critical of drug studies financed by pharmaceutical companies, they should critically evaluate the institutional affiliation of researchers publishing reports using sports injury surveillance data.

FUTURE DIRECTIONS

The wealth of concussion data collected by sports injury surveillance systems is undeniable. With the ability to monitor trends over time and compare populations internally and across systems, while upholding high quality data standards, sports injury surveillance systems have helped provide a better understanding of the incidence of concussion and its risk factors as well as the effectiveness of various interventions on reducing concussion incidence and severity. Nevertheless, future investments are required both to strengthen existing surveillance systems and to inform the development of future sports injury surveillance efforts (**Table 3**).

Increase Buy-In from Stakeholders

When data from sports injury surveillance systems are collected from the entire population of interest, a census is obtained. However, in many cases, only a sample of the population is collected, thus potentially limiting generalizability to the entire population. Currently, both HS RIO and NCAA-ISP have participation from only a small proportion of all schools eligible to participate. Thus, although HS RIO utilizes a stratified random selection approach for participation,[89] and NCAA-ISP solicits participation from all 3 divisions,[65] such strata likely do not control for all variables of importance (eg, staff resources). However, to allow for more strata, more participation by eligible data collection sites is required. Additionally, in both HS RIO and NCAA-ISP, participation levels vary across sports. Increased participation would help obtain more data for sports in which concussion incidence is lower or lower overall school participation hinders obtaining sufficient data. Although both the NFHS and NCAA have long supported HS RIO and NCAA-ISP, participation by eligible schools has always been voluntary. Without increased financial incentives or required participation, the best way to increase participation and thus, the generalizability of these datasets, likely lies with increased endorsement by regional stakeholders (eg, collegiate conferences and state high school athletic associations).

To increase participation, buy-in from a wide variety of stakeholders is necessary. The data collectors, in many cases, team or school sports medicine clinicians, need to be further educated about the benefits of participation and data collection. Coaches and athletic directors should also understand how such data can benefit their programs. The rapidly growing number of private sports organizations with internal sports injury surveillance systems should be encouraged to collaborate with external researchers to help disseminate data, compare findings across populations, and revise data collection tools in response to future research needs. Finally, researchers must aim to find ways to help provide such stakeholders with the resources that aid in better translating surveillance data to concrete prevention initiatives and interventions to prevent concussions and manage concussion recovery.

Common Data Elements

Although numerous sports injury surveillance systems collect data on concussions, the data elements collected vary widely from system to system. It is important to identify common data elements that can allow for comparisons of data among existing systems and that may help inform development of future systems. Such data points should pertain to athlete demographics, mechanism of concussion, symptomatology prevalence, return to play time, and symptom resolution time. The National Institutes of Health have developed common data elements for varying types of traumatic brain injury (TBI) in an effort to streamline the clinical aspects of such data collection to allow for more adequate comparison across studies, including those around concussion.[90] However, that effort demonstrates the difficulty of creating common data elements applicable to both the traditional health care setting (eg, emergency department, physician's office, concussion clinic) and the broader clinical settings currently covered by existing sports injury surveillance systems, as well as concussion that occur from sport- and non-sport-related mechanisms. Thus, while use of common data elements should be encouraged when feasible, an understanding of the primary purpose of the sports injury surveillance system and the needs of the stakeholders investing in the system must be allowed to drive data collection rather than an expectation to conform to any individual set of common data elements.

Additionally, continued efforts should be made to develop a consensus definition of concussion feasible across sports injury surveillance systems using varied data collectors to report concussion. Until such a consensus definition exists, researchers should clearly outline the definition for concussion used in all publications. It is important to note that, although common data elements would help increase comparability, it is unavoidable that differences among systems will exist. This may be attributable to differences in data collectors (eg, parents vs ATs vs team physicians), as well as the level of competition (professional team, where team medical staff are always present vs high school, where an AT may have to choose one sport to cover among multiple occurring simultaneously, vs youth sports league, where clinicians are rarely present). Disseminated research findings need to specify the limitations of the results based upon how injury was defined and how data were collected.

Exploring Novel Approaches

It is important for future research to consider novel approaches to addressing current limitations in data collection. One important consideration is that many of the current surveillance systems require additional entry beyond the medical records kept by the AT or physician. Utilizing existing electronic medical records, when available, is important in reducing the burden on the clinician and can aid in not only increased participation in surveillance systems, but also better tracking of outcomes. Because electronic medical record keeping systems are too expensive for many high schools, providing free/reduced fee access to high school ATs could increase participation in surveillance systems. When the presence of medical professionals is limited in a particular sports setting, considering other options for data collectors (eg, parents, coaches) could expand the populations included in sports injury surveillance systems. At the same time, with the abundance of individuals using handheld mobile devices,

Table 3
Strengths, limitations, and future directions for estimating concussion incidence via sports injury surveillance systems

Issue	Strengths	Limitations	Future Directions
Who collects the data?	Use of medical staff (eg, ATs, team physicians) educated and experienced to appropriately diagnose and manage concussion in the sports setting	Difficult to conduct surveillance where medical staff coverage is limited Medical staff may not have full authority (eg, medical decisions may be overridden by head coach)	Explore parents, athletes, and/or coaches as data collectors and the use of mobile-friendly Web-based tracking devices through validation research Use pre-existing electronic medical records to help ensure complete data entry
What sports are included?	Numerous sports captured across systems	Access to sports with lower visibility Access to youth sports without/with multiple national organizing bodies	Further buy-in from stakeholders to increase participation of sports with limited data Further buy-in from national sports governing bodies overseeing youth sports (eg, children aged 5–10)
Defining at-risk exposure time	Many established options available that can help reduce burden on data collector	Varying methods of capturing at-risk exposure time may impede comparability	Specify and define the at-risk exposure time measurement used
Defining injury/concussion	Use of medical staff (eg, AT, team physicians) may reduce need to provide specific definition	Varying definitions of concussion	Specify the injury/concussion definition used
Determining which measures of incidence to use	Most studies use injury rates, which allows for comparability across studies	Nonintuitiveness of certain measures Lack of published data using more intuitive measures	Specify and define the incidence measurements used Establish common analysis procedures

	Large samples, many of which are census data	Samples not generalizable across entire continuum of athletes participating in sport	Increase buy-in from stakeholders to increase participation Create unique athlete IDs to allow linkage of athlete data from 1 surveillance system to another as athletes move across the age continuum
Sampling challenges and generalizability			
Monitoring trends over time	Longitudinal effects of rule/policy changes	Incidence estimates may be associated with study period	Increase buy-in from stakeholders to increase participation
Evaluation of risk factors and interventions	Assess immediate effects of rule/policy changes	May be unable to directly examine the level of compliance with rule/policy changes	Consider surveillance alongside other research study designs to identify risk factors and develop and evaluate prevention strategies
Comparability across sports injury surveillance systems	Many common elements captured	Variations in data collection methods exist Levels of competitions have varying characteristics (eg, medical staff coverage, resource allocation), which surveillance efforts may not be able to fix	Examine manners to increase ability to compare studies, to standardize methodologies, but in the context of the purposes of the sports injury surveillance systems and the needs of the stakeholders investing in the systems
Access to data	Some systems allow external researchers to access data via simple data requests for no/low fee	Some data sources seldom publish data findings and are not available to external researchers	Increase buy-in from sports organizations overseeing systems

creating Web-based surveillance that is mobile-friendly may also aid data collection efforts. However, for such novel approaches to become integrated into the current structure of sports injury surveillance systems, it will be necessary to conduct validation research.

Going Beyond the Tip of the Iceberg

Although there is more known about the epidemiology and etiology of sport-related concussion today than ever before, only the tip of the iceberg has been uncovered. Surveillance is 1 component of injury prevention; it can help identify risk factors and assist in the development and evaluation of inventions to reduce injury frequency and severity.[91] Current ongoing sports injury surveillance, coupled with the commitment of federal agencies to develop surveillance mechanisms in other areas, will only continue to expand on this knowledge. General sports injury surveillance efforts have also driven more detailed studies, such as those under the NCAA-Department of Defense (DOD) Grand Alliance Project CARE (Concussion Assessment, Research and Education Consortium), that will further advance understanding of the etiology and outcomes following concussion. However, as the field continues to move forward, it is important to continue to work to streamline and align methodologies so that accurate comparisons can be made between studies.

SUMMARY

Understanding of concussion incidence through data captured by sports injury surveillance systems allows for bettered inform policy, organizational, and individual decision making about sport. It is important that all consumers of this information understand the methodologies and metrics of each surveillance system, including their strengths and limitations. The past few decades have seen dramatic shifts in concussion knowledge, moving beyond believing that loss of consciousness must occur with concussion, to understanding that concussion is more diffuse and nuanced. There is a better understanding that sports outside of football have higher than perceived concussion risk, and attained unprecedented levels of concussion education across broad non-clinical stakeholders (eg, sports policy makers, coaches, parents, athletes) have been attained. The next decade will hopefully show a continuing refinement of methods, a better understanding of the risk for concussion, and the discovery of how to best prevent these injuries across all sports at all levels.

REFERENCES

1. Guskiewicz KM, McCrea M, Marshall SW, et al. Cumulative effects associated with recurrent concussion in collegiate football players: the NCAA Concussion Study. JAMA 2003;290(19):2549–55.

2. Guskiewicz KM, Marshall SW, Bailes J, et al. Association between recurrent concussion and late-life cognitive impairment in retired professional football players. Neurosurgery 2005;57(4):719–26.

3. Guskiewicz KM, Marshall SW, Bailes J, et al. Recurrent concussion and risk of depression in retired professional football players. Med Sci Sports Exerc 2007; 39(6):903–9.

4. McCrea M, Guskiewicz KM, Marshall SW, et al. Acute effects and recovery time following concussion in collegiate football players: the NCAA Concussion Study. JAMA 2003;290(19):2556–63.

5. Institute of Medicine. Sports-related concussions in youth: improving the science, changing the culture. 2013. Available at: http://www.ninds.nih.gov/research/tbi/sports_concussion_report.pdf. Accessed September 29, 2016.
6. Bakhos LL, Lockhart GR, Myers R, et al. Emergency department visits for concussion in young child athletes. Pediatrics 2010;126(3):e550–6.
7. Jacobson NA, Buzas D, Morawa LG. Concussions from youth football results from NEISS hospitals over an 11-year time frame, 2002-2012. Orthop J Sports Med 2013;1(7). 2325967113517860.
8. Coronado VG, Haileyesus T, Cheng TA, et al. Trends in sports- and recreation-related traumatic brain injuries treated in US emergency departments: the National Electronic Injury Surveillance System-All Injury Program (NEISS-AIP) 2001-2012. J Head Trauma Rehabil 2015;30(3):185–97.
9. Buzas D, Jacobson NA, Morawa LG. Concussions from 9 youth organized sports results from NEISS hospitals over an 11-year time frame, 2002-2012. Orthop J Sports Med 2014;2(4). 2325967114528460.
10. Bryan MA, Rowhani-Rahbar A, Comstock RD, et al. Sports-and recreation-related concussions in US youth. Pediatrics 2016. http://dx.doi.org/10.1542/peds.2015-4635.
11. Langlois JA, Rutland-Brown W, Wald MM. The epidemiology and impact of traumatic brain injury: a brief overview. J Head Trauma Rehabil 2006;21(5):375–8.
12. Arbogast KB, Curry AE, Pfeiffer MR, et al. Point of health care entry for youth with concussion within a large pediatric care network. JAMA Pediatr 2016. http://dx.doi.org/10.1001/jamapediatrics.2016.0294.
13. Daneshvar DH, Nowinski CJ, McKee AC, et al. The epidemiology of sport-related concussion. Clin Sports Med 2011;30(1):1–17.
14. Meehan WP. d'Hemecourt P, Comstock RD. High school concussions in the 2008-2009 academic year mechanism, symptoms, and management. Am J Sports Med 2010;38(12):2405–9.
15. Dompier TP, Kerr ZY, Marshall SW, et al. Incidence of concussion during practice and games in youth, high school, and collegiate American football players. JAMA Pediatr 2015;169(7):659–65.
16. Kerr ZY, Zuckerman SL, Wasserman EB, et al. Concussion symptoms and return to play time in youth, high school, and college American football athletes. JAMA Pediatr 2016;170(7):647–53.
17. Kerr ZY, Marshall SW, Simon JE, et al. Injury rates in age-only versus age-and-weight playing standard conditions in American youth football. Orthop J Sports Med 2015;3(9). 2325967115603979.
18. Marar M, McIlvain NM, Fields SK, et al. Epidemiology of concussions among United States high school athletes in 20 sports. Am J Sports Med 2012;40(4):747–55.
19. Frommer LJ, Gurka KK, Cross KM, et al. Sex differences in concussion symptoms of high school athletes. J Athl Train 2011;46(1):76–84.
20. Rosenthal JA, Foraker RE, Collins CL, et al. National high school athlete concussion rates from 2005–2006 to 2011–2012. Am J Sports Med 2014;42(7):1710–5.
21. Lincoln AE, Caswell SV, Almquist JL, et al. Trends in concussion incidence in high school sports: a prospective 11-year study. Am J Sports Med 2011;39(5):958–63.
22. Schulz MR, Marshall SW, Mueller FO, et al. Incidence and risk factors for concussion in high school athletes, North Carolina, 1996–1999. Am J Epidemiol 2004;160(10):937–44.
23. Gessel LM, Fields SK, Collins CL, et al. Concussions among United States high school and collegiate athletes. J Athl Train 2007;42(4):495–503.

24. Powell JW, Barber-Foss KD. Traumatic brain injury in high school athletes. JAMA 1999;282(10):958–63.

25. Zuckerman SL, Kerr ZY, Yengo-Kahn A, et al. Epidemiology of sports-related concussion in NCAA athletes from 2009–2010 to 2013–2014: incidence, recurrence, and mechanisms. Am J Sports Med 2015;43(11):2654–62.

26. Covassin T, Moran R, Elbin R. Sex differences in reported concussion injury rates and time loss from participation: an update of the National Collegiate Athletic Association injury surveillance program from 2004–2005 through 2008–2009. J Athl Train 2016;51(3):189–94.

27. Wasserman EB, Kerr ZY, Zuckerman SL, et al. Epidemiology of sports-related concussions in National Collegiate Athletic Association athletes from 2009-2010 to 2013-2014: symptom prevalence, symptom resolution time, and return-to-play time. Am J Sports Med 2016;44(1):226–33.

28. Dick RW. A summary of head and neck injuries in collegiate athletics using the NCAA injury surveillance system. In: Hoerner EF, editor. Head and Neck Injuries in Sports. Philadelphia: American Society for Testing and Materials; 1994. p. 13–9.

29. Casson IR, Viano DC, Powell JW, et al. Twelve years of National Football League concussion data. Sports Health 2010;2(6):471–83.

30. Pellman EJ, Viano DC, Tucker AM, et al. Concussion in professional football: reconstruction of game impacts and injuries. Neurosurgery 2003;53(4):799–814.

31. Benson BW, Meeuwisse WH, Rizos J, et al. A prospective study of concussions among National Hockey League players during regular season games: the NHL-NHLPA concussion program. CMAJ 2011;183(8):905–11.

32. Green GA, Pollack KM, D'Angelo J, et al. Mild traumatic brain injury in major and minor league baseball players. Am J Sports Med 2015;43(5):1118–26.

33. Orchard JW, Seward H, Orchard JJ. Results of 2 decades of injury surveillance and public release of data in the Australian Football League. Am J Sports Med 2013;41(4):734–41.

34. Kemp SP, Hudson Z, Brooks JH, et al. The epidemiology of head injuries in English professional rugby union. Clin J Sport Med 2008;18(3):227–34.

35. Eirale C, Tol JL, Targett S, et al. Concussion surveillance: do low concussion rates in the Qatar professional football league reflect a true difference or emphasize challenges in knowledge translation? Clin J Sport Med 2015;25(1):73–4.

36. Kerr ZY, Roos KG, Djoko A, et al. Epidemiologic measures for quantifying the incidence of concussion in National Collegiate Athletic Association sports. J Athl Train 2016. http://dx.doi.org/10.4085/1062-6050-51.6.05.

37. Ekegren CL, Gabbe BJ, Finch CF. Sports injury surveillance systems: a review of methods and data quality. Sports Med 2016;46(1):49–65.

38. Balazs LGC, Brelin CAM, Wolfe CJA, et al. Variation in injury incidence rate reporting: the case for standardization between American and non-American researchers. Curr Orthopaedic Pract 2015;26(4):395–402.

39. Pryor RR, Casa DJ, Vandermark LW, et al. Athletic training services in public secondary schools: a benchmark study. J Athl Train 2015;50(2):156–62.

40. Lombardi NJ, Tucker B, Freedman KB, et al. Accuracy of athletic trainer and physician diagnoses in sports medicine. Orthopedics 2016;39(5):e944–9.

41. Yard EE, Collins CL, Comstock RD. A comparison of high school sports injury surveillance data reporting by certified athletic trainers and coaches. J Athl Train 2009;44(6):645–52.

42. Emery CA, Meeuwisse WH, Hartmann SE. Evaluation of risk factors for injury in adolescent soccer implementation and validation of an injury surveillance system. Am J Sports Med 2005;33(12):1882–91.

43. Schiff MA, Mack CD, Polissar NL, et al. Soccer injuries in female youth players: comparison of injury surveillance by certified athletic trainers and Internet. J Athl Train 2010;45(3):238–42.

44. Kerr ZY, Yeargin S, McLeod TCV, et al. Comprehensive coach education and practice contact restriction guidelines result in lower injury rates in youth American football. Orthop J Sports Med 2015;3(7). 2325967115594578.

45. National Collegiate Athletic Association. Student-athlete participation: 1981-82-2012-13. 2014. Available at: http://www.ncaapublications.com/productdownloads/PR2014.pdf. Accessed September 29, 2016.

46. National Federation of State High School Associations. Participation statistics. 2014. Available at: http://www.nfhs.org/ParticipationStatics/ParticipationStatics.aspx/. Accessed September 29, 2016.

47. Baugh CM, Kerr ZY. High school rowing injuries: National athletic treatment, injury and outcomes network (NATION). J Athl Train 2016;51(4):317–20.

48. Willigenburg NW, Borchers JR, Quincy R, et al. Comparison of injuries in American Collegiate football and club rugby a prospective cohort study. Am J Sports Med 2016;44(3):753–60.

49. Shields BJ, Smith GA. Epidemiology of cheerleading fall-related injuries in the United States. J Athl Train 2009;44(6):578–85.

50. Boyce R. Cheerleading in the context of Title IX and gendering in sport. Sport J 2008;11(3). Available at: http://thesportjournal.org/article/cheerleading-in-the-context-of-title-ix-and-gendering-in-sport/. Accessed April 22, 2017.

51. National Federation of High Schools. New rules for dance risk minimization among high school spirit rules changes. 2016. Available at: https://www.nfhs.org/articles/new-rules-for-dance-risk-minimization-among-high-school-spirit-rules-changes/. Accessed September 29, 2016.

52. NCAA. 2010-11 NCAA Division I manual. 2010. Available at: http://www.ncaapublications.com/productdownloads/D111.pdf. Accessed September 29, 2016.

53. Varnavas H. Should cheerleading be a sport? Ill Business Law J 2009;2009(1):40–8.

54. Eaton-Robb P. U.S. judge in Conn.: cheerleading not a sport. MSNBC.com 2010. Available at: http://www.msnbc.msn.com/id/38347400/?GT1=43001. Accessed September 29, 2016.

55. Currie DW, Fields SK, Patterson MJ, et al. Cheerleading injuries in United States high schools. Pediatrics 2015. http://dx.doi.org/10.1542/peds.2015-2447.

56. Zuckerman SL, Totten D, Rubel K, et al. 174 Mechanisms of injury as a diagnostic predictor of sport-related concussion severity in football, basketball, and soccer: results from a regional concussion registry. Neurosurgery 2016;63(Suppl 1):169.

57. Fuller CW, Ekstrand J, Junge A, et al. Consensus statement on injury definitions and data collection procedures in studies of football (soccer) injuries. Br J Sports Med 2006;40(3):193–201.

58. Fuller CW, Molloy MG, Bagate C, et al. Consensus statement on injury definitions and data collection procedures for studies of injuries in rugby union. Br J Sports Med 2007;41(5):328–31.

59. Biderman D. Football games have 11 minutes of action. 2010. Available at: http://online.wsj.com/article/SB10001424052748704281204575002852055561406.html. Accessed September 29, 2016.

60. Moyer S. In America's pastime, baseball players pass a lot of time. 2013. Available at: http://www.wsj.com/articles/SB1000142412788732374080457859793234 1903720. Accessed September 29, 2016.
61. Kerr ZY, Collins CL, Fields SK, et al. Epidemiology of player–player contact injuries among US high school athletes 2005–2009. Clin Pediatr (Phila) 2011; 50(7):594–603.
62. Li CY, Sung FC. A review of the healthy worker effect in occupational epidemiology. Occup Med 1999;49(4):225–9.
63. Stovitz SD, Shrier I. Injury rates in team sport events: tackling challenges in assessing exposure time. Br J Sports Med 2012;46(14):960–3.
64. Dick R, Agel J, Marshall SW. National Collegiate Athletic Association injury surveillance system commentaries: introduction and methods. J Athl Train 2007; 42(2):173–82.
65. Kerr ZY, Dompier TP, Snook EM, et al. National Collegiate Athletic Association injury surveillance system: review of methods for 2004–2005 through 2013–2014 data collection. J Athl Train 2014;49(4):552–60.
66. Kerr ZY, Hayden R, Dompier TP, et al. Association of equipment worn and concussion injury rates in National Collegiate Athletic Association football practices: 2004–2005 to 2008–2009 academic years. Am J Sports Med 2015;43(5): 1131–41.
67. McCrory P, Meeuwisse WH, Aubry M, et al. Consensus statement on concussion in sport: the 4th International Conference on Concussion in Sport, Zurich, November 2012. J Athl Train 2013;48(4):554–75.
68. Rauh M, Macera C, Marshall SW. Applied sports injury epidemiology. In: Magee D, Manske R, Zachazewski J, et al, editors. Athletic and sports issues in musculoskeletal rehabilitation. St Louis (MO): Elsevier Saunders; 2011. p. 730–72.
69. Kerr ZY, Register-Mihalik JK, Marshall SW, et al. Disclosure and non-disclosure of concussion and concussion symptoms in athletes: review and application of the socio-ecological framework. Brain Inj 2014;28(8):1009–21.
70. Kerr ZY, Register-Mihalik JK, Kroshus E, et al. Motivations associated with nondisclosure of self-reported concussions in former collegiate athletes. Am J Sports Med 2016;44(1):220–5.
71. Sullivan L, Thomas AA, Molcho M. An evaluation of Gaelic Athletic Association (GAA) athletes' self-reported practice of playing while concussed, knowledge about and attitudes towards sports-related concussion. Int J Adolesc Med Health 2016. http://dx.doi.org/10.1515/ijamh-2015-0084.
72. Register-Mihalik JK, McLeod TCV, Linnan LA, et al. Relationship between concussion history and concussion knowledge, attitudes, and disclosure behavior in high school athletes. Clin J Sport Med 2016. http://dx.doi.org/10.1097/JSM. 0000000000000349.
73. Torres DM, Galetta KM, Phillips HW, et al. Sports-related concussion: anonymous survey of a collegiate cohort. Neurol Clin Pract 2013;3(4):279–87.
74. Kroshus E, Kubzansky LD, Goldman RE, et al. Norms, athletic identity, and concussion symptom under-reporting among male collegiate ice hockey players: a prospective cohort study. Ann Behav Med 2015;49(1):95–103.
75. Llewellyn T, Burdette GT, Joyner AB, et al. Concussion reporting rates at the conclusion of an intercollegiate athletic career. Clin J Sport Med 2014;24(1):76–9.
76. Ekegren C, Gabbe B, Finch C. Injury surveillance in community sport: can we obtain valid data from sports trainers? Scand J Med Sci Sports 2015;25(3): 315–22.

77. Marshall SW, Guskiewicz KM, Shankar V, et al. Epidemiology of sports-related concussion in seven US high school and collegiate sports. Inj Epidemiol 2015; 2(13). http://dx.doi.org/10.1186/s40621-015-0045-4.

78. Powell JW, Dompier TP. Analysis of injury rates and treatment patterns for time-loss and non-time-loss injuries among collegiate student-athletes. J Athl Train 2004;39(1):56–70.

79. Kerr ZY. The NCAA injury surveillance program (Injury surveillance in high school and collegiate sport: what do we know? What don't we know?). Paper presented at: National Athletic Trainers' Association 66th Clinical Symposia and AT Expo; St Louis (MO); June 23–26, 2015.

80. Collins CL, Fletcher EN, Fields SK, et al. Neck strength: a protective factor reducing risk for concussion in high school sports. J Prim Prev 2014;35(5): 309–19.

81. Kerr ZY, Dalton SL, Roos KG, et al. Comparison of Indiana high school football injury rates by inclusion of the USA football "Heads Up Football" player safety coach. Orthop J Sports Med 2016;4(5). 2325967116648441.

82. Kroshus E, Daneshvar DH, Baugh CM, et al. NCAA concussion education in ice hockey: an ineffective mandate. Br J Sports Med 2014;48(2):135–40.

83. Kroshus E, Baugh CM, Hawrilenko M, et al. Pilot randomized evaluation of publically available concussion education materials: evidence of a possible negative effect. Health Educ Behav 2015;42(2):153–62.

84. Carey JL, Huffman GR, Parekh SG, et al. Outcomes of anterior cruciate ligament injuries to running backs and wide receivers in the National Football League. Am J Sports Med 2006;34(12):1911–7.

85. Kuhn AW, Zuckerman SL, Totten D, et al. Performance and style of play after returning from concussion in the National Hockey League. Am J Sports Med 2016; 44(8):2152–7.

86. Yengo-Kahn AM, Zuckerman SL, Stotts J, et al. Performance following a first professional concussion among National Basketball Association players. Phys Sportsmed 2016;44(3):297–303.

87. Wasserman EB, Abar B, Shah MN, et al. Concussions are associated with decreased batting performance among Major League Baseball players. Am J Sports Med 2015;43(5):1127–33.

88. Beyer JA, Rowson S, Duma SM. Concussions experienced by Major League Baseball catchers and umpires: field data and experimental baseball impacts. Ann Biomed Eng 2012;40(1):150–9.

89. Centers for Disease Control and Prevention (CDC). Sports-related injuries among high school athletes—United States, 2005–06 school year. MMWR Morb Mortal Wkly Rep 2006;55(38):1037–40.

90. National Institute of Neurological Disorders and Stroke. NINDS common data elements. 2016. Available at: https://www.commondataelements.ninds.nih.gov/TBI.aspx#tab=Data_Standards. Accessed September 29, 2016.

91. Van Mechelen W, Hlobil H, Kemper HC. Incidence, severity, aetiology and prevention of sports injuries. Sports Med 1992;14(2):82–99.

92. Aubry M, Cantu R, Dvorak J, et al. Summary and agreement statement of the first International Conference on Concussion in Sport, Vienna 2001. Br J Sports Med 2002;36(1):6–7.

93. Pellman EJ, Powell JW, Viano DC, et al. Concussion in professional football: epidemiological features of game injuries and review of the literature—part 3. Neurosurgery 2004;54(1):81–96.

94. Maddocks DL, Dicker GD, Saling MM. The assessment of orientation following concussion in athletes. Clin J Sport Med 1995;5(1):32–5.

95. Edelman M. Sports and the law: can sports 'cheer' their way into title IX compliance? Above the law 2009. Available at: http://abovethelaw.com/2009/02/sports-and-the-law-can-schools-cheer-their-way-into-title-ix-compliance/. Accessed April 22, 2017.

96. Hennefer A. Dance and cheerleading as competitive sports: making a case for OCR sport recognition and NCAA emerging sport designation. 2003. Available at: http://files.eric.ed.gov/fulltext/ED479762.pdf. Accessed April 22, 2017.

Sideline Sports Concussion Assessment

Kenneth Podell, PhD[a],*, Chase Presley, MS[b], Howard Derman, MD[a]

KEYWORDS

- Concussion • Sideline assessment • SCAT • Assessment

KEY POINTS

- The sideline concussion assessment is the first line of defense in preventing a player from sustaining more severe effects from concussion through the rapid and accurate detection of concussion during a practice or in competition.
- Sideline assessment of concussions is a complex multisystem assessment to detect whether an athlete is evidencing signs or symptoms of concussion and should be removed from practice or competition.
- Sideline concussion assessments are challenging given some of the environmental conditions, substitution rules of some sports, possibility of athletes underreporting symptoms, and the difficulties of defining a concussion.
- Concussions can evolve or worsen over time and serial assessment of concussions acutely is important and critical.

Concussions are one of, it not the, single most prominent medical issue in sports today. There are more than 8 million athletes participating in organized competitive sports at the high school and collegiate level annually with many playing in a contact sport.[1] One of the most difficult aspects of sports concussion is the initial diagnosis during a competition.[2,3] It is critical to identify a concussion that occurs during a competition as soon as possible and to be able to remove a player immediately because of the significant risk of short- and long-term neurologic consequences of playing concussed.[4]

Although the understanding of sports-related concussions (SRC) and diagnostic ability have improved tremendously over the past several years, the ability to accurately and quickly diagnose a concussion during competition is an extremely complex and challenging task[5] for several reasons: (1) players often underreport concussion

Disclosure Statement: The authors have nothing to disclose.
[a] Department of Neurology, Weill-Cornell Medical College, Houston Methodist Hospital, Houston Methodist Concussion Center, 6560 Fannin Street, Suite 1840, Houston, TX 77030, USA;
[b] Department of Neurology, Houston Methodist Hospital, Houston Methodist Concussion Center, 6560 Fannin Street, Suite 1840, Houston, TX 77030, USA
* Corresponding author.
E-mail address: kpodell@houstonmethodist.org

Neurol Clin 35 (2017) 435–450
http://dx.doi.org/10.1016/j.ncl.2017.03.003
0733-8619/17/© 2017 Elsevier Inc. All rights reserved.

neurologic.theclinics.com

symptoms during competition and feel pressured to continue playing while con-cussed[6–11] or simply may not be aware they sustained one; (2) most concussions do not involve loss of consciousness or any pathognomonic neurologic signs[12]; (3) there is not a single, truly objective measure of concussion[13]; and (4) constraints placed on the evaluation by the rules of the sport (limited substitution or time limits for evaluation) makes the task of accurately diagnosing concussion during a compe-tition that much more daunting. The current adage of "when in doubt, sit them out" is easy to apply to the youngest athletes, but it gets harder and more complicated as the competition and importance of the game (ie, higher level collegiate and professional) comes into play. This places a lot of pressure on the health care provider tasked with the responsibility of either detecting a possible on-field concussion during competition or practice (referred to as a spotter), or accurately diagnosing it once the player has been removed to be evaluated.

As described by McCrea and coworkers,[2] the last 20 years or so has seen a concerted effort to standardize the sideline assessment of concussion with the devel-opment of more objective, performance-based techniques that improve specificity and sensitivity. This article reviews the current state-of-the-art tools in acute assess-ment of concussion during athletic competitions on the sideline, bench, or on the pitch. We review the current standard of care, the components involved in the sideline assessment, and the sensitivity and specificity, and critique the current literature and make recommendations for future practice.

DEFINITION OF CONCUSSION

Before discussing how to diagnose an SRC it is important to have a clear definition of concussion. This is what makes having specificity and sensitivity in concussion diag-nosis difficult. Unlike many other neurologic disorders/diseases, concussions have no pure pathognomonic finding (short of loss of consciousness) or any true gold standard in making a diagnosis. The multifactorial signs and symptoms of concussion overlap with many other disorders that occur during athletic competitions (eg, heat stroke or dehydration). Therefore having a clear and accurate, and as objective as possible, definition of concussion can help improve the actual diagnosis.

Traumatic brain injury (TBI) is often considered a blunt trauma to the head causing acceleration/deceleration or torqueing (rotational shearing) of the brain resulting in one or more signs or symptoms, such as brief (<30 minutes) loss of consciousness, retro-grade or posttraumatic amnesias, confusion, disorientation, various somatic or phys-iologic symptoms (eg, sensory sensitivity, dizziness, impaired balance), and memory impairment.[14] TBI severity is defined along a continuum from mild to severe with mild TBI typically defined as a Glasgow Coma Scale (GCS) of 13 to 15 with loss of con-sciousness less than 30 minutes and posttraumatic amnesia of less than 24 hours.[15]

Oftentimes SRC and mild TBI are interchangeably used, however concussions are typically considered to be on the milder end of mild TBI[16] because there rarely is loss of consciousness (<10% of the time[17]) and rarely is there retrograde and posttrau-matic amnesias lasting a few hours. Some groups have altered the definition of con-cussions as it pertains to sports. For example, the fourth international conference on concussions in sports in 2012 defined a concussion as "a complex pathophysiological process affecting the brain, induced by biomechanical forces..." caused by a direct blow to, or "an impulsive" force, transmitted to the head.[3] Inclusive of this definition is unremarkable standard structural neuroimaging. However, others have noted subtle structural changes associated with concussions.[18,19] More recently, others have advocated for diagnosing concussions along a continuum of possible, probable, and definitive,[20] showing the complexity of coming up with a quick and accurate diagnosis of concussion.

SIDELINE ASSESSMENT

It is important to understand that the true goal of the acute assessment during a competition or practice is not simply to diagnosis a concussion. Rather it is an assessment to determine if it is safe for an athlete to return to play because of any possible injury/trauma to the head, brain, or neck and spine. Concussion sideline assessments are a complex evaluation because of not only the complexity and intricacies of concussions, but also because of a multitude of challenges and particulars that impact the actual sideline assessment of athletes. First and foremost, one must be competent in assessing the heterogeneous complex processes that involve multiple systems including spine, skull and face, ocular-motor, vestibular, and central nervous system/brain when doing a sideline assessment of concussion. One can easily see that a multimodal, multitier assessment must be done quickly within the constraints of being on the sideline, possibly having a player not being completely open about symptoms, time constraints, possible dehydration and heat, and the pressure of removing an athlete during a close game.

It all starts with written and detailed emergency action plans and concussion protocols. All organizations are expected to have emergency action plans to handle medical emergencies of any type. A written concussion protocol is the standard at the professional level for most major international sports and for all of the major professional sports in the United States, and is being developed in the National Collegiate Athletic Association.

The first and most critical component of a sideline concussion assessment is a written emergency action plan that details the procedures to deal with a medical emergency at the competition. The initial response to a player down on the field/pitch is always airway maintenance and cervical protection, breathing and ventilation, and circulation (bleeding control) (ABCs). This is followed by assessing for any spinal component, such as sensation, numbness, tingling, weakness, and movement of the extremities. Any loss of consciousness or acute seizure activity, particularly prolonged, should automatically call for the ABC assessment. Obviously, any difficulties with ABC or reported weakness or difficulties moving an extremity calls for cervical protection/immobilization and backboarding with transportation to a hospital[5,21,22] per the organization's written emergency action plan.

After the more critical issues have been ruled-out the goal then becomes diagnosing a concussion and the need for removal from play. Depending on the sport, the decision of determining the presence of a concussion may have to be done in a time-limited fashion while the player is still on the field (soccer and baseball, where the player cannot re-enter the game if removed) or on the sideline (football, ice hockey, and basketball) when one has more time and the player is eligible to return to competition if no concussion is diagnosed.

The role of serial follow-up evaluations once a player is diagnosed with a concussion is often missed or not performed. However, the standard of care calls for follow-up assessments with a player every 20 to 30 minutes for the first hour and then once over the next hour. If this is not possible, then a follow-up assessment should occur at least once more at the end of the competition and before the athlete is discharged to someone designated to watch the concussed athlete. The importance of serial assessments after a concussion is to protect from, or diagnose, a more serious emerging neurologic injury (eg, subdural or subarachnoid hemorrhage or parenchymal hematoma), and to prevent an athlete from returning to competition with a concussion possibly leading to a second and potentially more severe concussion (sometimes referred to as second impact syndrome)[23,24] or prolonged recovery, which occurs in concussed individuals who continue to play compared with being removed immediately.[25]

Pathognomonic Signs of In-Competition Acute Concussion

There are signs and symptoms considered pathognomonic in diagnosing a concussion on the sideline.

Loss of consciousness

Any loss of consciousness automatically calls for the implementation of the emergency action plan to rule out any serious cervical spine or neurologic injuries. Even though loss of consciousness in SRC occurs less than 10% of the time[17] it should be considered pathognomonic that a concussion occurred and the player should be removed from play with the full sideline assessment. A subsequent serial assessment should then be performed and the player must be ruled ineligible to return.

Presence of any retrograde or posttraumatic amnesia

Any retrograde amnesia, post-traumatic amnesia or confusion by an athlete likely indicates a concussion and requires the removal from play with a full concussion assessment should be performed to determine the presence of concussion.

Other signs

Imbalance, wobbly gait, missing the play or lining up improperly/being out of position, or erratic behavior can possibly be evidence of concussion and again a determination by the health care providers observing the game should be made to remove the player for an evaluation. Unfortunately, the magnitude of a "big hit" does not correlate with the occurrence of a clinical concussion[26] and cannot by itself determine that a concussion occurred. However, any player suspected of taking a "big hit" should be observed and possibly removed for an assessment to rule out concussion.

SIDELINE CONCUSSION ASSESSMENT TOOL-3

The Sideline Concussion Assessment Tool (SCAT), currently in its third revision (SCAT3)[27,28] (http://bjsm.bmj.com/content/47/5/259.full.pdf+html) is the standard of care in sideline concussion assessments. It is the most widely used sideline assessment tool internationally. For example, SCAT3 is used by the Federation of International Football Associations and the International Olympic Committee and is the central component (with some variations noted) of sideline assessment for all of the major sport leagues in the United States (Major League Baseball, National Hockey League [NHL], National Football League [NFL], Major League Soccer, and National Basketball Association) and National Collegiate Athletic Association. The SCAT arose out of the need for an objective measure of acute concussion, because a subgroup of athletes minimize or deny acute concussion symptoms.[29,30] McCrea and coworkers[31–34] where the first to develop and publish a brief cognitive assessment tool for sideline concussion management that has a brief neurologic screen, tests of verbal (immediate and delay) memory and concentration, and a physical exertion component.

In 2004, at the second International Conference on Concussion in Sport, the Standardized Assessment of Concussion (SAC) served as the core component with additions of the Post-Concussion Symptom Scale, sport-specific questions of orientation, on-field markers of concussion, along with a stepwise return to play[27] giving rise to the SCAT. The SCAT was revised in 2008 during the second meeting of the Concussion in Sport Group.[35] Additions to the SCAT-2 included the GCS, alternate word list, and modified balance error scoring system (mBESS). The SCAT3 was published in 2013 with only minor adjustments[36] along with a new child version (Child-SCAT3 for younger than 13 years of age).[3]

The SCAT3 in its current form is designed to assess and detect most aspects of acute concussion. However, the SCAT3 does not fully assess ocular-motor impairments (nystagmus only), which have become a common component of concussion assessments (discussed later). A comprehensive literature review of the SCAT[27] looked at the multiple components of the SCAT3. However, most research was performed with either the original SCAT or with the SCAT2. There are only a few larger studies that looked at the specificity and sensitivity of the SCAT2/3, per se, in detecting concussion.[37]

The importance of baseline assessment with the SCAT3 is debatable. Normative data (and reliable change indexes) exist at the high school, collegiate, and professional level (NHL),[37–40] but more recent research[37,41] shows that certain demographic factors (gender, level of competition, attention-deficit/hyperactivity disorder, learning disability, depression/anxiety, and verbal abilities) significantly alter at least one SCAT3 component, which influences interpretation of the SCAT3, at least at the high school and collegiate level. Of particular note, Chin and colleagues[37] supply normative conversion tables with reliable change indexes for interpreting significant change on SCAT2/3 with and without baseline. The SCAT3 test-retest reliability is variable,[37,39] which only complicates the interpretation of scores.

The SCAT3 is designed for use by a health care professional for athletes 13 years of age or older. It makes a specific statement indicating that it is not a "stand-alone" instrument, and "...should not be used solely to make, or exclude, the diagnosis of concussion in the absence of clinical judgment. An athlete may have a concussion even if their SCAT3 is 'normal.'" The SCAT3 also emphasizes monitoring of the athlete with repeat assessment during the acute phase, "Since signs and symptoms may evolve over time, it is important to consider repeat evaluation in the acute assessment of concussion," and monitor for deterioration over time. The SCAT3 also contains detailed instructions on administration for each of the component parts, which is useful in helping with standardized administration. The following is a description of the SCAT3 sections with added comments or suggestions to enhance the sideline assessment.

One caveat of administering the SCAT3 should be discussed. Optimally, the SCAT3 should be administered in a quiet, distraction-free environment such as the locker room. This is the recommendation for all of the major sporting leagues' concussion guidelines. This is to ensure accurate and reliable test findings. While certain situations may prevent this from happening extreme caution should be used when comparing serial SCAT assessments that were performed in different environments (eg, sideline and quiet locker room), as this difference could significant impact test scores.

Background

This section consists of general demographic information and six background questions that are best answered preseason or before the competition. For example, questions regarding psychiatric history, diagnoses of learning disability, dyslexia, or attention-deficit/hyperactivity disorder are best answered before the competition and would only complicate the acute sideline assessment of concussion.

Indications for Emergency Management

This section outlines four findings that may warrant activating the team's emergency action plan with "urgent transportation to the nearest hospital": (1) GCS less than 15

($\leq$14); (2) potential signs/symptoms of spinal injury; (3) progressive, worsening symptoms; and (4) new neurologic signs.

Potential Signs of Concussion

The SCAT3 uses a combination of signs and symptoms to detect concussion. This section highlights specific signs that are elicited and observed by the health care professional performing the sideline concussion assessment. Some of them are fairly objective (eg, loss of consciousness, visible facial injury, or loss of memory), whereas others are more subjective (eg, blank or vacant look). Other signs the health care provider should look for include unequal or poorly reactive pupillary response, discharge from the ears or nose (unrelated to deviated nasal septum), or evidence of a basilar skull fracture (Battle sign). All of these indicate the need for cervical stabilization and urgent transportation to the emergency department.

Glasgow Coma Scale

GCS is used to determine the presence of a more severe TBI and less for a diagnosis of concussion, per se. By definition, concussion falls in the GCS range of 13 to 15 and even then, most are a 14 or 15. Rarely is loss of consciousness (<10%) ever involved in concussion.[17]

Maddocks Score

The Maddocks score is a competition-specific measure of orientation. This helps with the diagnosis of concussion by addressing issues of retrograde amnesia. However, often concussed athletes are generally oriented.

Symptom Evaluation

This section consists of 22 concussion (and cervical)-related symptoms scored along a seven-point Likert scale (0–6) and follows the Post-Concussion Symptom Scale.[42] Although the SCAT3 concussion symptom scale is considered to have good "face validity" and is a generally reliable and sensitive measure of acute and residual concussion, like many other concussion symptom scales it has psychometric limitations and caveats of which the clinician should be aware.[43,44] The scale is strictly subjective and a small percentage of athletes underreport symptoms to stay in the game. The scale also collects the total number of symptoms acknowledged with a score of one to six (ie, x/22 symptoms reported, and the sum of the score for all of the symptoms).

One of the difficulties of relying strictly on symptom report has to do with understanding the cause and effect of symptom reporting to concussion. Many of the symptoms on any concussion symptom scale are phenotypic of concussion and nonconcussion-related problems, such as dehydration, overheating, and physical exertion.[45] Therefore, it takes experience understanding the pattern of symptom reporting and its relationship to other parts of the SCAT3 to accurately diagnose a concussion.

There are also Yes/No questions regarding exertional effects (physical and mental) on symptom reporting, because the SCAT3 (in particular the symptom scale) can be given serially to document progress and recovery.

Cognitive and Physical Evaluation

This section has two components: a cognitive assessment and a physical evaluation. The cognitive assessment component is directly from the SAC[46] and consists of general orientation; immediate memory (a five-item word-list with three learning trials); two measures of concentration (digit span backward [ranging from 3–6 digits] and months of the year in reverse order); and delayed memory, which is performed after the neck, balance, and coordination examinations. The SAC has good sensitivity in detecting acute concussion. However, the cognitive component may not be a useful tool for follow-up or serial evaluation because the SAC score tends to normalize within 48 hours postconcussion.[34] The physical evaluation section has three components: neck, balance, and coordination examinations.

Neck/Spine

Ruling out any spinal cord, peripheral nerve, or plexopathies is critical.[47] The neck examination assesses range of motion, pain, and tenderness along the base of the skull, cervical and full neck, and upper back. Along with range of motion, the subject should be asked about any pain, numbness, tingling, weakness, or dysesthesias they have in general, but also specifically during range of motion in all planes (laterally and flexion and extension). Focal spinal pain, with decreased range of motion, weakness, numbness or burning, electrical, and radiating symptoms should be considered a spinal fracture until proven otherwise with removal from play and the standard spinal precautions taken. Brachial plexopathies are often transient and unilateral symptoms of burning, electrical sensation, and numbness and often improve quickly. If residual, then suspicion for a spinal fracture is warranted with all of the necessary spinal precautions.

It is recommended to add extremity strength assessment if time permits during the first assessment and always during any serial assessment. We recommend grip, resistance to lateral arm raise, and flexion and extension of foreman (biceps and triceps) with elbow bent at 90°. Leg raises and hamstring curls are done to assess lower extremity strength, but often are cumbersome to do on the sideline (but easier to do in the locker room). Strength is typically graded from 0 to 5 but one is looking for weakness that can be bilateral or unilateral. One may also want to assess for facial muscle strength (eyelids, smile, and tongue protrusion). Any loss or significant asymmetry of strength indicates the need to assess reflexes. Reflex assessment may be difficult to perform immediately on the sideline because of environment or the athlete's equipment. But an assessment of reflexes should be carried out if there is any suspicion of upper or lower motor neuron impairment. Pupillary reflex assessment is also recommended. We acknowledge that this is difficult to do initially, especially in the bright sunlight and/or when the athlete has severe photophobia. But during serial examinations the pupillary reflex must be brisk and equal to bright light and any unilateral differences may suggest a significant neurologic dysfunction, such as increased intracranial pressure. Vital signs can also help monitor for intracranial pressure (hypertension with decreased pulse). Finally, a quick assessment of sensation (light touch and/or pinprick to the face and upper and lower extremities) is performed initially but definitely should be performed during serial assessments to help determine any spinal involvement.

Balance assessment

The balance examination has two components: the mBESS[48] and/or adding tandem gait. The tandem gait assessment is specific because it must be timed over a 3-m length with the best time of four trials used. One is looking for arms moving out to the side to counter imbalance, excessive hip or upper extremity movement, and inability to coordinate feet movement in the tandem stance.

The mBESS is challenging to administered because of the specialized footwear (cleats or skates) worn by most athletes and the surface being used. Balance is also affected by the surface. Imagine testing a football player with taped cleats on a concrete locker room floor versus artificial turf. Similarly, having the same athlete remove their shoes and the extra time it would take to retape the shoe can influence the balance assessment. Such subtle nuances need to be considered when performing an in-game concussion assessment.

Coordination

The coordination component is simply success of finger-to-nose repetition with the athlete using his or her index finger. Again, total number of repetitions in a given period of time (five correct repetitions in <4 seconds) is the criteria for success.

If an athlete demonstrates any of the following signs or symptoms (Red Flags) during the sideline assessment, including the subsequent serial assessments, the athlete should be urgently transported to the nearest emergency department for assessment and care:

- Worsening headache
- Nuchal rigidity
- Battle signs
- Developing blurred, double, or loss of vision
- Becomes drowsy, lethargic, or obtunded
- Develops or has worsening mental/cognitive abilities, such as unusual or agitated behavior, slurred speech, inability to answer simple questions, inability to recognize familiar people, confusion, worsening memory, or starts to repeat themselves
- Repetitive emesis ($\geq$2)
- Any signs of seizure activity
- Urinary or bowel incontinence

Additional Sections

Signs to watch for

This section includes a listing of eight different signs designed for the lay person watching the concussed athlete at home that may represent a neurologic emergency and require immediate and urgent care with transportation to a hospital emergency department.

Scoring summary

The rows represent the different sections of SCAT3 and the columns are different dates to help with serial assessment.

Return to play

This section gives an example of a typical return to play exertional exercise protocol that is considered the standard in returning athletes to competition.[3]

Concussion injury advice

This section, which is designed to be cut off and given to a responsible person monitoring the concussed athlete on discharge, has basic information about signs/symptoms to look for that might represent a neurologic emergency, which can evolve over time, and an area to add contact information for the person who performed the sideline assessment and any other detailed information that might be helpful. However, one piece of advice that we recommend adding to any take-home instructions is to include limiting any pain relief medication to acetaminophen only for the first 48 hours. It should be very clear that aspirin is not to be given at all within the first 48 hours and that the standard of care is also to not use nonsteroidal anti-inflammatory drugs within the first 48 hours because of the blood thinning properties of these medications worsening the small likelihood of any possible cerebral bleed.

Any abnormality or impairment on the SCAT3 or additional testing is considered indicative that the athlete suffered a concussion (or cervical/spinal injury). The standard of care calls for removing that athlete from the competition or practice and to perform serial assessments and monitor the athlete for any evolving or worsening neurologic/spinal injury.

Additional Tips

Performing a sideline concussion assessment is challenging given the conditions under which it must be done; the speed required to do the examination; and the need to make rapid, important medical decisions. Listed next are tips to improve one's ability to make the most accurate decisions:

1. Practice. It helps a great deal to practice performing the sideline concussion assessment. Developing a fluid, smooth rhythm makes the evaluation go quickly and accurately.
2. Know your athletes. It helps to know the athlete's baseline behavior.[47] For example, are they quick thinkers or are they aggressive during game time and always wanting to play? Imagine a player that denies symptoms and does well on the SCAT3 but was very slow to respond with a lot of "uhms" and "ahhs." This might be a subtle indication that they are concussed. Do they look confused? Similarly, imagine a player that does well on SCAT3 but their body language is different and they are not pressing you to go back into the game. Athletes typical feel the need to play but perhaps their body language says something different. This may be a sign of concussion or at the very least they are not ready to return.
3. Re-evaluate. Remember, one can always re-evaluate an athlete even if they passed a sideline concussion examination and were returned to play. There will be times when you evaluate a player for a suspected concussion but they do well on the sideline examination. If the decision was to return to play remember to watch the athlete play and be observant of how the athlete plays. If you suspect that the athlete is not playing the way he or she should then have the athlete pulled from the game or practice and re-evaluate. At the time of this publication the SCAT-5 (the version represents the Fifth International Consensus Conference on Concussion in Sport in Berlin, Germany, October 2016. Thus how it went from SCAT-3 - developed during the third meeting - to the fifth edition) was in its final revisions and to be published in the British Journal of Sports Medicine with the rest of the proceedings from the same conference. The SCAT-5 consisted of two versions: one for children 12 and under (SCAT-5 child) and the second for athletes above the age of 12. The SCAT-5 added a section of four elements to assess immediately after a concussion or on the side-line/pitch:
   • Red Flags that include nine signs or symptoms that if observed or reported by the athlete after a blow to the head or body requires the removal of the athlete from competition with a full concussion assessment using the SCAT.
   • Observable signs that indicate a possible concussion.
   • Quick memory or game orientation series of questions.
   • Glasgow Coma Scale and cervical spine assessment.
The rest of the SCAT-5 is highly similar to what was described in the SCAT-3 with the following differences:
   • Use of the SCAT on-field or in the office.
   • Expanded background information of the athlete.
   • Option of six different five-item, or a new expanded 10-item, word-lists.
   • Expanded digit span forward (up to six digits) and digit span backwards.
   • Expanded neurological screen.

- Expanded decision making section.

Lastly, the consensus conference also updated The Concussion Recognition Tool (CRT) designed to educate non-professionals in identifying concussions.

4. Consider an exertional challenge. If an athlete passes a sideline concussion assessment and you are considering returning them to the practice or competition consider doing an exertional challenge. You can have the athlete do some sprinting along with push-ups and sit-ups and then readminister portions of the SCAT (symptoms, balance, or any other components) to be sure that they do not become symptomatic and need to be removed. We also suggest giving them a series of commands to follow (eg, do three 20-yard sprints follow by 20 push-ups and 30 sit-ups) so you can also assess their memory. Observe the athlete during the exertional challenge and note their coordination, gait, and if they followed the instructions properly. All of this is valuable information when making a return to competition or practice decision.

5. Do not forget to monitor the athlete after diagnosing a concussion and performing serial assessments to ensure no neurologic emergency develops. Also, one can have an athlete sit for a while and reassess to determine if they can return to the competition.

6. Baseline mBESS should use the same surface and footwear that you might use during the sideline concussion assessment (ie, hard floor or field).

CHILD SIDELINE CONCUSSION ASSESSMENT TOOL-3

The Child-SCAT3[3] (http://bjsm.bmj.com/content/47/5/263.full.pdf+html) is based on expert consensus and was developed out of the understanding of the development factors that impact the assessment of concussion, especially sideline assessment.[49–54] The Child-SCAT3 maintains the general structure and components of the SCAT3, but alters the wording and symptoms of concussion, and even asks for parental input, to account for development differences. Nelson and colleagues[51] were the first to look at the initial psychometric properties of the Child-SCAT3 and found small to moderate age effects across all of the Child-SCAT3 components. Some gender differences were evident (females 10–13 years of age reporting more symptoms), whereas younger children, particularly those with more limited vocabulary skills, had a more difficult time expressing symptoms. Also, the SAC-C component had moderate age effects and suggests the importance of age-corrected normative data consistent with other development literature. The older subset of children 9 to 13 years of age showed moderate reliability in symptom reporting consistent with prior research of symptom reporting in youth athletes.[49]

KING-DEVICK TEST

The assessment of ocular-motor and vestibular-ocular deficits after concussion has become a topic of recent interest and research. Many believe that subtle ocular-motor changes occur after concussions and that with the proper techniques one can detect subtle changes following a concussion acutely and therefore have an objective technique that enhances diagnostic sensitivity. This is partly based on the idea that about 50% of the brain is involved in vision including brainstem, thalamic, cerebellum, and cortical regions,[55,56] which are vulnerable to acceleration/deceleration injury (occipital and frontal cortex) and sheer injury (frontal white matter and midbrain[57]) and that visual and ocular deficits have been detected following TBI.[58–60]

The King-Devick test (KD)[61] has been used to detect subtle visual scanning impairments following concussions acutely (and other neurologic disorders) and thus can help with sideline concussion diagnosis. It is a quick 2- to 3-minute visual scanning test (reading numbers from left to right of varying degrees of visual difficulty, such as spacing of the numbers). The dependent measure is the sum time it takes to read three test cards. Baseline assessment is required and any slowing (increased time) is considered diagnostic of a concussion. Healthy subjects improve (faster) their reading time by about 2 seconds on average and concussed athletes slow (longer) by about almost 5 seconds.[62] The test has shown good reliability (inter-class correlations of 0.95–0.97).[62] A recent meta-analysis[61] across multiple contact sports reported high sensitivity (86%) and specificity (90%). Studies show that the addition of KD with other common sideline assessment tools (SAC and BESS portions of SCAT) improved the detection of concussions[63] and possibly surpassed them in detection.[64] However, it should be noted that the comparison was with only sections of the SCAT and not the entire SCAT.

VESTIBULAR OCULAR MOTOR SCREEN

The Vestibular Ocular Motor Screen (VOMS)[65] is a recently developed screen for outpatient assessments of vestibular and ocular impairments. Given the recent evidence of vestibular-ocular deficits following concussions[66] it would seem helpful to do this type of assessment on the sidelines. Upward of 60% of concussed athletes presenting for outpatient assessment have an abnormal VOMS finding.[65] Impairment on portions of the VOMS has odds ratio ranging from 3.37 to 3.89 in predicting the presence of concussion in a pediatric sample presenting, on average, 7 days after a concussion. The VOMS, although not formally used on the sideline, might serve as a useful tool in the toolbox in more complicated, subtle cases. For example, in those cases where the SCAT3 is normal but a concussion is suspected, an assessment of vestibular-ocular functions can aid in decision making. Although empirical evidence is needed, the VOMS may be a useful adjunct in a sideline assessment, because it may have clinical utility in cases where it is difficult to definitely diagnose a concussion.

EVOLVING TECHNOLOGY AND TECHNIQUES

More and more technology is being developed and tested to improve sideline concussion detection. This can range from sophisticated medical devices that track eye movements using specialized equipment (goggles), virtual reality, and electroencephalogram to computerized neuropsychological tests on tablets. It is beyond the scope of this article to describe all of these in detail. However, it is noteworthy to describe the use of concussion spotters or "eyes-in-the-sky." These are trained individuals whose sole purpose is to detect possible concussions by observing the game live or in real time. The NFL and NHL have significantly upgraded/improved their programs. Each NFL game has an independent, athletic trainer whose sole job is to help detect possible concussions by monitoring the game. They look for signs that might suggest a player is concussed but was not identified on the field. They can watch the game live, through the television broadcast, with a 2-second delay, or have video to play back. The spotter can call down to either sideline to notify either team's medical staff to evaluate a player, and since 2016 they have the ability to stop the game (medical timeout) to have a player removed for a concussion evaluation.[67] Also, at each NFL game there is an unaffiliated neurotrauma consultant who serves as a consultant for either team, but also can ask to have a player removed to be evaluated for concussion.

Before 2016, the NHL had team-affiliated spotters at the games who could communicate with their respective teams to have a player removed voluntarily. However, in 2016 not only were there spotters at each game but there were spotters employed by the NHL located in either Toronto or New York City monitoring all of the games in real time. The spotters, starting in the 2016 to 2017 season, can mandate player removal for the concussion evaluation.[68] The added, incremental value of the concussion spotter over the sideline medical team still needs to be proven.

SUMMARY

The importance of in-competition or sideline concussion assessment cannot be stressed enough because it is the first line of defense against developing potentially possibly significant neurologic complications of the head, spine, and face. The ability to rapidly and accurately detect an in-competition or sideline concussion (whether in practice of game) is a challenging endeavor given the multitude of complexities that occur simultaneously, such as

- The evasive and often subtle deficits of concussion, which can evolve over time.
- The possibility of the athlete not being completely open and forthright about their symptoms.
- The need to make a rapid decision that is dictated by the rules of the sport (eg, not being allowed to substitute a player).
- Varying environmental factors of the situation.
- Similarity or overlap of symptoms with other co-occurring conditions, such as physical overexertion, overheating, and dehydration.

The SCAT3 has been adopted as the standard of care for detecting in-competition concussions. We believe that adding additional testing components to the SCAT that have proven reliability, sensitivity, and specificity (eg, KD) afford the best techniques for ensuring the health and safety of athletes at all levels of competition. We recommend that all organizations have detailed written concussion and emergency action plans and that they are objectively reviewed at the end and beginning of every season to improve the organization's response and assessment.

The sideline assessment has evolved over time. There has been substantial improvement in the understanding of concussions and large strides have been made in detecting concussions and spinal injuries during competitions and practices. There continue to be new products and techniques to help objectify the evaluation and improve sensitivity and specificity. However, until the empirical evidence demonstrates their use one should rely on a combination of objective tests and subjective reporting to diagnosis in-competition concussions.

REFERENCES

1. Kroshus E, Garnett B, Hawrilenko M, et al. Concussion under-reporting and pressure from coaches, teammates, fans, and parents. Soc Sci Med 2015;134:66–75.
2. McCrea M, Iverson GL, Echemendia RJ, et al. Day of injury assessment of sport-related concussion. Br J Sports Med 2013;47(5):272–84.
3. McCrory P, Meeuwisse WH, Aubry M, et al. Consensus statement on concussion in sport: the 4th International Conference on Concussion in Sport held in Zurich, November 2012. Br J Sports Med 2013;47(5):250–8.
4. McCrory P. Sports concussion and the risk of chronic neurological impairment. Clin J Sport Med 2011;21(1):6–12.
5. Putukian M, Raftery M, Guskiewicz K, et al. Onfield assessment of concussion in the adult athlete. Br J Sports Med 2013;47(5):285–8.
6. Baugh CM, Kroshus E, Bourlas AP, et al. Requiring athletes to acknowledge receipt of concussion-related information and responsibility to report symptoms: a study of

the prevalence, variation, and possible improvements. J Law Med Ethics 2014; 42(3):297–313.

7. Galetta KM, Morganroth J, Moehringer N, et al. Adding vision to concussion testing: a prospective study of sideline testing in youth and collegiate athletes. J Neuroophthalmol 2015;35(3):235–41.

8. McCrea M, Hammeke T, Olsen G, et al. Unreported concussion in high school football players: implications for prevention. Clin J Sport Med 2004;14(1):13–7.

9. Meehan WP, Mannix RC, O'Brien MJ, et al. The prevalence of undiagnosed concussions in athletes. Clin J Sport Med 2013;23(5):339–42.

10. Meier TB, Brummel BJ, Singh R, et al. The underreporting of self-reported symptoms following sports-related concussion. Aust J Sci Med Sport 2015;18(5): 507–11.

11. Register-Mihalik JK, Linnan LA, Marshall SW, et al. Using theory to understand high school aged athletes' intentions to report sport-related concussion: implications for concussion education initiatives. Brain Inj 2013;27(7–8):878–86.

12. Guskiewicz KM, Weaver NL, Padua DA, et al. Epidemiology of concussion in collegiate and high school football players. Am J Sports Med 2000;28(5):643–50.

13. Kutcher JS, Giza CC. Sideline assessment of sports concussion: the lure of simplicity. Neurology 2011;76(17):1450–1.

14. Thurman DJ, Alverson C, Dunn KA, et al. Traumatic brain injury in the United States: a public health perspective. J Head Trauma Rehabil 1999;14(6):602–15.

15. Kay T, Harrington DE, Adams R, et al. Definition of mild traumatic brain injury. J Head Trauma Rehabil 1993;8(3):86–7.

16. Harmon KG, Drezner JA, Gammons M, et al. American Medical Society for Sports Medicine position statement: concussion in sport. Br J Sports Med 2013;47(1): 15–26.

17. Meehan WP, d'Hemecourt P, Comstock RD. High school concussions in the 2008-2009 academic year mechanism, symptoms, and management. Am J Sports Med 2010;38(12):2405–9.

18. Barkhoudarian G, Hovda DA, Giza CC. The molecular pathophysiology of concussive brain injury. Clin Sports Med 2011;30(1):33–48.

19. Henry LC, Tremblay J, Tremblay S, et al. Acute and chronic changes in diffusivity measures after sports concussion. J Neurotrauma 2011;28(10):2049–59.

20. Kutcher JS, Giza CC. Sports concussion diagnosis and management. Continuum (Minneap Minn) 2014;20(6):1552–69.

21. Herring SA, Kibler WB, Putukian M. Sideline preparedness for the team physician: a consensus statement-2012 update. Med Sci Sports Exerc 2012;44(12): 2442–5.

22. Swartz EE, Decoster LC, Norkus SA, et al. Summary of the National Athletic Trainers' Association Position Statement on the Acute Management of the Cervical Spine-Injured Athlete. Phys Sportsmed 2009;37(4):20–30.

23. Cantu RC, Gean AD. Second-impact syndrome and a small subdural hematoma: an uncommon catastrophic result of repetitive head injury with a characteristic imaging appearance. J Neurotrauma 2010;27(9):1557–64.

24. McCrory P, Davis G, Makdissi M. Second impact syndrome or cerebral swelling after sporting head injury. Curr Sports Med Rep 2012;11(1):21–3.

25. Elbin RJ, Sufrinko A, Schatz P, et al. Removal from play after concussion and recovery time. Pediatrics 2016;138(3):e20160910.

26. Guskiewicz KM, Mihalik JP, Shankar V, et al. Measurement of head impacts in collegiate football players: relationship between head impact biomechanics and acute clinical outcome after concussion. Neurosurgery 2007;61(6):1244–53.

27. Yengo-Kahn AM, Hale AT, Zalneraitis BH, et al. The sport concussion assessment tool: a systematic review. Neurosurg Focus 2016;40(4):E6.

28. Okonkwo DO, Tempel ZJ, Maroon J. Sideline assessment tools for the evaluation of concussion in athletes: a review. Neurosurgery 2014;75:S82–95.

29. Krol AL, Mrazik M, Naidu D, et al. Assessment of symptoms in a concussion management programme: method influences outcome. Brain Inj 2011;25(13–14): 1300–5.

30. Kerr ZY, Register-Mihalik JK, Marshall SW, et al. Disclosure and non-disclosure of concussion and concussion symptoms in athletes: review and application of the socio-ecological framework. Brain Inj 2014;28(8):1009–21.

31. McCrea M, Kelly JP, Kluge J, et al. Standardized assessment of concussion in football players. Neurology 1997;48(3):586–8.

32. McCrea M, Kelly JP, Randolph C, et al. Immediate neurocognitive effects of concussion. Neurosurgery 2002;50(5):1032–42.

33. McCrea M, Kelly JP, Randolph C, et al. Standardized assessment of concussion (SAC): on-site mental status evaluation of the athlete. J Head Trauma Rehabil 1998;13(2):27–35.

34. McCrea M. Standardized mental status testing on the sideline after sport-related concussion. J Athl Train 2001;36(3):274–9.

35. McCrory P, Meeuwisse W, Johnston K, et al. Consensus statement on concussion in sport 3rd International Conference on Concussion in Sport held in Zurich, November 2008. Clin J Sport Med 2009;19(3):185–200.

36. Guskiewicz KM, Register-Mihalik J, McCrory P, et al. Evidence-based approach to revising the SCAT2: introducing the SCAT3. Br J Sports Med 2013;47(5): 289–93.

37. Chin EY, Nelson LD, Barr WB, et al. Reliability and validity of the sport concussion assessment tool–3 (SCAT3) in high school and collegiate athletes. Am J Sports Med 2016;44(9):2276–85.

38. Hänninen T, Parkkari J, Tuominen M, et al. Interpreting change on the SCAT3 in professional ice hockey players. J Sci Med Sport 2016;20(5):424–31.

39. Hänninen T, Tuominen M, Parkkari J, et al. Sport concussion assessment tool - 3rd edition: normative reference values for professional ice hockey players. Aust J Sci Med Sport 2016;19(8):636–41.

40. Zimmer A, Marcinak J, Hibyan S, et al. Normative values of major SCAT2 and SCAT3 components for a college athlete population. Appl Neuropsychol Adult 2015;22(2):132–40.

41. Putukian M, Echemendia R, Dettwiler-Danspeckgruber A, et al. Prospective clinical assessment using Sideline Concussion Assessment Tool-2 testing in the evaluation of sport-related concussion in college athletes. Clin J Sport Med 2015; 25(1):36–42.

42. Lovell MR, Iverson GL, Collins MW, et al. Measurement of symptoms following sports-related concussion: reliability and normative data for the post-concussion scale. Appl Neuropsychol 2006;13(3):166–74.

43. Alla S, Sullivan SJ, Hale L, et al. Self-report scales/checklists for the measurement of concussion symptoms: a systematic review. Br J Sports Med 2009;43(Suppl 1):3–12.

44. McLeod TCV, Leach C. Psychometric properties of self-report concussion scales and checklists. J Athl Train 2012;47(2):221–3.

45. Balasundaram AP, Sullivan JS, Schneiders AG, et al. Symptom response following acute bouts of exercise in concussed and non-concussed individuals: a systematic narrative review. Phys Ther Sport 2013;14(4):253–8.

46. McCrea M. Standardized mental status assessment of sports concussion. Clin J Sport Med 2001;11(3):176–81.
47. Anderson S, Schnebel B. Sideline neurological evaluation: a detailed approach to the sideline, in-game neurological assessment of contact sport athletes. Curr Pain Headache Rep 2016;20(7):46.
48. Guskiewicz KM. Assessment of postural stability following sport-related concussion. Curr Sports Med Rep 2003;2(1):24–30.
49. Davis GA, Purcell LK. The evaluation and management of acute concussion differs in young children. Br J Sports Med 2013;48(2):98–101.
50. Glaviano NR, Benson S, Goodkin HP, et al. Baseline SCAT2 assessment of healthy youth student-athletes: preliminary evidence for the use of the child-SCAT3 in children younger than 13 years. Clin J Sport Med 2015;25(4):373–9.
51. Nelson LD, Loman MM, LaRoche AA, et al. Baseline performance and psychometric properties of the child sport concussion assessment tool 3 (Child-SCAT3) in 5- to 13-year-old athletes. Clin J Sport Med 2016. http://dx.doi.org/10.1097/JSM.0000000000000369.
52. Sady MD, Vaughan CG, Gioia GA. Psychometric characteristics of the postconcussion symptom inventory in children and adolescents. Arch Clin Neuropsychol 2014;29(4):348–63.
53. Snyder AR, Bauer RM. A normative study of the sport concussion assessment tool (SCAT2) in children and adolescents. Clin Neuropsychol 2014;28(7):1091–103.
54. Valovich McLeod TC, Barr WB, McCrea M, et al. Psychometric and measurement properties of concussion assessment tools in youth sports. J Athl Train 2006;41(4):399–408.
55. Felleman DJ, Van Essen DC. Distributed hierarchical processing in the primate cerebral cortex. Cereb Cortex 1991;1(1):1–47.
56. Ventura RE, Balcer LJ, Galetta SL, et al. Ocular motor assessment in concussion: current status and future directions. J Neurol Sci 2016;361:79–86.
57. Nevin NC. Neuropathological changes in the white matter following head injury. J Neuropathol Exp Neurol 1967;26(1):77–84.
58. Ciuffreda KJ, Kapoor N, Rutner D, et al. Occurrence of oculomotor dysfunctions in acquired brain injury: a retrospective analysis. Optometry 2007;78(4):155–61.
59. Heitger MH, Jones RD, Macleod AD, et al. Impaired eye movements in post-concussion syndrome indicate suboptimal brain function beyond the influence of depression, malingering or intellectual ability. Brain 2009;132(10):2850–70.
60. Heitger MH, Jones RD, Anderson TJ. A new approach to predicting postconcussion syndrome after mild traumatic brain injury based upon eye movement function. Conf Proc IEEE Eng Med Biol Soc 2008;2008:3570–3.
61. Mayo Clinic. King-Devick test in association with Mayo Clinic. 2016. Available at: http://kingdevicktest.com/.
62. Galetta KM, Liu M, Leong DF, et al. The King-Devick test of rapid number naming for concussion detection: meta-analysis and systematic review of the literature. Concussion 2015;1(2). http://dx.doi.org/10.2217/cnc.15.8.
63. Marinides Z, Galetta KM, Andrews CN, et al. Testing is additive to the sideline assessment of sports-related concussion. Neurol Clin Pract 2014;5(1):25–34.
64. Leong DF, Balcer LJ, Galetta SL, et al. The King–Devick test for sideline concussion screening in collegiate football. J Optom 2015;8(2):131–9.
65. Mucha A, Collins MW, Elbin RJ, et al. A brief vestibular/ocular motor screening (VOMS) assessment to evaluate concussions: preliminary findings. Am J Sports Med 2014;42(10):2479–86.

66. Ellis MJ, Cordingley DM, Vis S, et al. Clinical predictors of vestibulo-ocular dysfunction in pediatric sports-related concussion. J Neurosurg Pediatr 2016; 19:38–45.
67. Vrentas J. The NFL's Eye in the Sky Sees Everything, Often More Than Once. 2014. Available at: http://www.si.com/2014/08/13/the-nfls-eye-in-the-sky-sees-everything-often-more-than-once.
68. Whyno S. Daly: NHL adding more concussion spotters for this season. 2016. Available at: http://www.usatoday.com/story/sports/nhl/2016/09/14/daly-nhl-adding-more-concussion-spotters-for-this-season/90381280/.

Neurosurgical Emergencies in Sport

Brian Sindelar, MD[a,b], Julian E. Bailes, MD[a],*

KEYWORDS

- Neurosurgical emergencies • Cerebral contusion • Epidural hematoma
- Subdural hematoma • Diffuse axonal injury • Second impact syndrome
- Severe traumatic brain injury • Spinal cord injury

KEY POINTS

- Proper education in the management of spinal cord and severe brain injuries can not only prevent mortality but can also reduce propagation of further neurogenic injury.
- Therefore, a standardized, coordinated approach based on clinical guidelines must be used, commencing with the athletic trainer and team physician and continued with the critical care and surgical attending physicians.
- This article is only a primer to the basic foundation to the acute management of the athlete with a neurosurgical emergency, and further reading is recommended for those tasked with managing such acute and complex patients.

INTRODUCTION

Of the limited, but available statistical information regarding sports morbidity and mortality, it has been reported that over the last 20 years there are roughly 4 annual fatalities, in football, mostly occurring at the high school level and caused by intracranial injuries.[1,2] Although mortality is a seemingly rare occurrence in sports, there is no governmental or central reporting agency following these events; therefore this figure may be subject to bias and is limited. Also, the main published data are obtained from only high school and collegiate football and include only the injuries that resulted in death, not including those that led to profound morbidity. Therefore, the incidence of morbidity and mortality in contact and noncontact sports at all levels of play may be even more prevalent than what has been published.

Severe brain and spinal cord injuries are medical and potentially surgical emergencies that require timely intervention in order to reduce worsening secondary injury. For this reason, it is important for all medical professionals managing athletic injuries to be knowledgeable in the clinical approach to this type of acute event. This article reviews

[a] Department of Neurosurgery, NorthShore University HealthSystem, 3rd Floor Kellogg, Evanston, IL 60201, USA; [b] Department of Neurosurgery, University of Florida, Gainesville, FL, USA
* Corresponding author.
E-mail address: jbailes@northshore.org

Neurol Clin 35 (2017) 451–472
http://dx.doi.org/10.1016/j.ncl.2017.03.006
0733-8619/17/© 2017 Elsevier Inc. All rights reserved.

neurologic.theclinics.com

the initial evaluation of the athlete that occurs on the field and also within the emergency department, with a focus on presenting clinical signs of a neurosurgical emergency. Then, a discussion of the different types of emergent cranial and spinal injuries will follow, ending with a basic overview of the medical management and specific indications for surgical intervention.

EVALUATION OF THE ATHLETE WITH A NEUROSURGICAL LESION
Emergency Action Plan

With the low incidence of neurosurgical lesions in athletics, complacency can easily occur among the athletic staff tasked at managing an acute emergency. Therefore, it is essential for a solid emergency action plan (EAP) that is routinely practiced at levels of competitive play, high school, collegiate, and professional.[3] Depending on the level of competitive play, this should be a coordinated effort between the team physician and/or athletic trainer.[4,5] This protocol not only delegates specific roles but also provides a coordinated direction to the treatment team. For example, the EAP will address who is charged with the initial assessment of the athlete and determine need for emergency medical services (EMS). This is only 1 example of the many specific medical and nonmedical tasks and responsibilities that can be predelegated in order to prevent treatment delay in a life-threatening situation (eg, an expanding subdural/epidural hematoma or malignant cerebral edema). Although appearing minute, these details exponentially waste valuable time when interjected into a high stress event where timely management reduces long-term neurologic deficits and mortality.

On-field Primary Assessment

A neurosurgical emergency is one that requires emergent medical and surgical intervention in response to a neurologic decline. For example, the traumatic onset of unconsciousness, lethargy, profound confusion, hemiparesis (weakness to one half of the body), or anisocoric pupils (unequal sizes) is ordinarily due to serious condition of an expanding space occupying lesion in the brain that warrants emergent care. Subdural hematomas and even epidural hematomas can present in asymptomatic patients, and in certain cases, may not warrant emergent intervention. Therefore, cranial and spinal neurosurgical emergencies present clinically with dramatic neurologic deficits potentially even affecting the athlete's respiratory and/or cardiac function.

Regardless of the play in which a player remains down after injury or subsequently collapses after reaching the sidelines, a rapid and focused primary evaluation of the athlete should be completed in order to rule out life-threatening injuries.[3,6,7] Upon approaching the athlete, his or her level of consciousness should be initially determined. If the patient is unresponsive, then EMS should be immediately contacted by another individual, followed by assessment of the patient's respiratory/cardiac functioning established by the algorithm outlined in either the Basic Life Support (BLS) or Advanced Cardiac Life Support (ACLS) Guidelines depending on the expertise of the available personelle.[8,9] This may require initiation of cardiopulmonary resuscitation (CPR) and the use of an automated external defibrillator (AED). If an athlete is conscious, communicative without any signs of respiratory distress (eg, use of respiratory accessory muscles, rapid or shallow breaths, discoloration of the lips), he or she is likely producing adequate respirations and does not warrant advanced airway maneuvers.

Regardless if the athlete is unconsciousness or conscious, if there are ineffective respirations to provide adequate systemic oxygenation (eg, cervical spine lesions at C3-5 effect diaphragm function), airway maneuvers should be performed with possible placement of an advanced airway depending on the knowledge of the present medical staff, or in conjunction with emergency medical personnel. Any contact sport athlete who is unconscious warrants concern for cervical spine injury; therefore, a jaw thrust should be performed rather than a head-tilt, chin-lift. If intubation is required, it is important to note that even perfect in-line cervical stabilization while mask ventilating a patient or performing intubation does result in significant cervical motion.[10] Depending on the clinical location and expertise, either nasal fiber optic bronchoscope or video laryngoscope intubation is preferred in order to reduce cervical motion.[10] Whether on the field, within the ambulance, or in the emergency department, the available equipment and training of the handler will ultimately dictate the specific type of airway that is placed.

The next step in the assessment of the athlete involves a brief neurologic examination. This is first initiated by giving the athlete a specific command followed by a gross motor examination of the upper and lower extremities. If there is a perceived brain injury, even this brief primary assessment allows the examiner to assign the athlete a score based on the Glasgow Coma Scale (GCS). The GCS is a clinical classification scheme used in traumatically injured patients that is determined by their level of alertness, mentation, and functional abilities that allows concise and rapid communication between medical providers denoting the severity of injury. This simple metric grades the athlete from 3 to 15 based on eye opening, verbal response, and motor activity **Table 1**. A score between 13 and 15 denotes a mild traumatic brain injury (TBI), between 9 and 12 moderate TBI, and less than 9 severe TBI.

Cervical Spine Precautions

As mentioned, any contact sport athlete who receives a direct cranial or indirect (body) blow causing a flexion, extension, or rotation of the head can be at risk for a cervical spine injury, and therefore determination of instability and need for immobilization should be made by the evaluating medical provider during the primary assessment.[11] Spinal immobilization is required in any athlete who is altered or obtunded, has neck or radicular pain, or neurologic abnormalities on examination.[6,12–14] Recently updated guidelines released by the National Athletic Trainer's Association recommend removal, first, of the player's equipment, helmet, and shoulder pads, while maintaining manual cervical stabilization.[15] This should only occur if there are a sufficient number of trained personnel available (roughly six) to safely perform these maneuvers without causing neck motion. In the scenario where this is not achievable (lack of proper equipment, training, or personnel), the athletic gear should remain in place and incorporated into the cervical spine immobilization, but the facemask should be removed to allow easy access to the athlete's airway **Fig. 1**.[16]

Table 1 The Glasgow Coma Scale			
	Eye Response	**Verbal**	**Motor**
1	Do not open	Nonverbal	No movement
2	Open to painful stimuli	Incomprehensible	Decerebrate posturing
3	Open to voice	Inappropriate words	Decorticate posturing
4	Open spontaneously	Confused	Withdraws to painful stimuli
5		Oriented	Localizes to painful stimuli
6			Follows commands

A score of 3-8 denotes a severe TBI, 9-12 a moderate TBI, and 13-15 mild TBI.

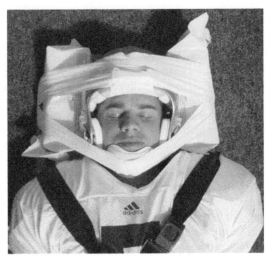

Fig. 1. Cervical spine immobilization in an athlete where lack of equipment or personnel requires athletic gear to remain in place. (*Reproduced from* Ghiselli G, Schaadt G, McAllister DR. On-the-field evaluation of an athlete with a head or neck injury. Clin Sports Med 2003;22(3):459; with permission from Elsevier.)

Once the equipment is removed properly, spinal immobilization requires manual in-line cervical stabilization, cervical collar application, followed by a team-assisted log-roll and placement onto a hard backboard. Foam blocks or sandbags are then placed on each side of the head with tape or elastic straps to then secure the head, blocks, and backboard in place. Once at the hospital, the athlete should be removed from the backboard as soon as possible to prevent skin breakdown, preferably in the emergency department after computed tomography (CT) imaging has been obtained.

Secondary Assessment

The primary assessment is required in order to immediately identify life-threatening situations in which emergent transportation to a trauma facility is required. If the player is found to be without any acute issues requiring immediate escalation in care, the player should be moved to the locker room for a further secondary assessment including a thorough clinical examination, review of subjective complaints, details of the injury, and potential administration of a sideline assessment tool to evaluate for a concussive injury.[3,5,17–24] Due to the scope of this article, the multimodal approach to diagnosis of a concussion will not be discussed, and other articles in this issue are recommended.

All athletes following a blunt injury require a detailed, serial neurologic examination in order to evaluate for any clinical signs of cranial or spinal pathology.[5,17–22,25] This examination should include an assessment of the athlete's mental status, cranial nerve examination (**Table 2**), motor strength testing focusing on specific myotomes (**Tables 3** and **4**), sensation (**Fig. 2**), and deep tendon reflexes. The athlete should also be log-rolled in order to allow spine palpation to assess for subjective tenderness or objective spinal deformities like step-down or interspinous widening. If a spinal cord injury is suspected based on clinical examination, a further detailed evaluation (occurring in the emergency department) would involve determination of the level of injury (most caudal segment where athlete has at least antigravity strength), completeness of injury (involving rectal examination for sensation, resting tone, and contractility),

Table 2
Basics of cranial nerve testing

Cranial Nerve	Name	Function	Clinical Testing
1	Olfactory	• Smell	• May test with coffee beans (clinic setting)
2	Optic	• Sight	• Test with the Snellen chart (clinic setting) or have patient count fingers at a distance
3	Oculomotor	• Controls inferior oblique, superior rectus, and inferior rectus muscle of the eye • Carries parasympathetic nerves to ciliary ganglion in eye that causes constriction of pupil (pupillary sphincter) • Also innervates the levator palpebrae superioris	• Test eye by instructing patient to look medially • Look for equal and bilateral pupillary response to light • Symmetric elevation of eye lid
4	Trochlear	• Controls superior oblique muscle of the eye	• Test by instructing patient to look medially and downward
5	Trigeminal	• Provides sensation (light touch, pain, temperature, and proprioception) to face in a forehead, midface, and mandibular distribution • Provides control of muscles of mastication	• Test by touching specific distribution on athlete's face • Test by instructing the patient to bite down and palpate contraction of masseter muscles
6	Abducens	• Controls lateral rectus muscle of the eye	• Test by instructing the patient to look laterally
7	Facial	• Muscles of facial expression	• Observe symmetry of face at rest then instruct patient to close eyes and also smile
8	Vestibulocochlear	• Provides balance and hearing	• Evaluate by dedicated audiology testing (clinic setting) or by producing sound (rubbing fingers together) next to athlete's ear and asking to localize sound
9/10	Glossopharyngeal and vagus	• Motor control of soft palate, pharynx, larynx • Sense of taste over posterior portion of tongue and pharynx • Also carries parasympathetic fibers to innervate parotid gland (9) and thoracic and abdominal viscera (10) • Regulates blood pressure/heart rate through aortic and carotid receptors (9&10)	• Test by inspecting posterior pharynx for a deviated uvula
11	Accessory	• Motor control of trapezius and sternocleidomastoid muscle	• Test muscle groups by having athlete shrug shoulders and turn head against resistance
12	Hypoglossal	• Motor control to tongue	• Tongue should be midline when instructed to protrude

Table 3
Standard clinical measurement of motor strength

Grade	Description
5/5	Full strength
4/5	Moves extremity against some resistance, but not full strength
3/5	Only antigravity strength
2/5	Moves extremity with gravity eliminated
1/5	Only twitch/contractility of muscle without extremity movement
0/5	No movement

and obtaining the rubric measurement of the ASIA (American Spinal Injury Association) Impairment Score.[26,27]

Herniation Syndromes

The Monroe-Kellie Doctrine states that the closed intracranial space is composed of brain parenchyma, cerebrospinal fluid, and blood in which any precipitous increase in any one of this constituents or additional space occupying lesion can lead to a detrimental rise in intracranial pressure leading to shifts in brain parenchyma, which in extreme is termed cerebral herniation.[28] Depending on the specific size, location, and rapidity of the process, hematomas (subdural, epidural, intraparenchymal) and cerebral edema can produce dangerous mass effect necessitating an emergent neurosurgical intervention.

Cerebral herniation is introduced within this article, because specific herniation syndromes produce classic clinical signs. The most common herniation syndromes are uncal, central, subfalcine, and tonsillar herniation.[29,30] Uncal herniation occurs with convexity or middle fossa lesions that push the medial edge of the temporal lobe, or uncus, over the edge of the tentorium. Early clinical findings are due to compression of the third cranial nerve causing an ipsilateral dilated or enlarged, blown, pupil. Further shift of the temporal lobe leads to mass effect on the ipsilateral cerebral peduncle (causing contralateral hemiparesis) and brainstem, specifically the reticular activating system (causing depressed consciousness, which if unrelieved, progresses

Table 4
Clinical testing of nerve root myotomes

Nerve Root	Motor Testing
C5	Deltoid
C5-6	Biceps
C6	Brachioradialis (wrist extension)
C7	Triceps
C8	Flexor digitorum (grip)
T1	Hand Intrinsics (finger abduction)
L2,3	Illiopsoas (hip flexor)
L3,4	Quadriceps (knee extension)
L5	Extensor hallucis longus (great toe extension)
S1	Gastrocnemius (plantar flexion)
S2-4	Bladder and anal sphincter

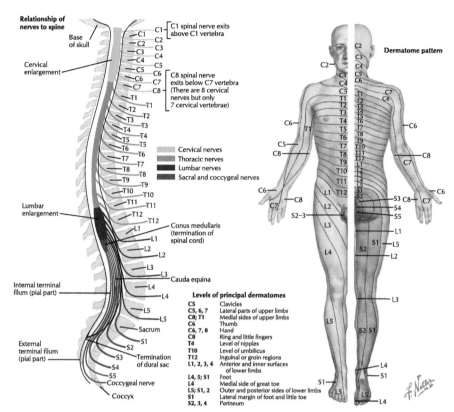

Fig. 2. Sensory dermatomes of the trunk, upper, and lower extremities. (*Courtesy of* Netter-images (image 19968); with permission from Elsevier.)

to coma or death). Central or transtentorial herniation is due to a supratentorial lesion that causes downward migration of the diencephalon through the tentorial incisura. This presents as early altered mental status, due to the diencephalic dysfunction, which can progress with oculomotor findings (Parinaud syndrome or midposition fixed pupils), posturing (decorticate or decerebrate), pituitary dysfunction (diabetes insipidus), and brainstem ischemia/death as mass effects cause a progression of diencephalic, midbrain, and lower pons dysfunction. Central herniation is a devastating injury with 60% mortality, where only 9% have good recovery.[31] Subfalcine or cingulate herniation is also due to a supratentorial mass lesion that is more lateralized, causing the cingulate gyrus to be pushed underneath the falx cerebri. Usually asymptomatic, significant shift can cause compression of the pericallosal arteries of the anterior cerebral artery leading to ischemia. Lastly, tonsillar herniation is secondary to a posterior fossa mass lesion, causing the cerebellar tonsils to herniate downward through the foramen magnum, compressing the medulla and leading to coma and often respiratory arrest (**Fig. 3**).[30]

NEUROSURGICAL CRANIAL EMERGENCIES

Any athlete participating in contact and even noncontact sports can be exposed to either direct or indirect (where a force is applied to the torso creating a whiplash type effect) cranial impacts that transmit energy intracranially due to the physiologic

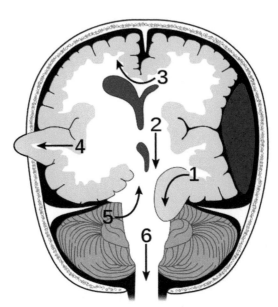

Fig. 3. Brain herniation in the setting of a space-occupying lesion. Cartoon depiction of a coronal brain image demonstrating (1) uncal (medial temporal lobe pushed over tentorial edge), (2) central (migration of the diencephalon through the tentorial incisura), (3) cingulate (cingulate gyrus pushed underneath the falx cerebri), (4) transcalvarial (extracranial cerebral migration through a bony iatrogenic or traumatic defect), (5) upward cerebellar (posterior fossa lesion causing the cerebellum to migrate upwards through the tentorial incisura), and (6) tonsillar (cerebellar tonsils pushed downwards through foramen magnum) herniation.

properties of the brain and cerebrospinal fluid.[11,21,32] Early preclinical animal and cadaveric studies by Holbourn, Ommaya, and Schneider have established the viscoelastic properties of the brain as its floating within the cerebrospinal fluid to create an uncoupled acceleration–deceleration event within the skull.[33–37] This movement of the brain, termed slosh (the dynamics of fluids within moving containers),[38,39] occurring at a microscopic levels leads to inertial axonal strain and diffuse axonal injury (DAI), but also more globally, can tear bridging blood vessels (creating subdural hematomas) or cause the brain to strike against the surface of the skull causing cerebral contusions.[33]

Skull fractures, on the other hand, are caused by a direct focal impact. Depending on the location or extent of displacement of a skull fracture, epidural hematomas, subdural hematomas, and parenchymal contusions can also occur in concert. Because of the large forces needed to fracture the cranial vault and improvements in protective head gear, the incidence of skull fractures in helmeted sports, like football and hockey, are increasingly rare. It is believed that the reduction in catastrophic head injuries in American football (average annual fatality from 1945 to 1975 was 9.5 players) is attributable to the technological advances in helmets.[1]

Types

Cerebral contusion/traumatic intracerebral hemorrhage

A hemorrhagic contusion/traumatic intracerebral hemorrhage (TICH) occurs due to the brain sloshing within the cranium, causing it to strike against the rigid edges of the skull directly adjacent to where the blow occurred, termed coup, and/or the opposite side, contrecoup. A TICH is demonstrated as a hyperdense lesion within the brain parenchyma on CT imaging, commonly occurring at the frontal or temporal poles **Fig. 4**. Depending on the size and location of the TICH, the patient may present either without symptoms, mild symptoms, or severe, profound neurologic deficits. Following the cerebral insult, worsening mass effect may occur due to delayed intracerebral hemorrhage and/or secondary cerebral edema; therefore continued clinical monitoring with serial examinations is required.[40] Commonly, small TICH may be managed nonoperatively if the patient remains neurologically stable without developing signs of increasing intracranial pressure (ICP). If the patient has increasing ICP that is refractory to medical therapy, a decline in neurologic clinical state, or the TICH volume is greater than 50 cm, then surgical decompression is warranted.[41]

Epidural hematoma

Typically, an epidural hematoma (EDH) occurs in the setting of a fracture involving the squamous portion of the temporal bone causing injury to the underlying middle meningeal artery. It can also occur from venous bleeding or from body edges, the latter more common in children. The classical presentation of an EDH involves a lucid interval caused by the usual lack of primary brain injury. This is followed by a dramatic decline in neurologic state as the systolic arterial pressure pushes blood into the space between the calvarium and dura matter resulting in a lateralized shift of the brain, uncal herniation, anisicoria, depressed consciousness, and potentially death. CT imaging of an EDH is significant for a hyperdense convex/lentiform-shaped lesion adjacent to the skull that does not extend beyond suture lines **Fig. 5**.[42] Any patient found to have an EDH with neurologic symptoms requires an emergent craniotomy for evacuation of the hematoma. Those

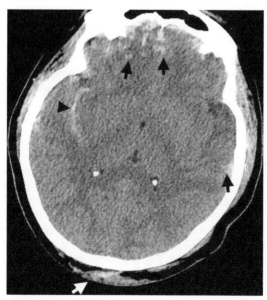

Fig. 4. Bifrontal hemorrhagic contusions seen on a noncontrast axial CT. Following a blow to the occiput, as indicated by soft tissue swelling (*white arrow*), characteristic contrecoup hemorrhagic contusions are seen in the inferior frontal and temporal lobes (*black arrows*). Also note the Subarachnoid hemorrhage (*arrowhead*) in the right Sylvian fissure, which is a poor prognostic indicator. (*Reproduced from* Kim JJ, Gean AD. Imaging for the diagnosis and management of traumatic brain injury. Neuotherapeutics 2011;8(1):45; with permission from Springer.)

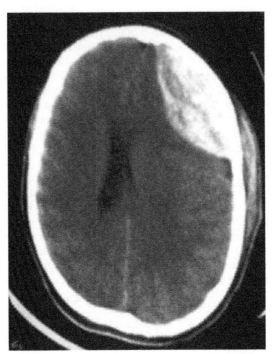

Fig. 5. Noncontrasted CT imaging demonstrating an epidural hematoma. (*Reproduced from* Davis G, Marion DW, Le Roux P, et al. Clinics in neurology and neurosurgery—extradural and subdural haematoma. Br J Sports Med 2010;44(16):1140; with permission from BMJ Publishing Group Ltd.)

athletes with a normal neurologic examination may be monitored closely, but surgery should still be considered in those asymptomatic individuals with a large EDH (>15 mm thickness or volume >30 cm^3) or significant mass effect (midline shift >5 mm).[43] Prompt recognition and management of an EDH reduce the mortality to 12%.[44]

Subdural hematoma
There exists bridging veins that traverse the subdural space to drain venous blood from the cerebrum to the dural sinuses. In the event of a large linear or rotational force, the motion of the brain away from the dura (that is fixed to the skull) can lacerate a bridging vein, causing venous blood to accumulate underneath the dura mater. Unlike EDHs, SDHs typically do not have a lucid interval, present with a poorer neurologic examination, and have worse outcomes due to the greater underling parenchymal injury. An SDH appears as a hyperdense concave/crescent-shaped lesion that is adjacent to the brain parenchyma on CT imaging **Fig. 6**. Prompt evaluation and determination for evacuation of an acute SDH are paramount in reducing mortality. One study demonstrated that SDHs were shown to have a reduced mortality, less than 30%, when evacuated within 4 hours of injury, while there was a dramatic increase in mortality, 90%, in those receiving surgery after 4 hours.[45] **Box 1** contains an overview of the indications for surgical intervention in an athlete found to have an acute SDH.[46]

Diffuse axonal injury
Rotational acceleration, specifically in the coronal plane, generates excessive strain upon the white matter and small blood vessels due to the differential motion of tissue

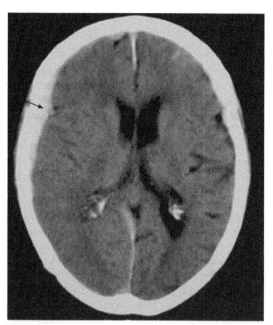

Fig. 6. Noncontrasted CT imaging demonstrating a 1 cm-thick right subdural haematoma (*arrow*) with underlying cerebral swelling. (*Reproduced from* Davis G, Marion DW, Le Roux P, et al. Clinics in neurology and neurosurgery—extradural and subdural haematoma. Br J Sports Med 2010;44(16):1140; with permission from BMJ Publishing Group Ltd.)

potentially causing axotomy and/or petechial hemorrhages.[37,47–51] Diffuse axonal injury (DAI) most commonly occurs at the gray–white matter junction and where long white matter tracts are located, like the corpus callosum, dorsolateral rostral brainstem, superior cerebellar peduncle, and internal capsule. With significant force, instant axonal tearing (primary axotomy) can occur, but more importantly this initiates a cascade of events associated with changes in lipid membrane permeability, ion shifts, excessive neurotransmitter release, mitochondrial dysfunction, changes in cerebral blood flow, hypoxia, impaired glucose metabolism, free radical formation, and activation of inflammatory cells.[52–58] This neuro-metabolic, chemical, vascular, and inflammatory state can result in either repair or secondary axotomy and wallerian degeneration of the axon. Due to the diffuse microscopic nature of this process, DAI is greatly underestimated by conventional imaging but can be seen, if hemorrhage is present, on T2 and SWI (susceptibility weight sequencing).[59,60] If hemorrhage is not

---

Box 1
Indications for surgical intervention for an acute subdural hematomas.

Neurologic deficit or decline in GCS by 2 points related to mass effect of SDH

Large size (>10 mm in thickness)

Significant mass effect (midline shift >5 mm)

Clinical signs of cerebral herniation (pupillary changes)

ICP refractory to medical treatments

present, the use of diffusion weighted imaging (DWI) is more sensitive for DAI compared with conventional CT and MRI.[60]

Second impact syndrome

The term second impact syndrome (SIS) has been adopted to classify a situation described in case reports in which a player sustains a minor head injury shortly after a diagnosed concussion, causing an exacerbated hyperemic state perpetuating diffuse malignant cerebral edema, herniation, and death in 50% of athletes.[61–67] It has been assumed that the cause of SIS is due to a persistent alteration in cerebral autoregulation days to months after the initial injury and that when exposed to a second impact, this dysautoregulation causes a robust hyperperfusion of the brain leading to profound cerebral edema.[62,63,68–75] Following the impact, it has been reported that the player will walk off the field and shortly thereafter collapse to the ground. On primary examination, the athlete is found to be unconscious demonstrating signs of cerebral herniation, blown/nonreactive pupils, and respiratory failure.[66,73] From the published case reports, neuroimaging of SIS is significant for diffuse cerebral edema that is out of proportion to any space occupying lesions that are present.[62,76–78]

It is important to note that SIS is an incredibly rare phenomenon in that in a team of 50 players, someone would need to coach 4100 seasons to see 1 case of SIS.[66] Interestingly, there is an absolute lack of literature regarding SIS in Australian football and professional boxing, sports known for their high concussion incidence.[64,73,79] This illustrates that head-to-head impacts with a helmeted cranium may be responsible for cases of SIS in American football compared with other sports. There have also been cases of SIS where there was not a documented initial concussion. Therefore, caution must be made in assigning a player with the diagnosis of SIS and consideration for the use of the term first impact syndrome in those players, where there was no previously documented concussion. A single, significant impact may theoretically trigger the pathophysiological state predicted to occur in SIS where there is vasomotor instability and vasodilation leading to aggressive cerebral edema, herniation, and potentially death.[2,80]

Skull fractures

As mentioned, skull fractures occur because of a large, focal, and direct blow to the cranium but are infrequently seen in helmeted sports because of the ability of helmets to dissipate the force over a larger surface area and their impact-resistant polycarbonate shell. Skull fractures are characterized as simple/complex, if there is skin overlying/not overlying the defect, and depressed or comminuted if there are bony fragments extending past the inner table of the cranium. Athletes will present with focal tenderness to the area along with findings of edema, ecchymosis, and potentially a gross deformity seen on clinical examination. Most simple, nondepressed skull

---

Box 2
Indications for surgical intervention of a skull fracture

Extensive depression (greater than the thickness of the calvarium)

Gross cosmetic deformity

Open, depressed fracture requiring surgical debridement

Neurologic deficit associated with depressed skull fracture or underlying hematoma

Dural laceration or cranial sinus injury

From Bullock MR, Chesnut R, Ghajar J, et al. Surgical management of depressed cranial fractures. Neurosurgery 2006;58(3 Suppl):S56–60; [discussion: Si–iv]; with permission.

fractures do not require surgical intervention and respond to analgesia prescribed for pain control **Box 2**.[81]

Cranial Neuroimaging Algorithm

Cranial imaging in those with a neurosurgical emergency is obvious, because most, if not all, neurosurgical emergencies cause a profound neurologic deficit. A noncontrasted CT scan of the head is the best imaging choice for any athlete presenting with an acute neurologic decline/deficit following trauma. This is because CT imaging is a rapid and reliable test for determining the presence of intracranial blood products, particularly hematomas.[13,82] For those athletes with less dramatic or even absent clinical examination findings, there have been multiple published guidelines recommending when to obtain a head CT, like the Canadian and New Orleans Head Injury/Trauma Rule (**Table 5**).[83–96] Consistent criteria among these guidelines is the absolute need to obtain cranial imaging in athletes with an abnormal neurologic examination, those with progressive worsening in subjective symptoms, or those with prolonged loss of consciousness after injury.[97,98] A clinical algorithm based on one of these criteria is advocated for in order to reduce unnecessary radiation exposure in a low-risk athlete, but also to properly predict even the presence of minute intracranial blood products, not always warranting surgical intervention, but likely reinforcing the need for clinical observation.

Initial Hospital Management

The primary goal of treatment of any focal or diffuse brain injury is to evaluate for the extent of injury, determine the role for surgical intervention, and initiate measures to reduce propagation of further brain injury. As previously discussed, focal lesions (EDH and SDH) displaying mass effect and neurologic signs require emergent surgical evacuation to avoid cerebral herniation. For less focal or diffuse injuries (like SIS, DAI, and occasionally TICH), the initial treatment is aggressive medical interventions that may require surgical intervention if these are unable to relieve ICP elevations.

Recent guidelines were released by the Brain Trauma Foundation in order to guide clinicians in the management of the patient with a severe TBI. The specific details of each recommendation extend beyond the scope of this article, and it is recommended that the reader reference the full publication for further information.[99] Prehospital and

Table 5	
Common guideline recommendations for obtaining cranial imaging after head trauma	
Guideline Source	**Recommendation**
Canadian head CT rule[89,90]	• GCS <15, >2 h after injury
	• Clinical suspicion for skull fracture
	• Prolonged emesis ($\geq$2 episodes)
	• Older age ($\geq$65 y old)
	• Prolonged amnesia of the event (>30 min)
	• High index of suspicion due to mechanism of injury
New Orleans rule[83]	In a patient with GCS of 15, obtain a head CT if he or she has one of the following:
	• Persistent headache
	• Emesis
	• Age >60
	• Alcohol or drug intoxication
	• Persistent anterograde amnesia
	• Visible trauma above the clavicles
	• Seizure episode

inpatient management goals should entail avoidance of hypoxia, hypotension (goal: systolic blood pressure $\geq$100 mm Hg for patients 50–69 years old or $\geq$110 mm Hg for patients 15–49 or >70 years old and CPP goal between 60–70 mm Hg), hypoglycemia, and hypocarbia (goal: normalcarbia pPCO$_2$ 35–45).[99–101] For pharmacologic therapies, the use of steroids in severe TBI has been shown to increase mortality and therefore is not recommended, but the use of antiepileptic agents, like dilantin or keppra, is recommended in order to reduce early post-traumatic seizures.[99–103]

All severe TBI patients should be considered for ICP monitoring based on specific clinical criteria with a treatment threshold of greater than 22 mm Hg, **Box 3**.[99] Measures for reducing elevations in intracranial pressure should follow a step-wise progression of simple measures such as raising the head of the bed, reducing any neck constriction (head midline, loosen cervical collar), followed by greater sedation and/or analgesia, ventricular drainage, mannitol/hypertonic saline, muscular paralysis, or barbiturate coma.[99–101]

If ICP is refractory to maximal medical therapy, then a decompressive craniectomy should be considered. In 2011, the "Decompressive Craniectomy in Diffuse Traumatic Brain Injury, or DECRA" was published demonstrating the limited benefit of surgical intervention for severe TBI, in which it was shown to reduce elevations in ICP and ICU hospital length of stay, but without any improvement in clinical outcomes at 6 months from surgery.[104] The results of this randomized controlled study have been questioned due to a significant difference in clinical examinations between the surgical and medical treatment arms, high cross-over rate, and poorly defined clinical management practices between institutions.[105] For this reason, a further randomized study was initiated, "Randomized Evaluation of Surgery with Craniectomy for Uncontrollable Elevation of Intracranial Pressure, or RESCUEicp," in order to address these criticisms.[106] This study randomized 408 patients with refractory ICP to either continued medical therapy or surgical intervention, to demonstrate that the group that received surgical decompression not only had a significant reduction in ICP, but also had a decreased mortality at 6 and 12 months.[107] Interestingly, within the surgical treatment arm, there was a greater proportion of patients in a vegetative state at 12 months, but there appeared to be a greater proportion of moderate-to-good recovery in those patients who received surgical intervention compared with those who did not. Because the Brain Trauma Foundation guidelines were released prior to the release of the RESCUEicp results, the guidelines stated "Bifrontal [decompressive craniectomy] is not recommended to improve outcomes as measured by the GOS-E score at 6 mo post-injury in severe TBI patients with diffuse injury and with ICP elevation…refractory to first-tier therapies. However, this procedure has been demonstrated to reduce ICP and to minimize days in the ICU."[99] With the publication of RESCUEicp demonstrating reduced mortality but varied outcomes depending on one's specific definition for good outcome, the decision to perform a decompressive craniectomy on a patient for refractory ICP is therefore to be decided through an honest, realistic discussion with the patient's family, taking into account the patient's clinical examination, comorbid medical conditions, age, and extracranial injuries in order to come to a joint conclusion.

Box 3
Indications for placement of an intracranial pressure monitor

GCS 3 to 8 with abnormal CT imaging

GCS 3 to 8 with normal CT imaging if $\geq$2 of the following:
- Age greater than 40 years old
- Unilateral or bilateral posturing
- Episode of systolic blood pressure less than 90 mm Hg

NEUROSURGICAL SPINAL EMERGENCIES
Spinal Cord Injury

There are numerous sports-related injuries involving the muscles/ligaments (sprains and strains), intervertebral discs (disc bulge), bony spine (transverse process, spinous process, vertebral compression fractures), or nerves (stingers, stretch injury to the brachial plexus causing unilateral burning, numbness, or pain to the arm) that may be evaluated by a neurosurgeon, but these are typically benign injuries prompting only conservative, nonsurgical therapy. Because of the nature of the article, the authors will focus solely on acute spinal cord injuries (SCI), because this is the main spinal emergency that a neurosurgeon can face in athletic competition prompting emergent surgical intervention.

Because the spinal cord ends at L1 or L2, typically, SCIs involve trauma to either the cervical (most common, roughly 60% of SCIs[108]) or thoracic spine. Not all SCIs require a bony fracture, but can also occur in the setting of only ligamentous disruption or spinal canal narrowing due to an acute or chronically herniated intervertebral disc or degenerative changes like ligamentous hypertrophy or osteophytic growth (cervical bone spurs) **Fig. 7**. These injuries are becoming increasingly less frequent due to the implementation of infractions in sports like hockey and football where spearing or cross-checking from behind is penalized.[1]

Spinal Imaging in the Athlete

The algorithm for spinal imaging in the athlete is determined by the presence of symptoms. The awake, asymptomatic athlete without neck pain (on full range of motion) or midline tenderness who does not have any neurologic symptoms or distracting injuries can be cleared clinically without obtaining any cervical spine imaging.[109,110] The awake athlete with either cervical, thoracic, or lumbar pain should receive a high-quality thin-cut noncontrasted CT scan to evaluate for spinal fractures.[109] If the patient

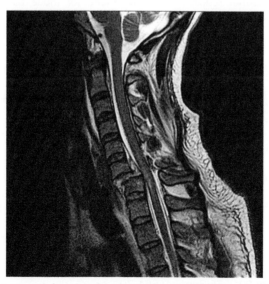

Fig. 7. C6-7 acute, traumatic herniated nucleus pulposus with a fracture–dislocation and spinal cord edema. (*Reproduced from* Bailes JE, Petschauer M, Guskiewicz KM, et al. Management of cervical spine injuries in athletes. J Athl Train 2007;42(1):126–34. Open Access.)

also has a neurologic deficit on examination, a noncontrasted MRI image should be obtained following the CT scan with location of image based on their presenting symptoms.

Management of Spinal Cord Injuries

Any athlete presenting with an SCI should have appropriate imaging obtained followed by consultation to a physician versed in managing such injuries, either neurologic or orthopedic surgeon. In the interim, the focus of treatment for any athlete with a suspected SCI is to prevent further neurologic deficits. Therefore, the athlete should remain in strict spinal precautions including cervical collar use (if cervical spine injury), flat bed rest, and log roll for transfers. Further, hypotension should be avoided with a goal mean arterial pressure of greater than 85 mm Hg.[111] Any player with a cervical or high thoracic spinal cord injury can present in neurogenic shock due to a loss of sympathetic tone to the vasculature. The athlete would clinically present with profound hypotension in the setting of warm and flushed skin. Fluids should be used cautiously only to replace losses, and the treatment of neurogenic shock is with vasopressors (ie, dopamine).[111] Currently, there is no Level 1 evidence to support the use of steroids in SCI; therefore steroids are not recommended.[112] Lastly, for the athlete with an SCI and an unstable spine, consultation with a spine surgeon will determine the timing and surgical approach needed for the specific injury.

SUMMARY

Proper education in the management of spinal cord and severe brain injuries can not only prevent mortality but can also reduce propagation of further neurogenic injury. Therefore, a standardized, coordinated approach based on clinical guidelines must be used commencing with the athletic trainer and team physician and continued with to the critical care and surgical attending physicians. This article is only a primer to the basic foundation to the acute management of the athlete with a neurosurgical emergency, and further reading is recommended for those tasked at managing such acute and complex patients.

REFERENCES

1. Boden BP, Breit I, Beachler JA, et al. Fatalities in high school and college football players. Am J Sports Med 2013;41(5):1108–16.
2. Bailes J, Patel V, Farhat H, et al. Football fatalities: the first impact syndrome. J Neurosurg Pediatr 2017;19(1):116–21.
3. Guskiewicz KM, Broglio SP. Sport-related concussion: on-field and sideline assessment. Phys Med Rehabil Clin N Am 2011;22(4):603–17, vii.
4. Herring SA, Kibler WB, Putukian M. Team physician consensus statement: 2013 update. Med Sci Sports Exerc 2013;45(8):1618–22.
5. Broglio SP, Cantu RC, Gioia GA, et al. National Athletic Trainers' Association position statement: management of sport concussion. J athletic Train 2014;49(2): 245–65.
6. Available at: https://www.nice.org.uk/guidance/cg176. Accessed November 9, 2016.
7. Putukian M, Kutcher J. Current concepts in the treatment of sports concussions. Neurosurgery 2014;75(Suppl 4):S64–70.
8. Chameides L, Samson R, Schexnayder S, et al, editors. Pediatric advanced life support: provider manual. Texas: American Heart Association Printing; 2011.

9. Sinz E, Navarro K, editors. Advanced cardiovascular life support: provider manual. Texas: American Heart Association; 2011.

10. Jung JY. Airway management of patients with traumatic brain injury/C-spine injury. Korean J Anesthesiol 2015;68(3):213–9.

11. McCrory P, Meeuwisse W, Aubry M, et al. Consensus statement on concussion in sport—The 4th International Conference on Concussion in Sport held in Zurich, November 2012. Phys Ther Sport 2013;14(2):e1–13.

12. Concussion (mild traumatic brain injury) and the team physician: a consensus statement. Med Sci Sports Exerc 2006;38(2):395–9.

13. Ropper AH, Gorson KC. Clinical practice. Concussion. N Engl J Med 2007; 356(2):166–72.

14. Putukian M. The acute symptoms of sport-related concussion: diagnosis and on-field management. Clin Sports Med 2011;30(1):49–61, viii.

15. National Athletic Trainer's Association. Appropriate prehospital management of the spine-injured athlete, updated from 1998 document. 2015. Available at: nata.org. Accessed November 9, 2016.

16. Ghiselli G, Schaadt G, McAllister DR. On-the-field evaluation of an athlete with a head or neck injury. Clin Sports Med 2003;22(3):445–65.

17. Putukian M, Raftery M, Guskiewicz K, et al. Onfield assessment of concussion in the adult athlete. Br J Sports Med 2013;47(5):285–8.

18. Guskiewicz KM, Broglio SP. Acute sports-related traumatic brain injury and repetitive concussion. Handb Clin Neurol 2015;127:157–72.

19. Committee on Sports-Related Concussions in Youth; Board on Children, Youth, and Families; Institute of Medicine; National Research Council. In: Graham R, Rivara FP, Ford MA, et al, editors. Sports-Related Concussions in Youth: Improving the Science, Changing the Culture. Washington, DC: National Academies Press; 2014. Available from: https://www.ncbi.nlm.nih.gov/books/NBK169016/.

20. Echemendia RJ, Giza CC, Kutcher JS. Developing guidelines for return to play: consensus and evidence-based approaches. Brain Inj 2015;29(2):185–94.

21. Giza CC, Kutcher JS, Ashwal S, et al. Summary of evidence-based guideline update: evaluation and management of concussion in sports: report of the Guideline Development Subcommittee of the American Academy of Neurology. Neurology 2013;80(24):2250–7.

22. Harmon KG, Drezner J, Gammons M, et al. American Medical Society for Sports Medicine position statement: concussion in sport. Clin J Sport Med 2013;23(1): 1–18.

23. Buckley TA, Burdette G, Kelly K. Concussion-management practice patterns of National Collegiate Athletic Association Division II and III athletic trainers: how the other half lives. J athletic Train 2015;50(8):879–88.

24. Willer B, Leddy JJ. Management of concussion and post-concussion syndrome. Curr Treat Options Neurol 2006;8(5):415–26.

25. McCrory P, Meeuwisse WH, Aubry M, et al. Consensus statement on concussion in sport: the 4th International Conference on Concussion in Sport, Zurich, November 2012. J athletic Train 2013;48(4):554–75.

26. Hadley MN, Walters BC, Aarabi B, et al. Clinical assessment following acute cervical spinal cord injury. Neurosurgery 2013;72(Suppl 2):40–53.

27. Kirshblum SC, Burns SP, Biering-Sorensen F, et al. International standards for neurological classification of spinal cord injury (Revised 2011). The Journal of Spinal Cord Medicine 2011;34(6):535–46. http://dx.doi.org/10.1179/204577 211X13207446293695.

28. Mokri B. The Monro-Kellie hypothesis: applications in CSF volume depletion. Neurology 2001;56(12):1746–8.

29. Blumbergs PC. Neuropathology of traumatic brain injury. In: Winn HR, editor. Youmans neurological surgery. 6th edition. Philadelphia: Saunders; 2011. p. 3288–99.

30. Blumenfeld H. Brain and environs: cranium, ventricles, and meninges. Neuroanatomy through clinical cases. 2nd edition. Sunderland (MA): Sinauer Associates, Inc. Publishers; 2010. p. 126–215.

31. Ropper A. Unusual spontaneous movements in brain-dead patients. Neurology 1984;34:1089–92.

32. Committee on Sports-Related Concussions in Youth; Board on Children, Youth, and Families; Institute of Medicine; National Research Council. In: Graham R, Rivara FP, Ford MA, et al, editors. Sports-Related Concussions in Youth: Improving the Science, Changing the Culture. Washington, DC: National Academies Press; 2014. 2, Neuroscience, Biomechanics, and Risks of Concussion in the Developing Brain. Available at: https://www.ncbi.nlm.nih.gov/books/NBK185339/.

33. McCrory P, Johnston KM, Mohtadi NG, et al. Evidence-based review of sport-related concussion: basic science. Clin J Sport Med 2001;11(3):160–5.

34. Ommaya AK. Head injury mechanisms and the concept of preventive management: a review and critical synthesis. J Neurotrauma 1995;12(4):527–46.

35. Stone JL, Patel V, Bailes JE. The history of neurosurgical treatment of sports concussion. Neurosurgery 2014;75(Suppl 4):S3–23.

36. Ommaya AK, Goldsmith W, Thibault L. Biomechanics and neuropathology of adult and paediatric head injury. Br J Neurosurg 2002;16(3):220–42.

37. Meaney DF, Morrison B, Dale Bass C. The mechanics of traumatic brain injury: a review of what we know and what we need to know for reducing its societal burden. J Biomech Eng 2014;136(2):021008.

38. Turner RC, Naser ZJ, Bailes JE, et al. Effect of slosh mitigation on histologic markers of traumatic brain injury: laboratory investigation. J Neurosurg 2012; 117(6):1110–8.

39. Smith DW, Bailes JE, Fisher JA, et al. Internal jugular vein compression mitigates traumatic axonal injury in a rat model by reducing the intracranial slosh effect. Neurosurgery 2012;70(3):740–6.

40. Gudeman SK, Kishore PR, Miller JD, et al. The genesis and significance of delayed traumatic intracerebral hematoma. Neurosurgery 1979;5(3):309–13.

41. Bullock MR, Chesnut R, Ghajar J, et al. Surgical management of traumatic parenchymal lesions. Neurosurgery 2006;58(3 Suppl):S25–46 [discussion: Si–iv].

42. Davis G, Marion DW, Le Roux P, et al. Clinics in neurology and neurosurgery—extradural and subdural haematoma. Br J Sports Med 2010;44(16):1139–43.

43. Bullock MR, Chesnut R, Ghajar J, et al. Surgical management of acute epidural hematomas. Neurosurgery 2006;58(3 Suppl):S7–15 [discussion: Si–iv].

44. Rivas JJ, Lobato RD, Sarabia R, et al. Extradural hematoma: analysis of factors influencing the courses of 161 patients. Neurosurgery 1988;23(1):44–51.

45. Seelig JM, Becker DP, Miller JD, et al. Traumatic acute subdural hematoma: major mortality reduction in comatose patients treated within four hours. N Engl J Med 1981;304(25):1511–8.

46. Bullock MR, Chesnut R, Ghajar J, et al. Surgical management of acute subdural hematomas. Neurosurgery 2006;58(3 Suppl):S16–24 [discussion: Si–iv].

47. Mihalik JP, Guskiewicz KM, Marshall SW, et al. Head impact biomechanics in youth hockey: comparisons across playing position, event types, and impact locations. Ann Biomed Eng 2012;40(1):141–9.

48. Crisco JJ, Wilcox BJ, Machan JT, et al. Magnitude of head impact exposures in individual collegiate football players. J Appl Biomech 2012;28(2):174–83.

49. Goldsmith W, Plunkett J. A biomechanical analysis of the causes of traumatic brain injury in infants and children. Am J Forensic Med Pathol 2004;25(2): 89–100.

50. Morrison AL, King TM, Korell MA, et al. Acceleration–deceleration injuries to the brain in blunt force trauma. Am J forensic Med Pathol 1998;19(2):109–12.

51. McKee AC, Stein TD, Kiernan PT, et al. The neuropathology of chronic traumatic encephalopathy. Brain Pathol (Zurich, Switzerland) 2015;25(3):350–64.

52. Choe MC, Giza CC. Diagnosis and management of acute concussion. Semin Neurol 2015;35(1):29–41.

53. Caskey RC, Nance ML. Management of pediatric mild traumatic brain injury. Adv Pediatr 2014;61(1):271–86.

54. Hovda DA. The neurophysiology of concussion. Prog Neurol Surg 2014;28: 28–37.

55. Giza CC, Hovda DA. The neurometabolic cascade of concussion. J athletic Train 2001;36(3):228–35.

56. Giza CC, Hovda DA. The new neurometabolic cascade of concussion. Neurosurgery 2014;75(Suppl 4):S24–33.

57. Nariai T, Inaji M, Tanaka Y, et al. PET molecular imaging to investigate higher brain dysfunction in patients with neurotrauma. Acta Neurochir Suppl 2013; 118:251–4.

58. Selwyn R, Hockenbury N, Jaiswal S, et al. Mild traumatic brain injury results in depressed cerebral glucose uptake: an (18)FDG PET study. J Neurotrauma 2013;30(23):1943–53.

59. Mittl RL, Grossman RI, Hiehle JF, et al. Prevalence of MR evidence of diffuse axonal injury in patients with mild head injury and normal head CT findings. AJNR Am J Neuroradiol 1994;15(8):1583–9.

60. Huisman TA, Sorensen AG, Hergan K, et al. Diffusion-weighted imaging for the evaluation of diffuse axonal injury in closed head injury. J Comput Assist Tomogr 2003;27(1):5–11.

61. Cantu RC. Second-impact syndrome. Clin Sports Med 1998;17(1):37–44.

62. Cantu RC, Gean AD. Second-impact syndrome and a small subdural hematoma: an uncommon catastrophic result of repetitive head injury with a characteristic imaging appearance. J Neurotrauma 2010;27(9):1557–64.

63. McQuillen JB, McQuillen EN, Morrow P. Trauma, sport, and malignant cerebral edema. Am J forensic Med Pathol 1988;9(1):12–5.

64. McCrory PR, Berkovic SF. Second impact syndrome. Neurology 1998;50(3): 677–83.

65. Kelly JP, Nichols JS, Filley CM, et al. Concussion in sports. Guidelines for the prevention of catastrophic outcome. JAMA 1991;266(20):2867–9.

66. Hebert O, Schlueter K, Hornsby M, et al. The diagnostic credibility of second impact syndrome: a systematic literature review. J Sci Med Sport 2016;19(10): 789–94.

67. Casa DJ, Guskiewicz KM, Anderson SA, et al. National athletic trainers' association position statement: preventing sudden death in sports. J athletic Train 2012;47(1):96–118.

68. Junger EC, Newell DW, Grant GA, et al. Cerebral autoregulation following minor head injury. J Neurosurg 1997;86(3):425–32.

69. Strebel S, Lam AM, Matta BF, et al. Impaired cerebral autoregulation after mild brain injury. Surg Neurol 1997;47(2):128–31.

70. Chan ST, Evans KC, Rosen BR, et al. A case study of magnetic resonance imaging of cerebrovascular reactivity: a powerful imaging marker for mild traumatic brain injury. Brain Inj 2015;29(3):403–7.

71. Mutch WA, Ellis MJ, Graham MR, et al. Brain MRI CO_2 stress testing: a pilot study in patients with concussion. PLoS One 2014;9(7):e102181.

72. Doshi H, Wiseman N, Liu J, et al. Cerebral hemodynamic changes of mild traumatic brain injury at the acute stage. PLoS One 2015;10(2):e0118061.

73. Bey T, Ostick B. Second impact syndrome. West J Emerg Med 2009;10(1):6–10.

74. Morris SA, Jones WH, Proctor MR, et al. Emergent treatment of athletes with brain injury. Neurosurgery 2014;75(Suppl 4):S96–105.

75. Bruce DA, Alavi A, Bilaniuk L, et al. Diffuse cerebral swelling following head injuries in children: the syndrome of "malignant brain edema". J Neurosurg 1981; 54(2):170–8.

76. Mori T, Katayama Y, Kawamata T. Acute hemispheric swelling associated with thin subdural hematomas: pathophysiology of repetitive head injury in sports. Acta neurochirurgica Suppl 2006;96:40–3.

77. Weinstein E, Turner M, Kuzma BB, et al. Second impact syndrome in football: new imaging and insights into a rare and devastating condition. J Neurosurg Pediatr 2013;11(3):331–4.

78. McLendon LA, Kralik SF, Grayson PA, et al. The controversial second impact syndrome: a review of the literature. Pediatr Neurol 2016;62:9–17.

79. McCrory P, Davis G, Makdissi M. Second impact syndrome or cerebral swelling after sporting head injury. Curr Sports Med Rep 2012;11(1):21–3.

80. Langfitt TW, Tannanbaum HM, Kassell NF. The etiology of acute brain swelling following experimental head injury. J Neurosurg 1966;24(1):47–56.

81. Bullock MR, Chesnut R, Ghajar J, et al. Surgical management of depressed cranial fractures. Neurosurgery 2006;58(3 Suppl):S56–60 [discussion: Si–iv].

82. Koo AH, LaRoque RL. Evaluation of head trauma by computed tomography. Radiology 1977;123(2):345–50.

83. Haydel MJ, Preston CA, Mills TJ, et al. Indications for computed tomography in patients with minor head injury. N Engl J Med 2000;343(2):100–6.

84. Kavalci C, Aksel G, Salt O, et al. Comparison of the Canadian CT head rule and the New Orleans criteria in patients with minor head injury. World J Emerg Surg 2014;9:31.

85. Stiell IG, Clement CM, Rowe BH, et al. Comparison of the Canadian CT head rule and the New Orleans criteria in patients with minor head injury. JAMA 2005;294(12):1511–8.

86. Smits M, Dippel DW, de Haan GG, et al. External validation of the Canadian CT Head Rule and the New Orleans Criteria for CT scanning in patients with minor head injury. JAMA 2005;294(12):1519–25.

87. Schachar JL, Zampolin RL, Miller TS, et al. External validation of the New Orleans criteria (NOC), the Canadian CT head rule (CCHR) and the National Emergency X-Radiography Utilization Study II (NEXUS II) for CT scanning in pediatric patients with minor head injury in a nontrauma center. Pediatr Radiol 2011;41(8): 971–9.

88. Korley FK, Morton MJ, Hill PM, et al. Agreement between routine emergency department care and clinical decision support recommended care in patients evaluated for mild traumatic brain injury. Acad Emerg Med 2013;20(5):463–9.

89. Stiell IG, Wells GA, Vandemheen K, et al. The Canadian CT Head Rule for patients with minor head injury. Lancet 2001;357(9266):1391–6.

90. Stiell IG, Lesiuk H, Wells GA, et al. The Canadian CT Head Rule Study for patients with minor head injury: rationale, objectives, and methodology for phase I (derivation). Ann Emerg Med 2001;38(2):160–9.

91. Jagoda AS, Bazarian JJ, Bruns JJ Jr, et al. Clinical policy: neuroimaging and decision making in adult mild traumatic brain injury in the acute setting. Ann Emerg Med 2008;52(6):714–48.

92. Osmond MH, Klassen TP, Wells GA, et al. CATCH: a clinical decision rule for the use of computed tomography in children with minor head injury. CMAJ 2010; 182(4):341–8.

93. Kuppermann N, Holmes JF, Dayan PS, et al. The diagnostic credibility of second impact syndrome: a systematic literature review. a prospective cohort study. Lancet 2009;374(9696):1160–70.

94. Mihindu E, Bhullar I, Tepas J, et al. Computed tomography of the head in children with mild traumatic brain injury. Am Surg 2014;80(9):841–3.

95. Faris G, Byczkowski T, Ho M, et al. Prediction of persistent post-concussion symptoms in youth using a neuroimaging decision rule. Acad Pediatr 2016;16(4):336–42.

96. Dunning J, Daly JP, Lomas JP, et al. Derivation of the children's head injury algorithm for the prediction of important clinical events decision rule for head injury in children. Arch Dis Child 2006;91(11):885–91.

97. Ellis MJ, Leiter J, Hall T, et al. Neuroimaging findings in pediatric sports-related concussion. J Neurosurg Pediatr 2015;16(3):241–7.

98. McCrea HJ, Perrine K, Niogi S, et al. Concussion in sports. Sports Health 2013; 5(2):160–4.

99. Carney N, Totten AM, O'Reilly C, et al. Guidelines for the management of severe traumatic brain injury, fourth edition. Neurosurgery 2016;80:6–15.

100. Brain Trauma Foundation, American Association of Neurological Surgeons, Congress of Neurological Surgeons. Guidelines for the management of severe traumatic brain injury. J Neurotrauma 2007;24(Suppl 1):S1–106.

101. American College of Surgeons. Best practices in the management of traumatic brain injury. Available at: https://www.facs.org/~/media/files/quality%20 programs/trauma/tqip/traumatic%20brain%20injury%20guidelines.ashx. Accessed November 9, 2016.

102. Roberts I, Yates D, Sandercock P, et al. Effect of intravenous corticosteroids on death within 14 days in 10008 adults with clinically significant head injury (MRC CRASH trial): randomised placebo-controlled trial. Lancet 2004;364(9442): 1321–8.

103. Beauchamp K, Mutlak H, Smith WR, et al. Pharmacology of traumatic brain injury: where is the "golden bullet"? Mol Med 2008;14(11–12):731–40.

104. Cooper DJ, Rosenfeld JV, Murray L, et al. Decompressive craniectomy in diffuse traumatic brain injury. N Engl J Med 2011;364(16):1493–502.

105. Honeybul S, Ho KM, Lind CR. What can be learned from the DECRA study. World Neurosurg 2013;79(1):159–61.

106. Hutchinson PJ, Corteen E, Czosnyka M, et al. Decompressive craniectomy in traumatic brain injury: the randomized multicenter RESCUEicp study (http:// www.rescueicp.com/). Acta neurochirurgica Suppl 2006;96:17–20.

107. Hutchinson PJ, Kolias AG, Timofeev IS, et al. Trial of decompressive craniectomy for traumatic intracranial hypertension. N Engl J Med 2016;375(12):1119–30.
108. Boran S, Lenehan B, Street J, et al. 10-year review of sports-related spinal injuries. Irish J Med Sci 2011;180(4):859–63.
109. Ryken TC, Hadley MN, Walters BC, et al. Radiographic assessment. Neurosurgery 2013;72(Suppl 2):54–72.
110. Hoffman J, Mower W, Wolfson A, et al. Validity of a set of clinical criteria to rule out injury to the cervical spine in patients with blunt trauma. National Emergency X-Radiography Utilization Study Group. N Engl J Med 2000;343:94–9.
111. Ryken TC, Hurlbert RJ, Hadley MN, et al. The acute cardiopulmonary management of patients with cervical spinal cord injuries. Neurosurgery 2013;72(Suppl 2):84–92.
112. Hurlbert RJ, Hadley MN, Walters BC, et al. Pharmacological therapy for acute spinal cord injury. Neurosurgery 2013;72(Suppl 2):93–105.

Blood-Based Biomarkers for the Identification of Sports-Related Concussion

Martina Anto-Ocrah, MPH[a,b,*],
Courtney Marie Cora Jones, PhD, MPH[a,b], Danielle Diacovo, BA[a],
Jeffrey J. Bazarian, MD, MPH[a,b,c,d,e]

KEYWORDS

- Sports-related concussion • Traumatic brain injury • Concussion • Biomarkers

KEY POINTS

- Sports-related concussion is common among athletes in the United States; however, current methods for sideline assessment are suboptimal because of their reliance on self-reported symptoms.
- Blood-based biomarkers have potential utility in sports-related concussion for diagnosis, prognostication, and identification of neurodegeneration.
- Several limitations exist in the current empirical literature that limit the current ability of biomarkers for use in this context; but with additional research and understanding of the neurobiological mechanisms, these limitations can be overcome.

INTRODUCTION

Sports-related concussions (SRCs) are common among athletes in the United States. The Centers for Disease Control and Prevention estimates that there are 1.6 to 3.8 million SRC per year[1] with the highest concussion rates found among contact sports, such as ice hockey, football, soccer, and basketball.[2] Most athletes who sustain an

Disclosure Statement: The authors have nothing to disclose.
[a] Department of Emergency Medicine, University of Rochester, School of Medicine and Dentistry, 265 Crittenden Boulevard, Box 655C, Rochester, NY 14642, USA; [b] Department of Public Health Sciences, University of Rochester, School of Medicine and Dentistry, 265 Crittenden Boulevard, Box 655C, Rochester, NY 14642, USA; [c] Department of Neurology, University of Rochester, School of Medicine and Dentistry, 265 Crittenden Boulevard, Box 655C, Rochester, NY 14642, USA; [d] Department of Neurosurgery, University of Rochester, School of Medicine and Dentistry, 265 Crittenden Boulevard, Box 655C, Rochester, NY 14642, USA; [e] Department of Physical Medicine and Rehabilitation, University of Rochester, School of Medicine and Dentistry, 265 Crittenden Boulevard, Box 655C, Rochester, NY 14642, USA
* Corresponding author. Department of Emergency Medicine, University of Rochester, School of Medicine and Dentistry, 265 Crittenden Boulevard, Box 655C, Rochester, NY 14642.
E-mail address: Martina_Anto-Ocrah@URMC.Rochester.edu

SRC recover within 7 to 10 days[3]; however, as many as 10% have prolonged postconcussion symptoms, such as headache and dizziness, which can persist much longer.[4–6]

There are multiple clinical definitions of concussion available; however, the 2 most widely used in the context of SRC are (1) the clinical definition of mild traumatic brain injury from the Centers for Disease Control and Prevention and (2) the definition of concussion from the "Consensus Statement on Concussion in Sport."[7] Both definitions include external force to the head that impairs neurologic functioning and the absence of structural damage to the brain on neuroimaging.

Sideline tools, such as the Standardized Assessment of Concussion[8] and the Sports Concussion Assessment Tool Versions 2 and 3,[3,7] are designed to assist coaches and certified athletic trainers to identify the neurophysiologic changes associated with concussion, such as loss of consciousness, amnesia, and confusion. Despite these standard tools, unrecognized or unreported concussions occur in more than half of high school football players.[9] This finding is evidenced by a recent study by Meehan and colleagues that found that one-third of athletes did not realize they had sustained a concussion and, thus, failed to report their injuries.[10] The reasons for this failure to diagnose SRC are multifactorial. Many of the current decision algorithms for diagnosis of concussion rely on patients' report of symptoms. However, this is often problematic, as assessments that rely on self-report assume the athletes' short-term memory is intact, although impairments in memory are one of the criteria for concussion diagnosis. Reliance on athletes' willingness to self-report also ignores the fact that, for many athlete populations, there is an incentive to hide or opt not to disclose symptoms because of a perceived or real fear of being removed from the team or engaging in sporting practices or contests. For many, the fear of being sidelined and restricted from play offsets the risk of not receiving treatment of the concussion injury.

Additionally, diagnosis of concussion in the emergency department is also problematic and faces similar challenges to sideline assessment. Studies have shown that health care providers failed to diagnose concussion in 56% to 89% of cases.[11–13] Accurate identification of concussion in the immediate postinjury period is critical, as failure to report and/or diagnose could result in long-lasting and catastrophic sequelae. Accurate and timely identification of SRC is important for (1) initiating a treatment protocol to limit the athlete's exposure to head hits and (2) for ensuring that the protocol is adhered to, to ensure full recovery. Full recovery for the athlete is essential to reducing excess concussion-related morbidity, such as second impact syndrome, which could be catastrophic.[7,14,15]

Because of the heavy reliance on self-report of symptoms in concussion diagnosis and the risks associated with missed concussion, there is a clear need to identify a time-sensitive and accurate method to identify SRC in the immediate postinjury period. Blood-based brain biomarkers (BBBMs) have been suggested as objective tools for the assessment of concussion diagnosis,[16–20] especially in this athlete population. BBBMs have the potential to aid not only in the diagnosis of concussion but also in the prognostication of symptom recovery and return to play (RTP) and identification of neurodegeneration.

In this document, the authors provide an overview of the empirical evidence related to the use of BBBMs in the athlete population for diagnosis of SRC, prognosis, and neurodegeneration from the injury. The authors also provide a summary of research challenges, gaps in the literature, and future directions for research.

NEUROBIOLOGY OF SERUM BIOMARKERS FOR TRAUMATIC BRAIN INJURY

The main structural correlate occurring after SRC is thought to be diffuse axonal injury (AI).[21] Biomechanical forces, such as head impacts, which occur during the course of sports, have been linked to white matter injury.[21–24] During concussion, stretch-induced calcium influx leads to axonal microtubule and neurofilament destruction and disruption of axonal transport leading to axonal swelling.[14,15] Proteins are released from the breakdown of neurons as well as from other supporting cells, such as astrocytes and oligodendrocytes.[25–27] Microtubule and neurofilament destruction releases a variety of proteins, which diffuse to the peripheral system through the blood-brain barrier.[26]

The traditional thinking has been that proteins released during AI diffuse into the space between brain cells (interstitial space), then into the fluid surrounding the brain (cerebrospinal fluid), and finally across the normally closed blood-brain barrier to reach the peripheral circulation, where they can be detected in a blood sample. Traditional thinking also held that a head blow hard enough to cause concussion also transiently opened the blood-brain barrier, allowing brain proteins to pass. As it turns out, how proteins get from the brain into the blood may be a bit more complicated, which has implications for the interpretation of BBBM results following suspected SRC. It now seems that there is an alternative route for brain proteins to gain access to the blood; it may sometimes be blocked during a concussion, preventing markers of brain damage from reaching the peripheral circulation. In this route, called the glymphatic pathway, brain proteins diffuse into the interstitial space and then into the brain's lymphatic system, which empties into the blood.[28,29]

Several BBBMs have been studied among the athlete population. **Table 1** outlines the 4 biomarkers that are discussed in this article in the context of SRC, their cerebral and extracerebral origins, and availability of an assay. *Tau* is a protein primarily localized in the axonal compartment of neurons. Extracerebral concentrations are indicated after acute traumatic brain injury in correlation to axonal trauma severity as well as in chronic degenerative disorders.[30] S100B is a calcium-binding protein that

Table 1
Blood-based brain biomarkers of sports-related concussion: source, indication, and significance

Marker	Cerebral Source	Noncerebral Sources	Assay Available
Tau	Axon	None	No
S100-B	Astroglial cells, oligodendrocytes	Expression also found in peripheral tissue, such as bone, injured skeletal muscles, adipocytes, and melanocytes	Yes, most widely used and accepted clinical biomarker
Glial fibrillary acidic protein	Astroglial cells	Has not been detected extracerebrally	No
αII-Spectrin N-terminal fragment	Neuron, abundantly expressed in axons and presynaptic terminals	Has not been detected extracerebrally	No
Neuron-specific enolase	Neuron	High sensitivity to hemolysis, however, and found in erythrocytes and endocrine cells	Yes

Adapted from Zetterberg H, Smith DH, Blennow K. Biomarkers of mild traumatic brain injury in cerebrospinal fluid and blood. Nat Rev Neurol 2013;9(4):201–10.

helps regulate intracellular levels of calcium. S100B is also expressed extracerebrally, in adipocytes and melanocytes, bone, and injured muscle tissue.[31,32] *all-spectrin N-terminal fragment* (SNTF) is a protein that is normally undetectable in axons but is generated following stretch injury by intra-axonal calcium and spectrin overload and subsequently accumulates in damaged axons.[31,33,34] *Neuron-specific enolase* (NSE) is a glycolytic enzyme enriched in neuronal cell bodies but is also present in erythrocytes and endocrine cells.[31,32]

OVERVIEW OF BLOOD-BASED BIOMARKERS OF SPORTS-RELATED CONCUSSION

Serum protein biomarkers have the potential to aid in the diagnosis of SRC, prognostication of postconcussive symptoms and delayed RTP, and identification of traumatically induced chronic neurodegeneration. Later, and also in **Table 2**, the authors provide an overview of the literature for each of these intended uses of the select BBBM.

Diagnosis of Sports-Related Concussion

In the context of SRC, BBBMs have been most frequently studied as an objective assessment for the diagnosis of concussion. Specifically, the ability of tau, S100B, and NSE to discriminate between concussed and nonconcussed athletes has been studied in a variety of sports, including ice hockey, boxing, American football, soccer, and basketball.[16,20,35–37]

Shahim and colleagues[20] (2014) compared serum levels of tau, S100B, and NSE in a group of 28 Swedish ice hockey players who sustained a concussion between September 2012 and January 2013. BBBM levels after injury were compared with preseason levels, before the start of the ice hockey season. In players who sustained head injury or concussion during the season, consecutive blood samples were collected at 1, 12, 36, and 48 hours as well as 144 hours after the injury or the date on which the player returned to unrestricted competition. Compared with preseason levels, concussed players had significantly elevated levels of tau and S100B but not NSE.

The highest biomarker concentrations of tau and S100B were measured 1 hour after concussion, and declined significantly during the first 12-hour period ($P<.001$). Although further declines between 12 and 144 hours in tau were not statistically significant ($P = .15$), the elevated levels of tau measured 144 hours after concussion were significantly greater than preseason levels ($P = .002$). Similarly, the levels of S100B peaked during the first hour after concussion and declined during the first 12-hour period ($P<.001$). Levels, however, remained higher than preseason concentrations. There were no statistically significant variations in NSE over time.[20]

Not surprisingly, levels of S100B and NSE, both of which have extracerebral sources (see **Table 1**) were elevated after a friendly game, whereby no concussions were sustained. This finding was corroborated in another study by Bouvier and colleagues[35] who reported a significant increase in S100B concentration within 2 hours after a sporting contest (without concussion) in a group of 39 male rugby players. This increase was correlated with the number of body collisions, not just concussion, during a match. Increasing S100B concentrations were significantly correlated with the number of jumps in a basketball game,[37] blows received during boxing,[38] headers made during a football match,[37] and collisions during an American football game.[39]

Although S100B has been clinically validated and is widely available outside of the US, its diagnostic utility may be potentially limited by these findings of extracerebral sources.[40] In 2014, a multi-institutional study involving 46 collegial athletes in

Germany (n = 30) and the United States (n = 16) compared elevations in S100B before concussion (baseline), after noncontact exertion, and after concussion.[16] The investigators conclude that the mean postexertion S100B was not significantly different from the preseason baseline levels (0.071 ± 0.03 μg/L vs 0.070 ± 0.03 μg/L, P = .87), but the mean 3-hour post-SRC S100B level was significantly higher than the preseason baseline value (0.099 ± 0.008 μg/L vs 0.058 ± 0.006 μg/L, P = .0002). S100B levels at postinjury days 2, 3, and 7 were significantly lower than the 3-hour level and not different than baseline. Both the absolute change and proportional increase in S100B 3 hours after injury were accurate discriminators of SRC from noncontact exertion without SRC (area under the curve 0.772 and 0.904, respectively). A 3-hour postconcussion S100B 0.122 mg/L and a proportional S100B increase of 45.9% greater than the baseline were both 96.7% specific for the diagnosis of SRC.

SNTF has also been proposed as a possible diagnostic tool for SRC, particularly for concussed athletes who may have negative neuroimaging but are at risk for developing white matter damage and lasting brain dysfunction.[19] In 28 ice hockey players who had sustained a concussion, Siman and team[19] report that compared with preseason levels, serum SNTF was significantly increased at 1 hour after injury and remained significantly elevated from 12 hours to 6 days after injury (P<.05) before declining to preseason baseline. Mean SNTF concentration was up to 2-fold higher at 1, 12, 36, and 144 hours after concussion, compared with preseason levels. Moreover, serum levels of SNTF after concussion were related to serum tau but not S100B. And unlike S100B, serum SNTF levels do not seem to be sensitive to exertion in the absence of concussion.[19] This finding would suggest that SNTF and tau may be elevated via the same pathway, whereas these BBBMs may have utility as an independent confirmatory assessment in the presence of elevated S100B levels.

Prognostication of Symptom Resolution and Return to Play

Serum biomarkers also have the ability to provide prognostication regarding postconcussion syndrome (PCS) and informing RTP decisions. The ability of S100B, SNTF, and tau to identify athletes who will have prolonged RTP has found promising results. In a small sample of 28 concussed ice hockey players who had sustained a concussion, Siman and colleagues[19] found that postconcussive symptoms resolved within a few days for 8 of the players but persisted in the remaining 20. Delayed RTP was defined as 6 days or longer, and BBBM levels of SNTF were compared with those athletes whose RTP was normal (<6 days). At times ranging from 1 hour to 6 days after concussion, serum SNTF was essentially unchanged from preseason baseline levels for the 8 players with rapidly resolving PCS.

In sharp contrast, for the 20 who had persistent PCS lasting 6 or more days, serum SNTF levels were higher by up to 2.5-fold from 1 hour to 6 days after injury, compared with concentrations either at preseason baseline or in players with less-severe PCS. The difference in serum SNTF concentration after concussion as a function of PCS severity was statistically significant at the 36-hour time point (P = .014) and from the mean at 12 and 36 hours (P = .004). Interestingly, serum tau levels were also higher in the subset of 20 athletes who had delayed RTP compared with the 8 cases with shorter-lasting PCS, with the difference at 12 hours being statistically significant (P = .039).[19] Furthermore, serum SNTF exhibited prognostic accuracy for concussion, especially as it related with delayed RTP with multivariable analyses, including both SNTF and tau, leading to improved prediction of beyond tau alone.

In the 2014 study of serum levels of tau, S100B, and NSE in 28 Swedish ice hockey players who sustained a concussion and underwent testing, Shahim and team[20] reported that of the 3 biomarkers only tau concentrations at 1 hour after concussion

Table 2
Blood-based biomarkers of sports-related concussion, by biomarker, time, and potential use

| | Time of Blood Sample (Since Injury) | | | | |
	1 h	<3 h	12 h	1–6 d	>1 wk
Diagnosis					
S100B	AUC: 0.67 (95% CI: 0.52–0.83)[20]	AUC (raw 3-h value): 0.77 (95% CI: 0.64, 0.91) AUC (proportional increase greater than baseline value): 0.90 (95% CI: 0.80, 1.0) Sensitivity: 94.1% (<0.0605 µg/L and S100B decrease less than −3.5% from baseline) Specificity: 96.7% (>0.122 µg/L and S100B increase >45.9% greater than baseline)[16]	ND	AUC: 0.92(95% CI: 0.84–1.00)[35] Sensitivity: 81% Specificity: 100% −Predictive value: 100% +Predictive value: 26% Mean value boxers[30]: 0.037 (+/−0.018) Mean value controls: 0.041 (+/−0.025)	Mean value boxers[30]: 0.043 (+/−0.024) Mean value controls: 0.041 (+/−0.025)
NSE	AUC: 0.55 (95% CI: 0.37–0.70)[20]	ND	ND	ND	ND
Tau	AUC: 0.80 (95% CI: 0.65–0.94)[20]	ND	ND	Mean value boxers[30]: 2.46 (+/−5.10) Mean value controls: 0.79 (+/−0.96)	Mean value boxers[30]: 1.43 (+/−2.51) Mean value controls: 0.79 (+/−0.96)
SNTF	AUC: 0.74 (95% CI: 0.61–0.86)[19]	ND	ND	AUC: 0.76 (95% CI: 0.63–0.90)[19]	ND
Prognostication					
S100B	AUC: 0.68 (95% CI: 0.50–0.87)[20]	ND	ND	AUC: 0.55 (95% CI: 0.33–0.78)[20]	ND
NSE	AUC: 0.54 (95% CI: 0.32–0.76)[20]	ND	ND	AUC: 0.65 (95% CI: 0.42–0.89)[20]	ND

Tau	AUC: 0.91 (95% CI: 0.81–1.00)[20] AUC: 0.87 (95% CI: 0.71–1.00)[20]	ND	AUC: 0.91 (95% CI: 0.78–1.00)[20]	AUC: 0.76 (95% CI: 0.58–0.94)[20]	ND
SNTF	ND	ND	ND	AUC: 0.85 (95% CI: 0.73–0.97)[19] AUC: 0.87 (95% CI: 0.79–0.96)[19]	ND
Neurodegeneration					
S100B	ND	ND	ND	ND	ND
NSE	ND	ND	ND	ND	ND
Tau	ND	ND	ND	ND	Higher levels compared with controls in the following regions[42]: Caudate: 1.48 vs 1.23 Putamen: 1.47 vs 1.20 Thalamus: 1.48 vs 1.29 Subthalamus: 1.45 vs 1.25 Midbrain: 1.31 vs 1.14 White matter: 1.15 vs 1.09 Amygdala: 1.30 vs 1.14
SNTF	ND	ND	ND	ND	ND

Abbreviations: AUC, area under the curve; CI, confidence interval; ND, no data; Time, time from injury to serum sample (in hours, unless otherwise specified).

predicted the number of days it took for the concussion symptoms to resolve and the players to return to unrestricted competition (r = 0.60; 95% confidence interval [CI], 0.23–0.90; P = .002). However, in a subsequent study, there was a significant correlation between the concentration of SNTF and the time to resolution of concussion symptoms (r = 0.75; 95% CI, 0.50–0.90; P<.001).[19] The concentration of NSE did not correlate with the resolution of concussion symptoms (r = 0.20; 95% CI, −0.20–0.55; P = .30). Further, the correlation persisted over time, with tau levels obtained 144 hours after injury remaining significantly elevated in players with PCS for more than 6 days compared with players with fewer days of PCS. There was no significant difference in the levels of S100B and NSE 144 hours after concussion in these 2 groups of players.[19]

Neurodegeneration

Chronic traumatic encephalopathy (CTE) has emerged as a potential long-term consequence of repeated concussions and/or subconcussive head hits among athletes.[41] One BBBM, tau, shows promise to identify those at high risk for CTE. Currently the only way to diagnose CTE is by postmortem examination of brain tissue. A method for antemortem diagnosis has not yet been developed, although PET-MRI scanning is currently under investigation.[42] Abnormal neuronal accumulations of the phosphorylated form of tau are thought to play a pathogenic role in CTE,[43,44] which has been reported in more than 150 deceased contact athletes[45] and in 4 military personnel exposed to multiple blast and nonblast head impacts.[46] After SRC, increases in plasma tau have been found within 12 hours among Olympic boxers and within 3 hours among professional ice hockey players.[20,30] Early post-SRC tau elevations predict prolonged postconcussive recovery.[47,48] Further, longer-term tau elevations have been found among 70 military personnel within 18 months of multiple deployment-related head injuries[49] and in 96 retired National Football League players (although concussion history is unavailable).[50] Thus, blood-based tau increases soon after SRC and is elevated months to years after multiple head impacts. Taken together, these studies suggest a possible link between elevated blood levels of tau and eventual accumulation of tau, which may be measurable via PET-MRI or serum sampling.

CHALLENGES AND FUTURE DIRECTIONS

The use of BBBMs in the athlete population is an evolving area of research with significant potential to influence the clinical care trajectories of those concussed playing their sport. There are several challenges that need to be addressed before BBBMs can be put to use on the sideline.

First, the serum kinetics and predictive power of these biomarkers in the initial minutes after injury is unknown. Most of the studies included in this review report the accuracy of marker concentrations 3 and 6 hours after injury, with a handful reporting values 1 hour after injury. However, to date, there are no data evaluating the use of BBBMs within the first 60 minutes of injury. This information is critically important if serum protein values are to be used on the sideline to make quick RTP decisions during a sporting contest. Additional research is needed to understand how soon after injury these proteins appear in the serum and how their diagnostic and predictive accuracy varies at these time points.

A related challenge involves the use of venous blood and the resulting serum or plasma to measure these markers. It may not be practical for contact sport teams to have a trained phlebotomist present at every game or practice in order to perform venipuncture within minutes of a potential SRC. Performing a finger stick, on the other hand, can be mastered with minimal training and practicably performed by an athletic trainer on the sideline, obviating a trained phlebotomist. Several handheld point-of-care test devices are currently being developed to measure brain proteins using capillary whole blood obtained from a finger stick, not venous blood.[51,52] If the future of sideline assessment includes the use of biomarkers, there is a clear need for a hand-held device with rapid turnaround time.

Another challenge is accounting for the increases in BBBM levels associated with body collisions[35,53] as well as with a variety of aerobic activities not involving collisions. These activities include sprinting for 6 minutes,[38] jogging 6 miles,[38] running a 15-mile half marathon,[38] swimming 4.5 miles,[54] cycling to 55% maximum oxygen consumption for 85 minutes,[55] running a 25-mile full marathon,[56] and running exertion-related increases in neuronal plasticity,[57,58] neurogenesis,[59] serotonin and astrocytic 5-hydroxytryptamine (serotonin) receptor activation (5-HT1A) receptor activation,[54,60] and neuroinflammation,[61,62] in conjunction with an exertion-related increase in blood-brain barrier permeability.[63–66] Additionally, BBBMs may be elevated in the presence of extracranial injuries and chronic neurologic disorders.[56,67,68] Thus, it is important to understand the various elements that may influence elevations in biomarker levels, beyond concussion, as well as the best way in which to control or adjust for such factors so as to maximize the discriminatory ability of these BBBMs.

Third, there is large interindividual variation in the serum levels of these proteins in normal, uninjured individuals.[16,20] This fact complicates efforts to find a single cutoff value that separates concussed from nonconcussed athletes. Several studies have shown that the discriminate or predictive ability of the biomarker improves when using an absolute increase from baseline versus only using samples obtained after injury.[16] Therefore, it is important to consider whether a preinjury baseline value is necessary in order to maximize the potential use of the biomarker. There may not be one uniform threshold value to which all athletes can be compared, but rather a personalized medicine approach in which each athlete is compared with his or her own baseline value in order to make an inference regarding concussion diagnosis or prognosis. Studies have also shown that baseline values of biomarker levels are highly variable across individuals and may be modified by other patient-level factors, including race.[69] Therefore, the magnitude of the increase relative to baseline on an individual level may be a more precise measure. However, this is an understudied area of research and should be explored further.

Fourth, the future of biomarkers and concussion will likely not rely on a single biomarker. Rather, a panel of biomarkers evaluating concurrently or sequentially will be needed to have desirable test characteristics. A combination of biomarkers may maximize sensitivity and specificity with little additional cost and/or burden to the clinical staff. The incremental value of biomarkers relative to clinical decision rules that rely on self-report has also not yet been evaluated. However, this is an area in which future research is warranted.

REFERENCES

1. Centers for Disease Control and Prevention. Nonfatal traumatic brain injuries related to sports and recreation activities among persons aged <19 years–United States, 2001-2009. MMWR Morb Mortal Wkly Rep 2011;60(39):1337–42.

2. Marar M, McIlvain NM, Fields SK, et al. Epidemiology of concussions among United States high school athletes in 20 sports. Am J Sports Med 2012;40(4): 747–55.

3. McCrory P, Meeuwisse W, Johnston K, et al. Consensus statement on concussion in sport: the 3rd International Conference on Concussion in Sport held in Zurich, November 2008. J Athl Train 2009;44(4):434–48.

4. Echemendia RJ, Putukian M, Mackin RS, et al. Neuropsychological test performance prior to and following sports-related mild traumatic brain injury. Clin J Sport Med 2001;11(1):23–31.

5. McCrea M, Guskiewicz K, Randolph C, et al. Incidence, clinical course, and predictors of prolonged recovery time following sport-related concussion in high school and college athletes. J Int Neuropsychol Soc 2013;19(1):22–33.

6. Ingebrigtsen T, Waterloo K, Marup-Jensen S, et al. Quantification of post-concussion symptoms 3 months after minor head injury in 100 consecutive patients. J Neurol 1998;245(9):609–12.

7. McCrory P, Meeuwisse WH, Aubry M, et al. Consensus statement on concussion in sport: the 4th International Conference on Concussion in Sport, Zurich, November 2012. J Athl Train 2013;48(4):554–75.

8. McCrea M, Kelly JP, Randolph C, et al. Standardized assessment of concussion (SAC): on-site mental status evaluation of the athlete. J Head Trauma Rehabil 1998;13(2):27–35.

9. McCrea M, Hammeke T, Olsen G, et al. Unreported concussion in high school football players implications for prevention. Clin J Sport Med 2004;14(1):13–7.

10. Meehan WP 3rd, Mannix RC, O'Brien MJ, et al. The prevalence of undiagnosed concussions in athletes. Clin J Sport Med 2014;23(5):339–42.

11. Delaney JS, Abuzeyad F, Correa JA, et al. Recognition and characteristics of concussions in the emergency department population. J Emerg Med 2005;29(2):189–97.

12. Powell JM, Ferraro JV, Dikmen SS, et al. Accuracy of mild traumatic brain injury diagnosis. Arch Phys Med Rehabil 2008;89(8):1550–5.

13. De Maio VJ, Joseph DO, Tibbo-Valeriote H, et al. Variability in discharge instructions and activity restrictions for patients in a children's ED postconcussion. Pediatr Emerg Care 2014;30(1):20–5.

14. Giza CC, Kutcher JS, Ashwal S, et al. Summary of evidence-based guideline update: evaluation and management of concussion in sports: report of the Guideline Development Subcommittee of the American Academy of Neurology. Neurology 2013;80(24):2250–7.

15. Harmon KG, Drezner JA, Gammons M, et al. American Medical Society for Sports Medicine position statement: concussion in sport. Br J Sports Med 2013;47(1):15–26.

16. Kiechle K, Bazarian JJ, Merchant-Borna K, et al. Subject-specific increases in serum S-100B distinguish sports-related concussion from sports-related exertion. PLoS One 2014;9(1):e84977.

17. Diaz-Arrastia R, Wang KK, Papa L, et al. Acute biomarkers of traumatic brain injury: relationship between plasma levels of ubiquitin C-terminal hydrolase-L1 and glial fibrillary acidic protein. J Neurotrauma 2014;31(1):19–25.

18. Papa L, Lewis LM, Silvestri S, et al. Serum levels of ubiquitin C-terminal hydrolase distinguish mild traumatic brain injury from trauma controls and are elevated in mild and moderate traumatic brain injury patients with intracranial lesions and neurosurgical intervention. J Trauma Acute Care Surg 2012;72(5):1335–44.

19. Siman R, Shahim P, Tegner Y, et al. Serum SNTF increases in concussed professional ice hockey players and relates to the severity of postconcussion symptoms. J Neurotrauma 2015;32:1294–300.

20. Shahim P, Tegner Y, Wilson DH, et al. Blood biomarkers for brain injury in concussed professional ice hockey players. JAMA Neurol 2014;71(6):684–92.

21. Meaney DF, Smith DH. Biomechanics of concussion. Clin Sports Med 2011;30(1): 19–31, vii.

22. Davenport EM, Whitlow CT, Urban JE, et al. Abnormal white matter integrity related to head impact exposure in a season of high school varsity football. J Neurotrauma 2014;31(19):1617–24.

23. Bazarian JJ, Zhu T, Zhong J, et al. Persistent, long-term cerebral white matter changes after sports-related repetitive head impacts. PLoS One 2014;9(4): e94734.

24. McAllister TW, Ford JC, Flashman LA, et al. Effect of head impacts on diffusivity measures in a cohort of collegiate contact sport athletes. Neurology 2014;82(1): 63–9.

25. Giza CC, Hovda DA. The neurometabolic cascade of concussion. J Athl Train 2001;36(3):228–35.

26. Giza CC, Hovda DA. The new neurometabolic cascade of concussion. Neurosurgery 2014;75(Suppl 4):S24–33.

27. Johnson VE, Stewart W, Smith DH. Axonal pathology in traumatic brain injury. Exp Neurol 2013;246:35–43.

28. Plog BA, Dashnaw ML, Hitomi E, et al. Biomarkers of traumatic injury are transported from brain to blood via the glymphatic system. J Neurosci 2015;35(2): 518–26.

29. Brinker T, Stopa E, Morrison J, et al. A new look at cerebrospinal fluid circulation. Fluids Barriers CNS 2014;11:10.

30. Neselius S, Zetterberg H, Blennow K, et al. Olympic boxing is associated with elevated levels of the neuronal protein tau in plasma. Brain Inj 2013;27(4):425–33.

31. Zetterberg H, Smith DH, Blennow K. Biomarkers of mild traumatic brain injury in cerebrospinal fluid and blood. Nat Rev Neurol 2013;9(4):201–10.

32. Olsson B, Zetterberg H, Hampel H, et al. Biomarker-based dissection of neurodegenerative diseases. Prog Neurobiol 2011;95(4):520–34.

33. Buki A, Povlishock JT. All roads lead to disconnection?–Traumatic axonal injury revisited. Acta Neurochir (Wien) 2006;148(2):181–93 [discussion: 193–4].

34. Siman R, McIntosh TK, Soltesz KM, et al. Proteins released from degenerating neurons are surrogate markers for acute brain damage. Neurobiol Dis 2004; 16(2):311–20.

35. Bouvier D, Duret T, Abbot M, et al. Utility of S100b serum level for the determination of concussion in male rugby players. Sports Med 2016. http://dx.doi.org/10. 1007/s40279-016-0579-9.

36. Mussack T, McIntosh TK, Soltesz KM, et al. Serum S-100B protein levels in young amateur soccer players after controlled heading and normal exercise. Eur J Med Res 2003;8(10):457–64.

37. Stalnacke BM, Tegner Y, Sojka P. Playing soccer increases serum concentration of the biochemical markers of brain damage S-100B and neuron-specific enolase in elite players: a pilot study. Brain Inj 2004;18(9):899–909.

38. Otto M, Holthusen S, Bahn E, et al. Boxing and running lead to a rise in serum levels of S-100B protein. Int J Sports Med 2000;21(8):551–5.

39. Marchi N, Bazarian J, Puvenna V, et al. Consequences of repeated blood-brain barrier disruption in football players. PLoS One 2013;8(3):e56805.

40. Schulte S, Rasmussen NN, McBeth JW, et al. Utilization of the clinical laboratory for the implementation of concussion biomarkers in collegiate football and the

necessity of personalized and predictive athlete specific reference intervals. EPMA J 2015;7:1.

41. McKee AC, Cantu RC, Nowinski CJ, et al. Chronic traumatic encephalopathy in athletes: progressive tauopathy after repetitive head injury. J Neuropathol Exp Neurol 2009;68(7):709–35.

42. Small GW, Kepe V, Siddarth P, et al. PET scanning of brain tau in retired national football league players: preliminary findings. Am J Geriatr Psychiatry 2013;21(2): 138–44.

43. Gavett BE, Stern RA, McKee AC. Chronic traumatic encephalopathy: a potential late effect. Clin Sports Med 2011;30(1):179–88, xi.

44. Omalu B, Bailes J, Hamilton RL, et al. Emerging histomorphologic phenotypes of chronic traumatic encephalopathy in American athletes. Neurosurgery 2011; 69(1):173–83 [discussion: 183].

45. Maroon JC, Winkelman R, Bost J, et al. Chronic traumatic encephalopathy in contact sports: a systematic review of all reported pathological cases. PLoS One 2015;10(2):e0117338.

46. Goldstein LE, Fisher AM, Tagge CA, et al. Chronic traumatic encephalopathy in blast-exposed military veterans and a blast neurotrauma mouse model. Sci Transl Med 2012;4(134):134ra60.

47. Shahim P, Linemann T, Inekci D, et al. Serum tau fragments predict return to play in concussed professional ice hockey players. J Neurotrauma 2016. http://dx.doi. org/10.1089/neu.2014.3741.

48. Gill J, Merchant-Borna K, Jeromin A, et al. Acute plasma tau relates to prolonged return to play after concussion. J Neurotrauma 2017;88(6):595–602.

49. Olivera A, Lejbman N, Jeromin A, et al. Peripheral total tau in military personnel who sustain traumatic brain injuries during deployment. JAMA Neurol 2015; 72(10):1109–16.

50. Belson K. Researchers make progress toward identifying C.T.E. in the living. New York Times 2016. Available at: http://www.nytimes.com/2016/09/27/sports/football/ cte-concussions-diagnose-in-living.html?_r=0. Accessed October 4, 2016.

51. PRNewswire, Abbott Joins forces with U.S. Department of Defense to develop portable blood tests for evaluating concussions. 2014. Available at: http:// abbott.mediaroom.com/2014-08-18-Abbott-Joins-Forces-with-U-S-Department- of-Defense-to-Develop-Portable-Blood-Tests-for-Evaluating-Concussions. Accessed October 7, 2016.

52. TBI, D.C.o.E.f.P.H., Portable field-based devices for the early diagnosis of mild TBI. 2010. Available at: http://www.dcoe.mil/content/navigation/documents/Portable% 20Field-Based%20Devices%20for%20the%20Early%20Diagnosis%20of%20mTBI. pdf. Accessed October 7, 2016.

53. Stalnacke BM, Ohlsson A, Tegner Y, et al. Serum concentrations of two biochemical markers of brain tissue damage S-100B and neurone specific enolase are increased in elite female soccer players after a competitive game. Br J Sports Med 2006;40(4):313–6.

54. Dietrich MO, Tort AB, Schaf DV, et al. Increase in serum S100B protein level after a swimming race. Can J Appl Physiol 2003;28(5):710–6.

55. Watson P, Black KE, Clark SC, et al. Exercise in the heat: effect of fluid ingestion on blood-brain barrier permeability. Med Sci Sports Exerc 2006;38(12):2118–24.

56. Hasselblatt M, Mooren FC, von Ahsen N, et al. Serum S100beta increases in marathon runners reflect extracranial release rather than glial damage. Neurology 2004;62(9):1634–6.

57. Knaepen K, Goekint M, Heyman EM, et al. Neuroplasticity - exercise-induced response of peripheral brain-derived neurotrophic factor: a systematic review of experimental studies in human subjects. Sports Med 2010;40(9):765–801.
58. Ding Q, Vaynman S, Souda P, et al. Exercise affects energy metabolism and neural plasticity-related proteins in the hippocampus as revealed by proteomic analysis. Eur J Neurosci 2006;24(5):1265–76.
59. Saur L, Baptista PP, de Senna PN, et al. Physical exercise increases GFAP expression and induces morphological changes in hippocampal astrocytes. Brain Struct Funct 2014;219(1):293–302.
60. Schulte S, Schiffer T, Sperlich B, et al. The impact of increased blood lactate on serum S100B and prolactin concentrations in male adult athletes. Eur J Appl Physiol 2013;113(3):811–7.
61. Spiropoulos A, Goussetis E, Margeli A, et al. Effect of inflammation induced by prolonged exercise on circulating erythroid progenitors and markers of erythropoiesis. Clin Chem Lab Med 2010;48(2):199–203.
62. Michetti F, Bruschettini M, Frigiola A, et al. Saliva S100B in professional sportsmen: high levels at resting conditions and increased after vigorous physical activity. Clin Biochem 2011;44(2–3):245–7.
63. Sharma HS, Cervos-Navarro J, Dey PK. Increased blood-brain barrier permeability following acute short-term swimming exercise in conscious normotensive young rats. Neurosci Res 1991;10(3):211–21.
64. Watson P, Shirreffs SM, Maughan RJ. Blood-brain barrier integrity may be threatened by exercise in a warm environment. Am J Physiol Regul Integr Comp Physiol 2005;288(6):R1689–94.
65. Koh SX, Lee JK. S100B as a marker for brain damage and blood-brain barrier disruption following exercise. Sports Med 2014;44(3):369–85.
66. Nierwińska KM, Malecka E, Chalimoniuk M, et al. Blood-brain barrier and exercise – a short review. J Hum Kinet 2008;19:83–92.
67. Savola O, Pyhtinen J, Leino TK, et al. Effects of head and extracranial injuries on serum protein S100B levels in trauma patients. J Trauma 2004;56(6):1229–34.
68. Pham N, Fazio V, Cucullo L, et al. Extracranial sources of S100B do not affect serum levels. PLoS One 2010;5(9):e12691.
69. Bazarian JJ, Blyth BJ, He H, et al. Classification accuracy of serum ApoA-I and S100B for the diagnosis of mild TBI and prediction of abnormal initial head CT scan. J Neurotrauma 2013. http://dx.doi.org/10.1089/neu.2013.2853.

Neuropsychological Screening of Sport-Related Concussion

Michael A. McCrea, PhD[a],*, Breton Asken, MS, ATC[b],
Lindsay D. Nelson, PhD[a]

KEYWORDS

- Concussion • Mild traumatic brain injury • Neuropsychological testing
- Sports injuries

KEY POINTS

- Neuropsychological assessment is a key component of the recommended multidimensional approach to evaluating athletes affected by sport-related concussion (SRC).
- There is not a "one-size-fits-all" solution to neuropsychological assessment of SRC; the scope of evaluation should be customized to the clinical setting and intended purpose.
- Neurocognitive testing should not be used as the sole basis for diagnosing concussion or determining when an athlete is fit for return to play after injury.
- Neurocognitive testing should be considered as 1 component of the multidimensional approach to concussion assessment.

INTRODUCTION

International consensus guidelines recommend a multidimensional approach to the assessment of sport-related concussion (SRC).[1–4] This framework is based on the theory that reliance on a single test or multiple measures in a single assessment domain will be less accurate than a multimodal assessment. At a minimum, this model integrates formal evaluation of injury signs and symptoms, neurologic status, postural stability, and neurocognitive functioning (**Fig. 1**). Over the past 30 years, neuropsychological assessment has been recognized as an important component in the multidimensional approach to evaluation of athletes affected by SRC.[5–7] The neuropsychological assessment typically involves multiple features, including survey of the somatic, cognitive, and emotional symptoms common after SRC, as well as formal

[a] Department of Neurosurgery, Medical College of Wisconsin, 8701 Watertown Plank Road, Milwaukee, WI 53226, USA; [b] Department of Clinical and Health Psychology, University of Florida, 1225 Center Drive, Room 3151, Gainesville, FL 32611, USA
* Corresponding author.
E-mail address: mmccrea@mcw.edu

Neurol Clin 35 (2017) 487–500
http://dx.doi.org/10.1016/j.ncl.2017.03.005
0733-8619/17/© 2017 Elsevier Inc. All rights reserved.

neurologic.theclinics.com

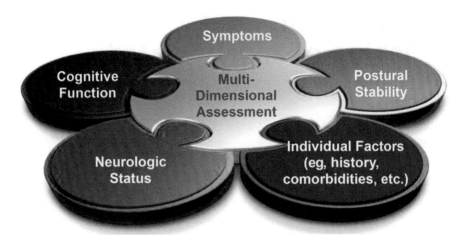

Fig. 1. Multidimensional approach to the assessment of sport-related concussion.

neurocognitive testing, which may be done using brief screening measures during the acute phase or more comprehensive neurocognitive tests in the clinic setting.

Self-report symptom checklists are a simple and convenient way to screen for common concussion symptoms, but their reliability and sensitivity can be limited because athletes may fail to recognize these symptoms, may be motivated to underreport symptoms to return to play more promptly, or they may report nonspecific symptoms for reasons other than concussion.[8,9] In addition to symptom assessment, objective, standardized measurement of cognitive functioning can be valuable for evaluating concussed athletes and informing return to play decisions. Among the major reasons for ascertaining whether athletes are clinically recovered before returning to competition is that repeat injuries seem to be most likely while athletes are early in their recoveries.[10]

Traditional approaches to more formal neuropsychological testing have targeted those domains of cognitive function most susceptible to change after concussion, often characterized by deficits in memory, attention, concentration, cognitive reaction time, cognitive processing speed, and executive cognitive functions.[11,12] The original neurocognitive testing movement focused largely on creating abbreviated batteries based on the existing literature using tests that demonstrated adequate reliability and validity for the assessment of traumatic brain injury.[13,14] A tiered set of brief test batteries emerged, ranging from neurocognitive screening tools fit for use on the sports sideline to more comprehensive testing protocols for the clinic setting. Over the last 10 to 15 years, computerized neurocognitive testing (CNT) has become especially popular in the sports medicine community.[15–17] There are now several CNT batteries commercially available and commonly used in the assessment of athletes with SRC.

This review provides a brief overview on the role of the neuropsychologist and neurocognitive assessment of SRC, with a particular focus on brief cognitive screening tools, traditional neuropsychological testing, and newer computerized neurocognitive assessment tools.

KEY ROLE OF THE NEUROPSYCHOLOGIST

Neuropsychologists have specialty training in the assessment of cognitive, behavioral, and emotional sequelae of traumatic brain injury and concussion, including SRC.[18]

Barth and colleagues[19] first introduced the use of neuropsychological tests to monitor the acute effects of SRC and recovery in collegiate athletes in the 1980s. Since the introduction of this movement, neuropsychologists have become an essential resource in the assessment and treatment of SRC.[20] As described by Barth and colleagues[21]:

> Clinical neuropsychologists use this knowledge in the assessment, diagnosis, treatment, and/or rehabilitation of patients across the lifespan with neurological, medical, neurodevelopmental and psychiatric conditions, as well as other cognitive and learning disorders. The clinical neuropsychologist uses psychological, neurological, cognitive, behavioral, and physiological principles, techniques, and tests to evaluate patients' neurocognitive, behavioral, and emotional strengths and weaknesses and their relationship to normal and abnormal nervous system functioning. (p. 16)

Neuropsychologists are also well-qualified to assess for preexisting factors, such as attention deficit hyperactivity disorder, learning disability, or other comorbidities that may affect cognitive test performance and complicate interpretation of cognitive test data, both at baseline and after concussion.

In addition to cognitive disturbance, individuals with SRC can present with psychological and neurobehavioral symptoms, such as depression, fear, anxiety, impulsivity, and other changes.[22] Athletes have been documented to respond differently to their injury than would nonathletes and can have difficulty coping with restriction in activity after SRC and other lifestyle changes during recovery.[23] Furthermore, there is a correlation between the presence of mood symptoms and recovery duration.[24–26] Neuropsychologists are highly trained in the assessment of these emotional factors that may be impacting cognitive functioning and injury recovery, and they are able to make appropriate recommendations for the treatment of mood symptoms if deemed necessary. This is often essential given the consistency with which data indicates strong associations between preexisting or cooccurring psychiatric symptoms and more complicated SRC recovery.[27–30]

Neuropsychologists have played an important role in the development of national and international consensus guidelines for assessment of SRC.[1] The American Academy of Neurology[4] and the American Medical Society for Sports Medicine[3] cite the usefulness of neuropsychological testing in identifying the presence of concussion and concluded that neuropsychological testing may be especially helpful in informing return to play decisions in high-risk athletes with prior concussion. In line with these views, professional organizations such as the National Football League, Major League Baseball, National Hockey League, and Major League Soccer all include neuropsychological assessment in their concussion management protocols.

The role of the neuropsychologist is also widely recognized in public policy and legislation around recommended best practice for the evaluation and management of SRC. Several states have enacted legislation mandating that student athletes with SRC be removed from play until cleared by a health care provider, a guideline that now has growing empirical support supplementing expert consensus opinion.[31,32] It is the official position of the main governing bodies in neuropsychology, the American Academy of Clinical Neuropsychology, the American Board of Neuropsychology, the Society for Clinical Neuropsychology of the American Psychological Association, and the National Academy of Neuropsychology, that neuropsychologists be included among the health care professionals authorized to participate in SRC evaluation and management.[18]

Conventional Approaches to Neurocognitive Testing

For decades, neuropsychologists have used traditional "paper and pencil" testing methods in the assessment of patients affected by traumatic brain injury of all levels of severity. Given their usefulness in measuring functions affected by acute head injury (eg, new learning and memory, attention, processing speed, and executive functioning), many of those measures were adapted for assessment of athletes with SRC. Most of these measures have demonstrated acceptable psychometric properties and are at least moderately sensitive to acute SRC.[33] Traditional measures also served as validation tools for more modernly developed CNTs. Several sporting organizations previously used either "fixed batteries" or "flexible batteries," allowing the neuropsychologist latitude for developing an individualized approach to athlete assessment,[14] particularly in the postinjury setting. This testing format has a number of advantages over computerized testing. One-on-one testing may maximize participant performance (eg, clinicians can respond to participants' needs for breaks or provide instructional clarification), allows for incorporation of behavioral observations and qualitative interpretation of individual-specific test strategies, and provides the examiner opportunities for expanding or reducing the test battery in a way that most efficiently and comprehensively assesses the patient's cognition. A negative attribute of traditional neuropsychological testing, however, is the amount of time and expertise needed to test athletes.[34,35] This limitation was the impetus for development of computerized test batteries.

Computerized Neurocognitive Testing

Several companies have devised CNTs for SRC assessment because performing a traditional neuropsychological assessment on large groups of athletes in a timely manner is not feasible for neuropsychologists or adequately trained sports medicine practitioners. Commercially available CNTs in the United States include ANAM (Automated Neuropsychological Assessment Metrics), Cogstate (Axon Sports), Concussion Vital Signs, and ImPACT (Immediate Postconcussion and Cognitive Testing Test Battery), with ImPACT being the most widely used.[15,16] Since their appearance in the 1990s, CNTs have become considerably more popular with sports medicine professionals, such as athletic trainers, owing to their ease of administration (eg, multiple athletes can be baseline tested simultaneously) and transportability (with easy access through the Internet or computer hard drive). Other purported advantages of CNTs over traditional paper and pencil neuropsychological tests include the availability of alternate forms (to reduce practice effects), ability to administer and interpret tests in the absence of neuropsychologists, maximally standardized test administration, precise quantification of reaction time, and availability of centralized data repositories.[36,37] Although strongly discouraged, nonneuropsychologists often assume the role of interpreting CNTs, making them more appealing in many sports medicine settings.[15]

There can be disadvantages inherent to cognitive assessment via CNT.[38] For example, environmental distractions (especially when testing several athletes at once in the same room), difficulty understanding test instructions, and computer issues may introduce error into the measurement of cognitive functioning and result in a higher number of invalid test results[39] or cognitive profiles unrepresentative of the athlete's true ability. Another criticism of CNTs is that studies of reliability and validity of these measures have been highly variable, with all CNTs containing some subtest and summary scores that do not meet acceptable levels of psychometric quality.[15]

A systematic review of measurement error in ImPACT, for example, concluded overall poor to moderate reliability and cautioned clinicians against relying too heavily on scores as criteria for diagnosing SRC or determining medical clearance.[40] CNTs also often lack norms corresponding with specific demographic groups and sensitivity to inadequate effort. However, it should be noted that most traditional neuropsychological measures also have psychometric limitations especially in the context of SRC assessment.[33,34] Finally, there has been concern about nonneuropsychologists, such as athletic trainers and team physicians, who are not trained in psychometrics or the nuance of cognitive functioning, interpreting CNT test data,[35] particularly in the context of athletes with comorbid medical conditions affecting neurocognitive functioning. Neuropsychologists offer expertise in evaluating test performance beyond the composite outcome scores readily available on each CNT printout. Relevant skills include consideration of psychometric issues, individual patient considerations that complicate neuropsychological assessment, and considering performance variability among individual subtests that make up composite scores for a given cognitive domain.

Another limitation of the literature on CNTs has been the lack of data directly comparing the different CNT batteries in terms of their reliability and sensitivity to SRC. We recently filled this gap with Project Head to Head, a prospective study of the psychometric properties and performance of 3 CNTs (Axon Sports, ANAM, and ImPACT) in the context of SRC assessment.[41] Overall, the findings supported earlier reviews of smaller scale studies and studies of individual CNTs.[15] In particular, these 3 CNTs showed similar and modest test–retest reliability in a healthy athlete sample (generally below levels considered acceptable for using test scores to make clinical decisions for individual patients). Furthermore, the sensitivity of the CNTs to SRC was similarly modest across batteries, with moderate to large (SRC vs control group) differences in performance observed within 24 hours of injury but minimal sensitivity to SRC at day 8 and later follow-up time points. In other words, at 1 week or more after injury, the false-positive rates of all 3 CNTs (ie, percentage of healthy, uninjured athletes classified as "impaired") was equivalent to the hit rates (ie, percentage of concussed athletes classified as "impaired"). Overall, the data implied that the degree to which CNTs help to identify clinical impairment owing to SRC is relatively modest and their peak usefulness is likely within a very acute postinjury window. The modest sensitivity of CNTs to SRC is thought to arise from a combination of the limited stability of these neurocognitive measures (and/or the cognitive constructs tapped by these measures) and the rapid natural course of clinical recovery from SRC. Although these findings do not provide strong support for the use of CNTs in the assessment of athletes with SRC, it is important to recognize that the limitations of this and other studies on SRC (eg, broad clinical definitions of SRC leading to heterogeneity within samples) could bias findings in ways that are currently difficult to pinpoint.

THE ROLE OF NEUROPSYCHOLOGY AFTER SPORT-RELATED CONCUSSION

Because recovery from SRC is complex and depends on individualized preinjury, injury-specific, and postinjury factors, there are multiple time points at which a neuropsychologist may intervene before or after injury. However, such complexity precludes a "one size fits all" method for SRC management, and practical considerations must also be made. Points when a neuropsychologist may intervene include at baseline (before the commencement of activity), immediately after injury, and in the subacute and chronic recovery phases (**Fig. 2**). The specific role of the neuropsychologist is variable with each time point, and consideration of the necessity

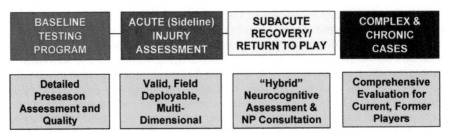

Fig. 2. Multitiered approach to neuropsychological (NP) assessment of sport-related concussion.

for explicit neuropsychological involvement is important. These assessment points are discussed in detail.

Baseline Neurocognitive Testing

Since the introduction of the Sport as Laboratory Assessment Model in the 1980s,[19] preseason baseline testing teams of athletes has become commonplace, particularly among collegiate and professional athletes. In this model, an athlete is tested before the season and retested after suspected injury to determine if he or she has experienced a statistically reliable functional decline. Basic baseline testing components include a symptom scale, cognitive assessment(s), postural stability, and increasingly common use of oculomotor and vestibular tests. Neurocognitive testing may be administered using paper and pencil, computerized, or mixed formats. The combination of CNT assessment with a brief screening tool (eg, Sports Concussion Assessment Tool, third edition [SCAT3]) is currently the default choice of many sports medicine staffs. This method theoretically has a greater sensitivity to true cognitive changes because the individual serves as his or her own performance reference, which controls for factors such as preexisting cognitive limitations like attention deficit hyperactivity disorder or learning disability. Neuropsychologists may play an important role in coordinating the baseline cognitive testing plan and interpreting the validity of baseline profiles of individuals with complicated medical histories.

Despite benefits of the use of baseline testing, there are a number of potential issues that may limit its value. For example, there are several factors that complicate the interpretation of repeated testing, including practice effects, even if alternate forms are used.[42] Measures with poor reliability have greater measurement error, which translates to (1) larger changes in cognitive scores needed for postinjury performance to be statistically different from baseline and (2) increased regression to the mean, a phenomenon in which extreme test scores 1 one test period tend to revert toward the mean of the normative group at repeat testing.[43] Poor reliability also dictates poor validity, limiting clinical confidence that the test accurately depicts cognitive functioning. Simultaneous testing of multiple athletes, perhaps one of the primary perceived benefits of CNT use, is susceptible to environmental distractors and computer problems, which may invalidate data. Logistical and motivational differences in the preinjury and postinjury setting are paramount considerations when using baseline assessments. Athletes are often tested alone after injury relative to potential complicating factors of mass baseline testing, creating difficulty in comparing scores. Arguably the most debated and concerning issue surrounding baseline testing is the contrast in performance motivation at baseline versus postinjury. At the extreme, clinical lore describes the phenomenon of "sandbagging" or intentionally performing below true abilities during preseason testing. Data suggest that successfully accomplishing sandbagging on CNTs (ie, purposefully performing poorly but still achieving a "valid" test score) is difficult[44]; however, approximately one-half of athletic trainers using ImPACT report not screening baseline assessments for validity.[45] Irrespective of concerns of sandbagging, internal motivational factors are vastly different at baseline versus after injury. Athletes often complete baseline testing in the context of broader preparticipation examinations with little (if any) incentive to extend maximum effort. It is likely that a significant number of baseline scores underestimate cognitive function owing to suboptimal, but not intentionally poor, effort. This contrasts with the postinjury test setting, where both internal and external motivational factors are readily apparent and will induce maximum effort. As such, accurately interpreting cognitive changes from baseline necessitates involvement from neuropsychologists trained in evaluating performance within the context of these competing factors.

Given some of the complicating factors in interpreting change from baseline performance, methods have been proposed to reduce some individual and measurement error. For example, 2 baseline assessments can be collected with the latter serving as a "true" baseline to reduce the influence of practice effects.[43] This approach is highly impractical, however, in most settings and rarely, if ever, used. Statistical methods exist for calculating change that statistically account for measurement error and regression to the mean,[46,47] and multiple regression formulas predicting postinjury performance may also be helpful in accounting for individual variables such as age, education, socioeconomic status, and history of prior head injury.[48] CNTs often use reliable change indices based on test–retest performance for the algorithm underlying determination of clinically and statistically relevant changes in cognitive scores.[49] But, despite their apparent sophistication, the potential sensitivity of reliable change indices is nevertheless limited by suboptimal stability of individual test scores on CNTs.[41]

In contrast with baseline testing, another method of determining cognitive impairment after SRC is the use of normative data, as is common practice in the field of neuropsychology at large. Using this approach, clinicians describe test performance in reference to a nonclinical sample of individuals who completed the test and established the normative distribution of scores. Commonly used normative reference groups include age-, sex-, race/ethnicity-, and/or education-matched groups. However, in SRC management, normative reference groups are typically limited to age- and sex-matched performance distributions. These distributions determine the patient's "expected" level of functioning. Then, test scores that fall statistically below one's expected functioning (often operationalized as 1 to 2 standard deviations below the normative mean) are examined in more detail. When using normative comparisons, input from neuropsychologists is essential for considering a patient's history, including medical, psychological, psychosocial, developmental, and educational factors, and determining if a decrease from estimated premorbid function has occurred. A well-trained neuropsychologist looks for patterns in test data indicative of dysfunction in distinct neural circuits and does not overinterpret individual impaired scores in isolation, because most individuals who complete a comprehensive neuropsychological examination will obtain at least 1 low score, with the likelihood of this occurring increasing with the number of tests given.[50] Additionally, neuropsychologists can examine the appropriateness of the normative reference group relative to the individual being tested and decide whether using a given normative distribution is sensible (eg, scores from a patient within a unique demographic category compared with a normative sample with no demographically similar representatives).

One criticism of using norm-based methods is illustrated in the work of Schatz and Robertshaw,[51] who demonstrated that this method may lead to false-positive errors in individuals whose normal baseline cognitive functioning is below average and to greater false-negative errors in above-average athletes. Regardless of the normative comparison limitations, it has been argued that if using normative data is as effective as baseline testing, the time, financial, and interpretative complications that come with baseline testing could be avoided. However, few studies have been conducted to compare the ability of these 2 methods to sensitively and specifically detect the cognitive effects of SRC. There are mixed findings from the studies that have examined this, with some indicating application of normative cut scores to postinjury scores produces comparable sensitivity to baseline-adjusted methods,[52,53] whereas others suggest slightly increased diagnostic accuracy for some individuals when baseline information is available.[54] This information, in addition to the findings of Schatz and Robertshaw, indicate that baseline testing may not be necessary for identifying impairment unless there is reason to believe the individual falls atypically above or below the normative sample at baseline for a number of reasons (eg, intellectual giftedness, attention deficit hyperactivity disorder, a learning or developmental disorder, emotional disturbance). The unfortunate reality is that neuropsychologists are currently underused in many of the areas where they may provide incremental expertise in the baseline test setting, such as determination of test validity, appropriateness of normative reference groups, and interpreting performance within the context of both CNT psychometrics and potentially complicated individual medical histories.

Acute Postinjury Assessment

Over the past 10 years or more, several standardized tests have been developed to aid in acute concussion assessment.[55] Concussion symptom checklists systematically document the presence and severity of concussion symptoms, and provide a method for tracking changes in symptom levels via serial assessment over the course of the patient's recovery.[55] A number of these tools are available for clinical use in a variety of settings (eg, hospital emergency department, outpatient clinic, sports medicine).[56–58]

In addition, several functional tests have been validated for use in the assessment of acute concussion.[55] These measures may form a more accurate and reliable assessment than simply relying on a patient's self-reporting of symptoms. Standardized tools are intended to provide a more objective, performance-based method of detecting the acute effects of injury and determining if a patient should be removed from activity. Given the high motivation to perform well enough to return to play, lower than expected performance on these more functional measures (whether in reference to baseline or normative scores) should significantly increase clinical suspicion of neurologic dysfunction. These tests provide important data on symptoms and functional impairments that clinicians can incorporate into their diagnostic formulation, but should not solely be used to diagnose concussion or drive clinical decision making, because even acute concussion-like signs and symptoms are nonspecific to SRC (eg, similar effects of dehydration, excessive fatigue, exertional headache). The specific tests selected to form the multidimensional assessment approach not only need to be reliable and valid, but also may vary depending on the situational constraints of the clinical environment, population, and the experience of the assessor. Considering mechanisms preceding potential SRC will also aid in estimating to what degree observed signs or symptoms are a consequence of recent brain injury or longstanding (see **Fig. 1**).

In the setting of SRC, the SCAT3 from the fourth Consensus Statement on Concussion in Sport[1] provides a multimodal assessment model that integrates several assessments recommended by the American Academy of Neurology into a singular assessment package.[1,4] The SCAT3 has a graded symptom checklist, the Standardized Assessment of Concussion, and a modified version of the Balance Error Scoring System all embedded in a unified, multidimensional assessment tool appropriate for use in a competitive sporting environment, such as a sideline or locker room. The individual components of the SCAT3 (symptom checklist, Standardized Assessment of Concussion, Balance Error Scoring System) have all been well-validated in the acute assessment of athletes affected by sports concussion, but further research is required to determine the overall usefulness of the integrated SCAT3.[55,59]

A critical review of the literature on the effectiveness of sideline measures[55] illustrated that clinical sequelae of concussion vary across individuals and therefore are best assessed using a multifactorial approach such as that used by the SCAT3. A critically important note regarding the sideline assessment of SRC is that these measures can be adequately administered and interpreted by sports medicine clinicians, such as certified athletic trainers, and the role of the neuropsychologist in the acute recognition and diagnosis of SRC is rather limited. Neuropsychologists rarely, if ever, develop the sorts of relationships with athletes commonly achieved by athletic trainers and team physicians. Athletes will likely be more comfortable and trusting of their familiar sports medicine clinicians, and neuropsychologists must understand and appreciate the limitations of their contributions in this specific setting.

Subacute and Chronic Assessment

As time progresses from the point of SRC diagnosis, the potential role and importance of the neuropsychologist increases. Although sideline measures are very useful for early diagnosis and subsequent tracking of changes in symptoms, cognition, and balance in the first few days after SRC, their brevity results in more psychometric limitations than longer tests (eg, restricted range of scores on the Standardized Assessment of Concussion, which will limit its maximal reliability and validity). However, the typical athlete experiences symptom resolution and completes a graduated return to athletic activity within 2 weeks after injury. The SRC signs and symptoms often follow an uncomplicated trajectory of daily improvement when appropriately managed with supervised return to physical and cognitive activity. In cases of "typical" SRC, the role of the neuropsychologist is once again limited and injury management is appropriately overseen by certified athletic trainers and team physicians. CNTs are often used in these cases to determine readiness for return to participation (based on performance relative to norms or baseline), and the neuropsychologist may assist in the interpretation of unclear test results or patients with complicated medical histories. Notably, there is debate over the most beneficial timing of CNT administration, because some clinicians prefer CNTs as a serial tool for diagnosis and tracking cognition throughout the recovery process, whereas others restrict use to a "final clearance" mechanism. As noted, using CNTs outside of the acute injury window may limit their sensitivity and specificity to SRC effects, and a neuropsychologist could provide important insight to interpreting performance amid these psychometric limitations. Whatever the preferred strategy, inappropriate or unnecessary direct involvement of the neuropsychologist may introduce iatrogenic sources of concern on the part of the athlete, which could delay symptom resolution owing to disproportionate focus and worry relative to the severity of his or her injury. Conversely, neuropsychologists become supremely important in the context of atypical or unexpected recovery trajectories.

Athletes experiencing prolonged symptomatology after SRC (ie, the elusively defined "postconcussion syndrome") represent a heterogeneous and complicated patient population for both sports medicine clinicians and neuropsychologists alike. This "miserable minority" includes an array of athletes who have returned to baseline or normative expectations on functional testing but continue reporting symptoms, athletes who report being asymptomatic but continually fail to achieve adequate performance on functional tests, or both report symptoms and exhibit poor performance on neurocognitive testing. When the symptoms-only patient presents, a neuropsychology referral can be beneficial for refining etiologic attribution of symptoms. Neuropsychologists can assess for and will give due consideration to multifactorial influences, such as preexisting neurodevelopmental disorders, psychiatric symptoms, and/or a predisposition to maladaptive adjustment after a stressful event such as an SRC that potentially removes an athlete from sport and academic participation for an extended time. Some athletes may not have identifiable preinjury risk factors but develop difficulties, for example, with anxiety, depression, or sleep quality after their injury, which perpetuate and/or exacerbate SRC symptomatology. Determining the "chicken and the egg" in these scenarios becomes increasingly challenging over time. Regardless, such ancillary interactions are important targets for treatment in cases of prolonged recovery. Prolonged symptomatology should also be considered within the broader understanding of base rates and nonspecificity of postconcussive symptoms. The possibility of a "good old days" bias, wherein patients incorrectly assume any and all current symptoms are directly related to their SRC despite their nonspecificity, should also be considered in this context.[60]

In instances where an athlete reports being asymptomatic but fails to return to baseline or normative standards on CNT performance, more comprehensive neuropsychological testing (eg, traditional assessments) may be warranted to define more conclusively the source of underlying impairment and better understand the patient's strengths and weaknesses across a broad range of neurocognitive domains. Comprehensive neuropsychological evaluations are rarely indicated but are occasionally invaluable for either identifying lingering problems or providing reassurance of cognitive normalcy to the patient. Additionally, neuropsychologists working in athletics should become intimately familiar with their team(s)' chosen CNT so score interpretation can go beyond the composite values, which frequently mask the finer details of underlying weaknesses. The competent neuropsychologist investigates multiple potential sources of cognitive dysfunction and determines whether poor performance is indeed the direct result of residual organic brain damage suffered during the SRC. The "neurobiopsychosocial" model proposed by McCrea and coworkers[61] provides a framework for better understanding prolonged recovery and also helps clinicians to understand weighing the risks and rewards of continued removal from athletic and/or academic involvement. Importantly, neuropsychologists and sports medicine clinicians must be aware that current standard of care assessments measure clinical recovery only and may not accurately measure the presumably extended physiologic disturbances. Ultimately, the complicated SRC patient benefits most from a multidisciplinary management approach including the sports medicine staff, neuropsychologist, neurologist, and physical/vestibular therapist, with degree of involvement depending on subjective and objective symptom profiles.

SUMMARY

Neuropsychologists are a valuable part of sports medicine teams for the evaluation and management of SRC across many stages of injury, including baseline assessment of at-risk athletes, acute and subacute evaluation, tracking recovery to inform return to play decisions, and treatment of individuals who experience prolonged recovery. There is not a "one size fits all" solution to neurocognitive assessment of SRC. Rather, a multitiered model is recommended, ranging from brief cognitive screening tools for the acute evaluation, intermediate conventional and computerized batteries for subacute evaluation and determining fitness for return to activity, and more comprehensive approaches for evaluation of athletes with complicated or persistent symptoms after SRC. Most important, neurocognitive testing should be viewed as 1 component of the multidimensional approach to concussion assessment, and should not be used as the sole basis for diagnosing concussion or determining when an athlete is fit for return to play after injury. Practitioners involved in neurocognitive test administration and interpretation should be aware of the myriad sources of influence on neurocognitive test performance and the psychometric issues important to appropriately interpret test data for individual cases. Going forward, there is a need for further refinement of neurocognitive assessment measures to maximize their contribution to the overall evaluation and management of athletes affected by SRC.

REFERENCES

1. McCrory P, Meeuwisse WH, Aubry M, et al. Consensus statement on concussion in sport: the 4th International Conference on Concussion in Sport held in Zurich, November 2012. Br J Sports Med 2013;47(5):250–8.
2. Broglio SP, Cantu RC, Gioia GA, et al. National Athletic Trainers' Association position statement: management of sport concussion. J Athl Train 2014;49(2): 245–65.
3. Harmon KG, Drezner JA, Gammons M, et al. American Medical Society for Sports Medicine position statement: concussion in sport. Br J Sports Med 2013;47(1): 15–26.
4. Giza CC, Kutcher JS, Ashwal S, et al. Summary of evidence-based guideline update: evaluation and management of concussion in sports: report of the Guideline Development Subcommittee of the American Academy of Neurology. Neurology 2013;80(24):2250–7.
5. McCrory P, Meeuwisse W, Aubry M, et al. Consensus statement on concussion in sport–the 4th International Conference on Concussion in Sport held in Zurich, November 2012. Clin J Sport Med 2013;23(2):89–117.
6. Echemendia RJ, Iverson GL, McCrea M, et al. Advances in neuropsychological assessment of sport-related concussion. Br J Sports Med 2013;47:294–8.
7. Moser RS, Iverson GL, Echemendia RJ, et al. Neuropsychological evaluation in the diagnosis and management of sports-related concussion. Arch Clin Neuropsychol 2007;22(8):909–16.
8. McCrea M, Hammeke T, Olsen G, et al. Unreported concussion in high school football players: implications for prevention. Clin J Sport Med 2004;14(1):13–7.
9. Iverson GL, Silverberg ND, Mannix R, et al. Factors associated with concussion-like symptom reporting in high school athletes. JAMA Pediatr 2015;169(12): 1132–40.
10. Guskiewicz KM, McCrea M, Marshall SW, et al. Cumulative effects associated with recurrent concussion in collegiate football players: the NCAA Concussion Study. JAMA 2003;290(19):2549–55.
11. Kelly JP, Rosenberg JH. Diagnosis and management of concussion in sports. Neurology 1997;48(3):575–80.

12. McCrea M, Kelly JP, Randolph C, et al. Immediate neurocognitive effects of concussion. Neurosurgery 2002;50(5):1032–40 [discussion: 1040–2].
13. Barth JT, Harvey DJ, Freeman JR, et al. Sport as a laboratory assessment model. In: Webbe F, editor. The handbook of sport neuropsychology. New York: Springer; 2010. p. 75–89.
14. Lovell MR, Collins MW. Neuropsychological assessment of the college football player. J Head Trauma Rehabil 1998;13(2):9–26.
15. Resch JE, McCrea MA, Cullum CM. Computerized neurocognitive testing in the management of sport-related concussion: an update. Neuropsychol Rev 2013; 23(4):335–49.
16. Meehan WP 3rd, d'Hemecourt P, Collins CL, et al. Computerized neurocognitive testing for the management of sport-related concussions. Pediatrics 2012;129(1): 38–44.
17. Covassin T, Elbin R 3rd, Stiller-Ostrowski JL. Current sport-related concussion teaching and clinical practices of sports medicine professionals. J Athl Train 2009;44:400–4.
18. Echemendia RJ, Iverson GL, McCrea M, et al. Role of neuropsychologists in the evaluation and management of sport-related concussion: an inter-organization position statement. Clin Neuropsychol 2011;25(8):1289–94.
19. Barth JT, Alves WM, Macciocchi SN, et al. Mild head injury in sports: neuropsychological sequelae and recovery of function. In: Levin H, Eisenberg J, Benton A, editors. Mild head injury. New York: Oxford University Press; 1989. p. 257–75.
20. Webbe FM, Zimmer A. History of neuropsychological study of sport-related concussion. Brain Inj 2015;29(2):129–38.
21. Barth JT, Pliskin N, Axelrod B, et al. Introduction to the NAN 2001 definition of a clinical neuropsychologist. NAN Policy and Planning Committee. Arch Clin Neuropsychol 2003;18(5):551–5.
22. Putukian M, Echemendia RJ. Psychological aspects of serious head injury in the competitive athlete. Clin Sports Med 2003;22(3):617–30, xi.
23. Smith AM, Scott SG, Wiese DM. The psychological effects of sports injuries. Coping. Sports Med 1990;9(6):352–69.
24. Mooney G, Speed J, Sheppard S. Factors related to recovery after mild traumatic brain injury. Brain Inj 2005;19(12):975–87.
25. Satz P, Forney DL, Zaucha K, et al. Depression, cognition, and functional correlates of recovery outcome after traumatic brain injury. Brain Inj 1998;12(7): 537–53.
26. Ponsford J, Cameron P, Fitzgerald M, et al. Predictors of postconcussive symptoms 3 months after mild traumatic brain injury. Neuropsychology 2012;26(3): 304–13.
27. Jotwani V, Harmon KG. Postconcussion syndrome in athletes. Curr Sports Med Rep 2010;9(1):21–6.
28. Lange RT, Iverson GL, Rose A. Depression strongly influences postconcussion symptom reporting following mild traumatic brain injury. J Head Trauma Rehabil 2011;26(2):127–37.
29. Nelson LD, Tarima S, LaRoche AA, et al. Preinjury somatization symptoms contribute to clinical recovery after sport-related concussion. Neurology 2016; 86(20):1856–63.
30. Waljas M, Iverson GL, Lange RT, et al. A prospective biopsychosocial study of the persistent post-concussion symptoms following mild traumatic brain injury. J Neurotrauma 2015;32:534–47.

31. Asken BM, McCrea MA, Clugston JR, et al. "Playing through it": delayed reporting and removal from athletic activity after concussion predicts prolonged recovery. J Athl Train 2016;51(4):329–35.

32. Elbin R, Sufrinko A, Schatz P, et al. Removal from play after concussion and recovery time. Pediatrics 2016;138(3):e20160910.

33. Randolph C, McCrea M, Barr WB. Is neuropsychological testing useful in the management of sport-related concussion? J Athl Train 2005;40(3):139–52.

34. Iverson GL, Schatz P. Advanced topics in neuropsychological assessment following sport-related concussion. Brain Inj 2015;29(2):263–75.

35. Harmon KG, Drezner J, Gammons M, et al. American Medical Society for Sports Medicine position statement: concussion in sport. Clin J Sport Med 2013;23(1): 1–18.

36. Collie A, Darby D, Maruff P. Computerised cognitive assessment of athletes with sports related head injury. Br J Sports Med 2001;35(5):297–302.

37. Rahman-Filipiak AAM, Woodward JL. Administration and environment considerations in computer-based sports-concussion assessment. Neuropsychol Rev 2014;23:314–34.

38. Bauer RM, Iverson GL, Cernich AN, et al. Computerized neuropsychological assessment devices: joint position paper of the American Academy of Clinical Neuropsychology and the National Academy of Neuropsychology. Arch Clin Neuropsychol 2012;27(3):362–73.

39. Schatz P, Neidzwski K, Moser RS, et al. Relationship between subjective test feedback provided by high-school athletes during computer-based assessment of baseline cognitive functioning and self-reported symptoms. Arch Clin Neuropsychol 2010;25(4):285–92.

40. Alsalaheen B, Stockdale K, Pechumer D, et al. Measurement error in the Immediate Postconcussion Assessment and Cognitive Testing (ImPACT): systematic review. J Head Trauma Rehabil 2016;31(4):242–51.

41. Nelson LD, LaRoche AA, Pfaller AY, et al. Prospective, head-to-head study of three computerized neurocognitive assessment tools (CNTs): reliability and validity for the assessment of sport-related concussion. J Int Neuropsychol Soc 2016; 22(1):24–37.

42. Benedict RH, Zgaljardic DJ. Practice effects during repeated administrations of memory tests with and without alternate forms. J Clin Exp Neuropsychol 1998; 20(3):339–52.

43. Collie A, Maruff P, Makdissi M, et al. Statistical procedures for determining the extent of cognitive change following concussion. Br J Sports Med 2004;38(3): 273–8.

44. Schatz P, Glatts C. "Sandbagging" baseline test performance on ImPACT, without detection, is more difficult than it appears. Arch Clin Neuropsychol 2013;28(3): 236–44.

45. Covassin T, Elbin RJ 3rd, Stiller-Ostrowski JL, et al. Immediate post-concussion assessment and cognitive testing (ImPACT) practices of sports medicine professionals. J Athl Train 2009;44(6):639–44.

46. Jacobson NS, Truax P. Clinical significance: a statistical approach to defining meaningful change in psychotherapy research. J Consult Clin Psychol 1991; 59(1):12–9.

47. Chelune GJ, Naugle RI, Luders H, et al. Individual change after epilepsy surgery: practice effects and base-rate information. Neuropsychology 1993;7(1):41–52.

48. Temkin NR, Heaton RK, Grant I, et al. Detecting significant change in neuropsychological test performance: a comparison of four models. J Int Neuropsychol Soc 1999;5(4):357–69.

49. Iverson GL, Lovell MR, Collins MW. Interpreting change on ImPACT following sport concussion. Clin Neuropsychol 2003;17(4):460–7.

50. Schretlen DJ, Testa SM, Winicki JM, et al. Frequency and bases of abnormal performance by healthy adults on neuropsychological testing. J Int Neuropsychol Soc 2008;14(3):436–45.

51. Schatz P, Robertshaw S. Comparing post-concussive neurocognitive test data to normative data presents risks for under-classifying "above average" athletes. Arch Clin Neuropsychol 2014;29(7):625–32.

52. Echemendia RJ, Bruce JM, Bailey CM, et al. The utility of post-concussion neuropsychological data in identifying cognitive change following sports-related MTBI in the absence of baseline data. Clin Neuropsychol 2012;26(7):1077–91.

53. Schmidt JD, Register-Mihalik JK, Mihalik JP, et al. Identifying impairments after concussion: normative data versus individualized baselines. Med Sci Sports Exerc 2012;44(9):1621–8.

54. Roebuck-Spencer TM, Vincent AS, Schlegel RE, et al. Evidence for added value of baseline testing in computer-based cognitive assessment. J Athl Train 2013; 48(4):499–505.

55. McCrea M, Iverson GL, Echemendia RJ, et al. Day of injury assessment of sport-related concussion. Br J Sports Med 2013;47(5):272–84.

56. Lovell MR, Iverson GL, Collins MW, et al. Measurement of symptoms following sports-related concussion: reliability and normative data for the post-concussion scale. Appl Neuropsychol 2006;13(3):166–74.

57. Guskiewicz KM, Register-Mihalik J, McCrory P, et al. Evidence-based approach to revising the SCAT2: introducing the SCAT3. Br J Sports Med 2013;47(5): 289–93.

58. Eyres S, Carey A, Gilworth G, et al. Construct validity and reliability of the Rivermead post-concussion symptoms questionnaire. Clin Rehabil 2005;19(8): 878–87.

59. Chin EY, Nelson LD, Barr WB, et al. Reliability and validity of the Sport Concussion Assessment Tool–3 (SCAT3) in high school and collegiate athletes. Am J Sports Med 2016;44:2276–85.

60. Iverson GL, Lange RT, Brooks BL, et al. "Good old days" bias following mild traumatic brain injury. Clin Neuropsychol 2010;24(1):17–37.

61. McCrea M, Broshek DK, Barth JT. Sports concussion assessment and management: future research directions. Brain Inj 2015;29(2):276–82.

Sport-Related Headache

Sylvia Lucas, MD, PhD, FAHS[a],*, Heidi K. Blume, MD, MPH[b]

KEYWORDS

- Concussion • Postconcussive syndrome • Posttraumatic headache
- Sports concussion • Migraine • Tension-type headache

KEY POINTS

- Headache is the primary symptom reported after concussion.
- Cumulative incidence and prevalence of posttraumatic headache is higher in those exposed to a mild TBI than to a moderate to severe TBI.
- Migraine or probable migraine is the most common headache phenotype after any severity TBI using primary headache disorder criteria.
- In pediatric studies, female sex, higher number of postconcussive symptoms, prior concussions, adolescent age, and headache after injury may be associated with increased risk of headache and prolonged postconcussive syndrome.
- Management of PTH is empiric with no evidence-based treatment protocols. Expert opinion suggests treating PTH according to its clinical characteristics.

INTRODUCTION

Headache occurring in the setting of sports or other recreational activities may be a primary or secondary headache. Primary headache disorders, such as migraine, are clinical syndromes that have no structural, infectious, or metabolic cause, and thought to have an underlying genetic basis with various individual internal or external triggers. Secondary headaches, such as posttraumatic headache (PTH), have a temporal relationship between a causative factor, such as a traumatic brain injury (TBI), and onset of the headache. The most common headache encountered in pediatric sports is migraine triggered by dehydration, fatigue, stress, or other factors encountered by the players.[1] Exercise can also be characterized as a "trigger" for adults, although it is difficult to assign any particular physiologic stressor, such as dehydration, as a unique causative factor. This review of sport-related headache focuses on secondary headache, particularly postconcussive headache or PTH, because of the increasing

---

[a] Department of Neurological Surgery, University of Washington Medical Center, Seattle Sports Concussion Program, Harborview Medical Center, Box 359924, 325 Ninth Avenue, Seattle, WA 98104, USA; [b] Division of Child Neurology, Seattle Children's Hospital and Research Institute, University of Washington, 4800 Sand Point Way, MS: M/S MB 7.420, Seattle, WA 98105, USA
* Corresponding author.
E-mail address: lucass@uw.edu

Neurol Clin 35 (2017) 501–521
http://dx.doi.org/10.1016/j.ncl.2017.03.012

attention that has been directed toward TBI in military, professional, and school-related organizations during the last several years. Indeed, every state in the United States now has legislation passed requiring evaluation of possible concussion before an athlete can re-enter play, so knowledge of concussion and postconcussive symptoms is particularly important.[2]

Although headache is the primary symptom reported after concussion,[3] the inherent difficulty in estimating headache incidence is two-fold. The first is that this symptom may not be recognized as a unique symptom within a constellation of symptoms after injury. It may be difficult to isolate headache symptoms from others following a concussion, such as dizziness, imbalance, photophobia, and nausea. Headache may be a part of "feeling bad" or "hitting my head," without recognition of its features. Many who experience headache after brain injury only seek attention if the symptoms are prolonged or interfere with quality of life. The second difficulty with estimating headache incidence is underreporting concussion, the presumptive cause. Athletes may underreport or may not recognize the symptoms of concussion and the American Medical Society for Sports reports that 50% of concussions may go unreported.[4] Personnel associated with sports or responsible for player safety may also have a significant role in reporting concussion. If physicians are observing sports events, a higher rate of concussion is reported.[5]

Methods of obtaining data on concussion vary across ascertainment settings, such as field sidelines, outpatient clinics, or population-based surveillance studies. In surveillance studies or large population-based studies, a structured clinical interview provides the most comprehensive clinical data but is not practical. Surveys provide most data on large groups of athletes with and without physician observation during activity. However, a significant number of concussions are not reported by athletes, trainers, or coaches, and surveillance studies may be based on International Classification of Diseases codes, which may not be accurate. One study in Minnesota found that mild TBI (mTBI) codes in an emergency department (ED) setting were 98% specific and 46% sensitive for mTBI.[6]

Given these difficulties in obtaining data on concussions, the estimate of 1.6 to 3.8 million sports-related concussions per year in the United States seems likely[7] and in range of 3.2 million TBIs reported to the Centers for Disease Control and Prevention by EDs, hospitals, and other reporting agencies.[8]

Although the exact numbers of concussions are unknown, the numbers of children and adults playing organized or unorganized sports is huge. The National Council on Youth Sports estimates at least 44 million boys and girls participate in sports in this country and more than 170 million adults. There are no large prospective studies on incidence of sports-related concussion, and the risk pool may vary with the sport played and the probability of contact particularly with high speed or high impact contact.

EPIDEMIOLOGY OF POSTTRAUMATIC HEADACHE

Many studies of symptoms following brain injury have been undertaken. However, variability in case ascertainment, TBI subgroup severity, subject selection and inclusion criteria bias, and variable follow-up times make the comparison and interpretation of studies difficult. Lack of objective findings, limitations in self-reporting of symptoms, secondary gain issues, and litigation concerns often discount patient reports. Therefore, despite the prominence of headache symptoms after mTBI, some biases and design variables may underlie the historically wide range of PTH prevalence of 30% to 90%.[3,9,10]

Key epidemiologic studies from adult (civilian) and pediatric populations are listed in **Tables 1** and **2**. In the largest, prospective civilian study to date, 452 subjects admitted to inpatient rehabilitation services following a moderate to severe TBI were followed over 1 year. Most subjects were males injured in vehicle-related accidents with an average age of 44 years. Initial evaluation was performed in hospital, with telephone follow-up at 3, 6, and 12 months.[11] Of these 452 subjects, 71% reported headache during the first year. The prevalence was 46% at the initial inpatient interview, and remained high with 44% reporting headache 1 year after TBI. Most PTH developed within 3 months of injury, although 28% of headaches developed after the initial

Table 1
Recent adult civilian posttraumatic headache studies

First Author, Year, Country	Number Enrolled	Study Design	Population	Key Results
Dikmen et al,[76] 2010, US	732	Prospective case control	>16 Any TBI	Any HA the week before time period: Prevalence: 1 mo post-TBI = 55% 1 y post-TBI = 26%
Faux & Sheedy,[77] 2008, Australia	100	Prospective case control; ED	>16 moderate-severe TBI	Prevalence at time of injury = 100% At 1 mo = 30% At 3 mo = 15%
Hoffman et al,[11] 2011, US	452	Prospective in-person enrollment Telephone interview 3, 6, 12 mo	>16 moderate-severe TBI	Cumulative incidence at 1 y = 71% Prevalence baseline = 47% At 1 y = 44%
Lieba-Samal et al,[29] 2011, Austria	100	Prospective, telephone interview	Age 18–65 Excluded whiplash, MOH, pre-existing chronic PTH	Prevalence acute PTH at 7–10 d = 66% All resolved by 3 mo Migraine/probable migraine = 35%
Lucas et al,[13] 2014, US; Lucas et al,[26] 2012, US	452 212	Prospective in-person enrollment; telephone interview 3, 6, 12 mo	>16 moderate-severe TBI >16 mTBI	Moderate-severe TBI baseline migraine/ probable migraine = 52% 1 y = 54% mTBI cumulative incidence = 92% Migraine/probable migraine at 3 mo = 49% At 1 y = 49%
Stovner et al,[30] 2009, Lithuania	217	Prospective ED cohort, case control; questionnaire at 3 mo, 1 y	Age 18–60 LOC <15 min	Prevalence HA 3 mo = 66% 1 y = 65% Migraine 3 mo = 19% 1 y = 21%

Abbreviations: HA, headache; LOC, loss of consciousness; MOH, medication overuse headache.

Table 2
Epidemiology of pediatric postconcussion headache, selected studies

Authors, Year, Country	Number in Study	Study Design	Population	Key Results
Meehan et al,[17] 2010, US	544 concussed high school athletes	Retrospective review	RIO Database, 2008–2009, high school athletes	• 17% sports concussions with sx ≥1 wk, 1.5% with sx >1 mo • 94% with headache
Marar et al,[78] 2012, US	1936 concussed high school athletes	Retrospective review	RIO Database 2008–2010, high school athletes	• 40% with sx ≤3 d • 94% with headache
Chrisman et al,[18] 2013, US	1412 concussed high school athletes	Retrospective review	RIO Database 2006–2009, high school athletes	• 16% with sx >1 wk, • 1.4% with sx ≥1 mo • 96% with headache • ≥4 initial sx associated with higher risk of sx >1 wk
Mihalik et al,[20] 2013, US	296 concussed athletes	Cohort	Concussed athletes Age 12–25, enrolled by team providers	• 1 d postinjury: 18% migraine, 59% headache, 23% no headache • Posttraumatic migraine sx in first week after injury associated with prolonged recovery • Females twice more likely to report post-traumatic migraine sx than males
Kontos et al,[19] 2013, US (Pennsylvania)	138 concussed high school football players	Prospective cohort	High school football players	• In first week postconcussion: 41% migraine, 46% headache, 14% no headache • Group with migraine sx had deficits on cognitive testing and longer sx duration compared with those with headache alone and no headache
Meehan et al,[79] 2013, US (Boston, Pittsburgh)	182 patients with sports concussion		Sports concussion clinic Age 7–26	• 26% with sx >28 d • Total PCSS score associated with prolonged recovery
Eckner et al,[80] 2016, US (Michigan)	115 sports concussion 106 orthopedic	Questionnaire, prospective, in specialty sports medicine clinic	Sports medicine clinic 12–24 y	• History of migraine more common in those with sports concussion than those with orthopedic sports injury, this was not significant after controlling for past hx of concussion

Study	Sample	Design	Setting/Age	Findings
Miller et al,[81] 2016, US (Alabama)	294 concussion	Case-control study of sports-related concussion	Concussion clinic Age 4–18 y	• 36% with "delayed recovery" >28 d • Female sex, SCAT2 <80, ADHD, nonhelmeted sport were associated with symptom duration >28 d
Corbin-Berrigan & Gagnon,[82] 2016, Canada	213 concussion	Retrospective cohort design	Concussion clinic Age 5–18	• 47% prolonged recovery >28 d • PCSS score at 10 d associated with delayed recovery
Howell et al,[83] 2016, US (Boston)	318: concussion 68: 8–12 y 250: 13–18 y	Retrospective cohort	Sports concussion clinic Age 8–18	• 30% of children, 35% of teenagers with sx ≥28 d • In teenagers prolonged recovery associated with high initial somatic sx burden
Barlow et al,[21] 2010, Canada (Calgary)	670 with mTBI 171 ECI	Prospective cohort	ER/hospital 1 mo–18 y	• 58% of mTBI vs 38% of ECI sx >1 mo • 13.7 of mTBI age >6 y with sx at 3 mo vs 1% of ECI group • 58% of mTBI group with headache 1 mo postinjury • 2.3% of mTBI group had sx at 12 mo • In mTBI group, those with sx at 100 d had 40% risk of being symptomatic the next month
Kuczynski et al,[22] 2013, Canada (Calgary)	mTBI: 670 ECI: 120 TBI clinic (>3 mo of PTH): 44	Cohort and retrospective review	mTBI and ECI in ER TBI clinic Age: 6–18	• 8% of mTBI group with sx 3 mo after injury • 54% of those w headache had migraine • 75% of those with sx 6 mo postinjury and 100% with sx 12 mo postinjury report headache • Clinic group post-mTBI: 61% with daily headache, 39% with migraine, 9% chronic tension headache, primary stabbing headache, occipital neuralgia also seen • Treatment of clinic group: 64% successful treatment with medications, melatonin and amitriptyline in particular; other treatments helped some

(continued on next page)

Table 2
(continued)

Authors, Year, Country	Number in Study	Study Design	Population	Key Results
Eisenberg et al,[84] 2013, US (Boston)	280 mTBI in ER	Prospective cohort	mTBI in ER Age 11–22	• 77% sx on Day 7, 32% with sx on Day 28, 15% with sx on Day 90 • 85% with headache initially after injury • Neither migraine nor family hx of migraine associated with recovery time
Eisenberg et al,[24] 2014, US (Boston)	207–280	Prospective cohort	mTBI in ER Age 11–22	• % headache worse than baseline: Day 7, 69%; Day 28, 25%; Day 90, 5%
Kirk et al,[23] 2008, UK	117 w TBI	Cohort	TBI admitted to hospital 2003–2005 Age: 3–15 y	• 6.7% had PTH when asked 8 wk postinjury • Headache resolved in 3–27 mo, average is 13 mo
Zemek et al,[42] 2016, Canada	2584	Prospective, multicenter cohort study	mTBI in ER Age 5–17	% with sx at 28 d (PPCS): • Age: 17% of age 5–7, 26% of age 8–12, 40% age 13–18 had PPCS • Sex: 23% of males, 41% of females had PPCS, 43% of those with migraine hx had PPCS, 28% of those without migraine hx had PPCS • Developed a risk score to predict risk of PPCS: female sex, age of 13–18 y, migraine history, prior concussion with symptoms >1 wk, headache, sensitivity to noise, fatigue, answering questions slowly, and ≥4 errors on the Balance Error Scoring System tandem stance
Blume et al,[25] 2012, US Washington	mTBI: 402 OI: 122	Prospective cohort study	mTBI in ER Age 5–17	• Headache more common 3 mo postinjury for those with mTBI vs OI, 43% vs 26%, RR, 1.7 • Headache risk higher in girls (59% vs 24%; RR, 2.4) and teenagers (46% vs 25%; RR, 1.8)

Abbreviations: ADHD, attention-deficit/hyperactivity disorder; ECI, extracranial injury; hx, history; OI, orthopedic injury; PCSS, postconcussive severity scale; RR, relative risk; SCAT2, Sport Concussion Assessment Tool 2; sx, symptoms.

evaluation, occurring at 6 and even 12 months after injury. A significant number of headaches developed after the 7-day window requirement in the International Classification of the Headache Disorders (ICHD) II criteria (used for this study) defining PTH.[12]

In a subsequent study of mTBI, the same research group using similar headache assessment tools followed 212 subjects admitted to the hospital with mTBI, and other, primarily orthopedic, injuries. Within 1 week after TBI, this group was evaluated in hospital, with telephone follow-up at 3, 6, and 12 months. There was a higher cumulative incidence of headache at 91% for mTBI than for the moderate to severe study at 1 year. Prevalence of new or worse headache in this cohort was 54% within 1 week of injury, and remained high at 58% 12 months postinjury.[13] Other studies have also noted a higher prevalence of PTH after mTBI compared with more severe TBI.[9,14–16]

PREVALENCE OF HEADACHE FOLLOWING PEDIATRIC CONCUSSION

Using the RIO database of sports injuries reported by high school athletic trainers in the United States, several authors have found that headache was reported by 94% to 96% of those who reported concussion but only 17% reported any symptoms lasting longer than 1 week after concussion.[17,18] In a study of 138 concussed high school football players Kontos and colleagues[19] found that in the week after concussion 41% had symptoms of "posttraumatic migraine" (headache with nausea and either phonophobia or photophobia), 46% had headache, and 14% were headache free. In 2013 Mihalik and colleagues[20] found that of 296 concussed athletes ages 12 to 25 enrolled into the study by a team doctor or trainer, on Day 1 after concussion, 18% had migraine, 59% had headache, and 23% did not have any headache (see **Table 1**). Although only a fraction of children with mTBI evaluated in the emergency room (ER) experienced a sports-related concussion, and most children with sports concussion are not seen in the ER, we may use data from the ER evaluation of pediatric mTBI to help understand PTH following sports-related concussion. Barlow and colleagues[21] found that 58% reported new headache 1 month after injury and 7.8% had new headache 3 months after injury. PTH was present in 75% of those with any postconcussion symptoms at 6 months and 100% of those with postconcussion symptoms at 1 year after injury.[22] Kirk and colleagues[23] found that 9.4% had new or worse headache for longer than 3 months mTBI. Eisenberg and coworkers[24] found that 85% had new headache the time of injury, 69% had headache 1 week after injury, 25% had headache 4 weeks after injury, and 5% had headache 3 months after injury. Blume and colleagues[25] found that headache was more common 3 months after injury for those with mTBI than those with arm injury (43% vs 26%; relative risk, 1.7; 95% confidence interval [CI],1.2–2.3), and that headache risk following mTBI was higher for girls (59% vs 24%; relative risk, 2.4; 95% CI, 1.4–4.2) and adolescents (46% vs 25%; relative risk, 1.8; 95% CI, 1.1–3.1).

CHARACTERIZATION OF POSTTRAUMATIC HEADACHE

There is no single clinical type of PTH. Although PTH is among the most prevalent of the secondary headache disorders as currently classified in the ICHD-III:12, there are no clinical characteristics that differentiate PTH from other primary or secondary headaches. Most PTHs are indistinguishable from descriptions of primary headaches, although some are not classifiable using ICHD of primary headache disorders. Some simple differentiating features of the primary headache disorders migraine and tension-type headache (TTH) may be clinically useful and are featured in **Table 3**. The importance of headache description is not only useful for diagnosis and treatment,

Table 3
Useful criteria to differentiate common PTH types

Migraine	Tension-Type
Moderate to severe	Mild to moderate
Unilateral (60%)	Bilateral
Pulsatile, throbbing, pounding	Tight, squeezing, viselike
Worse with physical activity	Not worse with physical activity
Nausea and/or vomiting	No nausea or vomiting
Photophobia and phonophobia	Photophobia or phonophobia sometimes noted

This simplified adaptation is from the primary headache classification disorders of migraine and tension-type headache found in the International Classification of Headache Disorders, 3rd edition (beta version). Cephalalgia 2013;33(9):629–808.

but the headache qualities, such as throbbing or pulsating, are fundamental features supporting theories of headache physiology following TBI. Treatment guidance may change as characteristics of the headache change; for example, may clinicians note that while a headache may be continuous and of high intensity early after a concussion, intensity may decrease over time or the headache may become episodic. Clinically, it is important to note that there may be a headache continuum so that the value in applying primary headache features to a PTH is not to define it (eg, as a primary headache disorder with "mixed features" of migraine and TTH), but to recognize the clinical features to assist in targeting treatment.

In adult populations, some studies reported that the headaches meeting TTH criteria were the most prevalent type of PTH,[3] although in some early reports ICHD diagnostic criteria were not used. Recent studies support migraine or probable migraine as the most common PTH type. In the largest, longitudinal study of PTH to date of headache following moderate to severe brain injury, the most common PTH type was migraine or probable migraine. This headache type was found in more than 52% of those reporting headache at baseline evaluation, and in 54% of those with headache at 1 year. In individuals without a prior history of headache, migraine/probable migraine was found in 62% of those reporting headache at baseline, and in 53% at 1 year.[26]

Migraine/probable migraine was also the most common headache type in a large prospective study of headache after mTBI.[13] These two headache types were found in 49% of subjects, with headache at 3, 6, and 12 months after injury and TTH never exceeding 40% over that year. Three quarters of the study population were males injured primarily in vehicle accidents. The migraine or probable migraine headache type seen after TBI was much more frequent than would be expected for primary migraine or probable migraine in males in the general population.[27] Cervicogenic headaches made up 10% or fewer headaches that were classifiable in these studies, of interest given the high number of vehicle accidents. In a smaller series of 41 patients in whom headache classification after mTBI was reported, migraine followed by TTH were the most common headache types found.[28]

Another prospective study of 100 adults presenting to a trauma surgery department with mTBI found migraine or probable migraine to be the most common headache type, followed by TTH or probable TTH using ICHD-II criteria.[29] In prior studies[30–32] in which TTH was the most common PTH after mTBI, some potential study factors underlying differences might be that one study was based on clinical samples with a long interval between injury and clinical evaluation,[31] and another study was a retrospective chart review.[32] Some studies report more than one headache type, whereas in the two large prospective studies discussed previously,[11,13,26] only the most severe headache type that a subject reported at each time period was determined. Thus, if both a migraine and TTH were present over that year at the same time, migraine headaches would be the reported headache. Even if a TTH was present more often than a migraine type, the more severe headache would be the one reported.

Headache frequency is higher in those who have more severe PTH. Comparing civilians who had PTHs that resembled migraine or probable migraine with those with PTH that resembled TTH or cervicogenic headache, those with migraine-like headaches were most likely to describe headaches occurring several days a week or daily.[13,17] In fact, 23% of individuals sustaining moderate to severe TBI reported headache frequency of several times a week or daily at all time-points up to 1 year after TBI. Following mTBI, for those who experienced headache several times a week or daily, 62% of the headache types were migraine in this high-frequency group at 1 year.[13] In contrast, 4% to 5% of those with headache in the general population report chronic daily headache (CDH).[33] Head and neck injury accounts for approximately 15% of CDH cases.[34]

In their study and classification of headache after pediatric mTBI Kuczynski and colleagues[22] found that headache was one of the most common symptoms for those with postconcussion syndrome (PCS), because headache was present for 75% of those with symptoms at 6 months and 100% of those with symptoms 1 year after injury. This was one of the only studies to date to examine PTH treatment in pediatrics. They found that for the population of children seen in the TBI clinic with headache for greater than 3 months after injury, 61% had daily headache, 39% had migraine, 9% had chronic tension headache, but 39% of the headaches were unclassifiable. Less common headache types, such as vestibular headache, stabbing headache, and occipital neuralgia, were also seen following TBI. In a large ED cohort of children, migraine was found to be the most common headache type, reported in 55% of those children who had headache after mTBI.[22]

Rare cases of PTH in the adult population are similar to other primary headaches: cluster[35]; hemicrania continua[36]; chronic paroxysmal hemicrania[37]; and short-lasting, unilateral, neuralgiform headache attacks with conjunctival injection and tearing (SUNCT syndrome[38]).

Some PTH patterns are associated with specific craniocerebral injuries, most likely to be found following moderate to severe TBI.[39] Leakage of cerebrospinal fluid (CSF) can produce low-CSF-pressure headaches. Postcraniotomy headaches can complicate postsurgical treatment of TBI. No significant correlation has been demonstrated between acute neuroimaging abnormalities and presence or absence of PTH in a study of moderate to severe TBI over 1 year.[40]

RISK FACTORS FOR PROLONGED SYMPTOMS FOLLOWING PEDIATRIC CONCUSSION

A growing number of studies are attempting to identify factors associated with prolonged PCS so that the most vulnerable children may be assessed and treated early to mitigate disability and provide relief. Studies of sports concussion and mTBI indicate that female sex, higher number of somatic or total number of symptoms, prior concussions, adolescent age, and headache and/or migraine after injury may be associated with increased risk of headache and prolonged PCS.[41] The largest study to date is a Canadian multicenter study of children with mTBI evaluated in the ER. They found that that pre-existing risk factors and symptoms immediately following injury were associated with elevated risk for persistent symptoms 28 days after injury. The pre-existing risk factors included adolescent age (age 5–7, odds ratio [OR], 1.0, age

8–12, OR, 1.54 [95% CI, 1.09–2.19]; age 13–17, OR, 2.31 [95% CI, 1.62–3.32]), female sex (OR, 2.23; 95% CI, 1.78–2.82), prior concussion with symptoms greater than 1 week (OR, 1.53; 95% CI, 1.10–2.13), and personal history of physician-diagnosed migraine (OR, 1.73; 95% CI, 1.24–2.43). The most important symptoms at evaluation (within 48 hours of injury) included "answering questions slowly" (OR, 1.37; 95% CI, 1.08–1.74), four or more errors on Balance Error Scoring System tandem stance (OR, 1.31; 95% CI, 1.04–1.66), headache (OR, 1.66; 95% CI, 1.11–2.48), sensitivity to noise (OR, 1.47; 95% CI, 1.15–1.87), and fatigue (OR, 1.84; 95% CI, 1.37–2.46). This group devised a scale to estimate the risk of prolonged PCS (including headache) in pediatric patients with mTBI or concussion in the acute phase as follows: age, 8 to 12 = 1 point, 13 to 17 = 2 points; female sex = 2 points; prior concussion with symptoms more than 1 week = 1 point; migraine history = 1 point; answering questions slowly = 1 point; four or more errors on Balance Error Scoring System tandem stance = 1 point; headache = 1 point; sensitivity to noise = 1 point; and fatigue = 2 points. Low risk was defined as less than or equal to three total points, medium risk four to eight points, and high risk nine or more points.[42] Although this scale needs further validation it may be helpful for researchers and clinicians to identify those teenagers and children at highest risk for disability following concussion who could benefit from early intervention.

MANAGEMENT OF POSTTRAUMATIC HEADACHE

Following a brain injury, those who sustain a moderate to severe injury, or who have coexisting other severe physical injuries, are likely to have those injuries addressed before evaluating headache. If the headache persists, or causes significant pain, disability, or inability to function, medical attention is then considered. Difficulty with concentration or attention to work or school may be secondary to a constant headache, or part of the PCS, or both, leading to significant work-loss and social functioning. Fear of the headache pain and its unpredictability, or fear that the headache reflects significant underlying brain injury from the concussion, also may bring those with headache to the attention of practitioners. Many people initially see their primary care providers, or sports medicine specialists if an injury is sports related. If prolonged treatment and rehabilitation is necessary for associated musculoskeletal injuries, a physiotherapist may be the specialist providing care. A headache specialist is usually seen well after injury for refractory headache.

The management of PTH is empiric. To date, no controlled clinical trials are available to direct treatment of PTH. In a review of interventions for PTH,[43] there were no class I studies and only one class II study in 23 subjects for management of PTH using manual spine therapy versus cold packs, finding that the group receiving spine therapy had a decrease in headache intensity 5 weeks after treatment but the treatment effect was lost after 8 weeks.[44] In a retrospective case series of 28 children and adolescents with a mean age of 15 years, peripheral nerve blocks demonstrated a good therapeutic effect in 93%, with 71% reporting immediate relief from PTH with a mean decrease in headache intensity of 94%.[45]

No medication studies greater than a class III study have been published. In a retrospective study of 100 patients after mTBI with CDH, headache frequency and severity were measured after at least 1 month of treatment with valproic acid. Analgesic, nonsteroidal anti-inflammatory drug (NSAID), chiropractic, and physical therapy treatments were allowed during this treatment intervention. After treatment, 44% of subjects had a 24% to 50% improvement, and another 16% had more than 50% improvement.[46] A subgroup analysis of subjects in a larger prospective study of amitriptyline for depression[47] compared 10 patients with depression and headache after mTBI versus trauma without mTBI. Those who did not have mTBI (n = 512) did better on headache severity and depression scores than those with mTBI (n = 510). In 20 subjects with at least a 3-month history of headaches, a topical compounded ketoprofen was used. Although results showed headache index decreased over 1 month, there was no subgroup analysis in the three trauma-related headaches in this study.[48] Anecdotal reports of successful treatment of acute PTH with sumatriptan or dihydroergotamine after concussion support the use of migraine-specific therapies.[49,50]

In one retrospective study of active duty service members with mTBI and PTH, triptans were effective as acute agents treating a predominantly migraine phenotype. Topiramate was an effective prophylactic agent, associated with a significant reduction in headache frequency, but overall the number of patients using different medications was small, which prevented treatment recommendations. A relatively high nonresponder rate was noted, and only 35% of soldiers were considered responders to preventive medication.[51]

Headaches after mTBI are not well managed. Many of those with headache are likely to self-treat and use over-the-counter (OTC) pain medication. In a prospective study of 212 subjects with mTBI and a high headache prevalence, never less than 58% of subjects at 3, 6, and 12 months after injury, more than 70% of those with headache at any time-period reported self-treating with acetaminophen or an NSAID for headache.[13] Less than 5% of this group used triptans, even though the predominant headache type was migraine, and only 19% found complete relief after taking their usual medication.[52]

Expert opinion suggests treating PTH according to its clinical characteristics using the primary headache disorder classification criteria.[53–55] Based on the close phenotypic similarity of some PTH to primary headache, one approach to treatment is to use primary headache characterization of the PTH as migraine, probable migraine, TTH, or other primary disorder. The most important factor in using this approach is to gauge the severity of the headache. Acute treatment of a PTH is crucial if the headache is severe or disabling. Some common medications used in the acute treatment of migraine-type headache are shown in **Table 4**.

Most headaches fluctuate in intensity over time after injury, allowing for patient identification of a time window for acute treatment. If the headache is continuous, preventive therapy may allow identification of severe worsening within a more constant lower intensity headache, so that medication overuse is avoided. A list of preventive therapies that are commonly used to treat frequent migraine is shown in **Table 5**.

The goal of acute PTH treatment is to educate those with headache to treat early with effective therapy once a treatment window is identified. Many patients wait to see if their headache worsens, or choose OTC products because of cost or lack of access to medical care. If their usual pattern is that of migraine, and if simple analgesic agents or other OTC products do not effectively treat their PTH, then migraine-specific therapy is recommended. Two treatment approaches are used for migraine headache.

Overuse of abortive medication may contribute to persistence of headache after injury through the development of medication overuse headache, also known as rebound headache. Few epidemiologic data are available on the extent of this problem. Although it is extremely important to recognize the possibility of medication overuse headache, especially given the high rate of use of OTC products by those who have sustained a TBI,[52] it is important to examine the development of persistent headache and associated medication use and consider changing or withdrawing suspected medication before concluding that PTH is worsened or prolonged because of medication overuse. Education regarding medication overuse is beneficial, and

Table 4
Acute medications for posttraumatic headache migraine-type

Medication Class	Brand Name	Dose
Triptans		
Almotriptan	Axert (Ortho-McNeil, Janssen, Titusville, NJ)	Tablet 6.25, 12.5 mg
Eletriptan	Relpax (Pfizer, New York, NY)	Tablet 20, 40 (80 outside the US) mg
Frovatriptan	Frova (Endo, Newark, DE)	Tablet 2.5 mg
Naratriptan	Amerge (GlaxoSmithKline, Middlesex, UK)	Tablet 1, 2.5 mg
Rizatriptan	Maxalt (Merck, Kenilworth, NJ)	Tablet 5, 10 mg ODT 5, 10 mg
Sumatriptan	Imitrex (US) Imigran (EU) (GlaxoSmithKline, Middlesex, UK) Sumavel (Zogenix, San Diego, CA)	Tablet 25, 50, 100 mg Nasal spray 5, 10 mg Subcutaneous 4, 6 mg Needleless 6 mg
Sumatriptan/naproxen	Treximet (GlaxoSmithKline, Middlesex, UK)	Tablet 85/500 mg
Zolmitriptan	Zomig (Astra-Zeneca, London, UK)	Tablet 2.5, 5 mg ZMT 2.5, 5 mg Nasal spray 5 mg
Dihydroergotamine		
Dihydroergotamine mesylate injection	DHE-45 (Bedford Labs, Bedford, OH)	1 mg/mL
Dihydroergotamine mesylate spray	Migranal (Valeant, Montreal, Canada)	4 mg/mL
NSAIDs		
Diclofenac	Voltaren (Novartis, Basel, Switzerland)	Tablet 25, 50 mg Powder for oral solution 50 mg Slow release 75, 100, 150 mg
Ibuprofen	Advil (Pfizer, New York, NY)	200 mg
Indomethacin	Indocin (Iroko, Philadelphia, PA)	25 mg, 50 mg, 75 mg ER, rectal 50 mg, suspension 25 mg/5 mL
Ketorolac	Toradol (Roche, Basel, Switzerland)	Tablet 10 mg Injection 30 mg/mL
Naproxen	Aleve (Bayer, Leverkusen, Germany)	Tablet 220 mg

This table is not a comprehensive list of all medications in categories, or all manufacturers. All are available as generic medications by multiple manufacturers.

the use of a diary or other record of medication use is helpful to the practitioner and patient. It is also important to consider possible cognitive limitations of those who have sustained a TBI, and whether assistance from caregivers or family members may be needed when PTH management is discussed.

MANAGEMENT OF PEDIATRIC POSTTRAUMATIC HEADACHE

The management of pediatric PTH shares similarities with the management of adult PTH, but the major differences are that children attend school, a family unit is involved,

Table 5
Preventive medications used in migraine treatment

Category	Class	Medication	Daily Dose Range, mg	Comments on Adverse Effects
Antidepressant	TCA	Amitriptyline	10–100	Sedation, dry mouth, urinary retention
	SSRI	Fluoxetine	10–60	Weight gain, sexual dysfunction
	SNRI	Duloxetine	30–120	Weight gain, sexual dysfunction, sweating
Antiepilepsy		Valproic acid	500–1500	Weight gain, hair loss, stomach upset
		Topiramate	75–100	Tingling, cognitive dysfunction, weight loss
		Zonisamide	100–400	Weight loss, altered taste
		Gabapentin	900–3600	Sedation, dizziness, poor absorption
		Lamotrigine	50–200	Sedation, dizziness
		Levitiracetam	500–1000	Sedation, dizziness
Cardiovascular	β-Blockers	Propranolol	40–240	Fatigue, lightheadedness
		Metoprolol	25–100	Fatigue, lightheadedness
		Nadolol	40–120	Fatigue, lightheadedness
	Calcium channel blockers	Verapamil	120–360	Constipation, ankle edema
		Amlodipine	5–10	ankle edema
		Flunarazine	10–20	Drowsiness, weight gain
Other		OnabotulinumtoxinA	100–155 units	Pain at injection site, muscle weakness
		Cryproheptadiene	4–12	Sedation, weight gain
		Magnesium	600	Poorly absorbed, laxative effect
		Tizanidine	4–16	Sedation

This is not a comprehensive list, but represents the most common medications used in frequent migraine prevention, approved and nonapproved by the Food and Drug Administration for this purpose.
Abbreviations: SNRI, serotonin norepinephrine reuptake inhibitor; SSRI, selective serotonin reuptake inhibitor; TCA, tricyclic antidepressant.

and adolescents have a longer recovery period following concussion than adults.[56] The acute management of concussion and imaging criteria are discussed elsewhere in this issue (see Kenneth Podell and colleagues article, "Sideline Sports Concussion Assessment" and Brian Sindelar and Julian E. Bailes's article, "Neurosurgical Emergencies in Sport," in this issue). During the initial assessment of a patient with headache following concussion, it is important to obtain a thorough medical history, including family history of pain and headaches, information about past concussions, and headache history before the head injury because concussion may exacerbate an underlying primary headache disorder. One should consider other potential causes of secondary headaches that would be managed differently than PTH, including intracranial thrombosis, vascular dissection, endocrine abnormalities, eating disorder, infection, dental disease, pregnancy, drug use, and so forth. The examination should include a thorough assessment of the head, neck, mouth, and eyes, and a complete neurologic examination with assessment of balance, speech, and memory. Laboratory studies may be requested if there is suspicion for another disorder, but are not typically helpful for uncomplicated PTH, although in the future biomarkers may be of use (see Martina Anto-Ocrah and colleagues article, "Blood-based Biomarkers for the Identification of Sports-Related Concussion," in this issue). There are no clear guidelines for the use of neuroimaging for those with persistent PTH. Certainly those with new abnormalities on neurologic examination, with rapidly worsening headaches, headache waking them from sleep, or new headache in an immunocompromised patient should raise concerns and prompt neuroimaging. MRI scans are currently being done frequently for children and teenagers with prolonged PTH; however, they are most often unrevealing. Screening for comorbid conditions, such as anxiety and depression, is essential because pre-existing mental health disorders or mood changes related to concussion or change in athletic status may exacerbate headache pain and disability, and it is difficult to alleviate pain without addressing these factors.

MEDICATIONS FOR THE TREATMENT OF PEDIATRIC POSTTRAUMATIC HEADACHE

There are few studies of the use of medications to treat pediatric PTH. Barlow's group[21] described the use of traditional migraine medications in persistent pediatric PTH, and in this group of 44, a total of 64% had successful treatment of their headache with medications that included amitriptyline, melatonin, nortriptyline, flunarizine, and topiramate, but melatonin and amitriptyline were associated with the highest success rate at 75% and 68%, respectively. Most experts agree that it is reasonable to consider treatment of PTH with agents that fit the phenotype of the headache. Thus, for persistent migrainous PTH it is reasonable to consider medications and supplements that are used for migraine.[57–59] In addition, it may be reasonable to consider using supplements with few side effects that may be helpful for the management of PTH, such as melatonin or magnesium, for patients who are at high risk for persistent PCS who have frequent or disabling headaches within a few weeks of the concussion.

There has been interest in the use of omega-3 fatty acids, particularly docosahexaenoic acid (DHA), because these have been used to treat persistent postconcussion symptoms and migraine for some time. In animal models, supplementation with omega-3 fatty acids before concussion seemed to reduce signs of neuronal injury and improve neuronal function.[60–62] One of the few human studies of DHA supplementation for concussion in humans randomly assigned 81 American football athlete volunteers on National Collegiate Athletic Association Division 1 college teams to varying doses of DHA or placebo (2 g/d, 4 g/d, 6 g/g, or corn oil). The authors recently published that, irrespective of dose, "supplemental DHA likely attenuated neurofilament light (a biomarker of axonal injury) levels," which rose during the active football season,[63] with the implication that DHA may be neuroprotective if taken before injury. Dietary supplementation with omega-3 fatty acids has been studied in CDH not related to trauma, and found to reduce headache pain.[64] However, neither of these studies involved pediatric patients. Thus, DHA or other omega-3 fatty acids may be useful tools in the management of persistent PTH, but more research is needed to determine the optimal formulation and dose for children and teenagers and to determine how effective it is when taken after injury.

Other therapy for persistent PTH should include interventions for concussion, such as subthreshold exercise; alteration of activity to avoid further head injury; adequate and appropriate hydration, nutrition, and sleep; and management of mood disorders. Biofeedback and physiotherapy have also been used for the management of PTH. There are no studies of these therapies in children with PTH, but aside from time and cost, they likely have few adverse effects and have been helpful for some children.

ABORTIVE THERAPIES

Once hemorrhage has been excluded it is reasonable to use NSAIDs or acetaminophen to manage episodic headaches. There are several reports of successful management of episodic migrainous PTH with triptans.[49,51,65] Although triptan use has not been formally studied in PTH, rizatriptan has been approved for the abortive treatment of migraine for those age 6 and up, and almotriptan has been approved for those 13 and older.

SCHOOL AND POSTTRAUMATIC HEADACHE

Returning to school and a full academic load following concussion is challenging for those with prolonged PTH.[66,67] It is important to work with the family and school to develop a plan that helps to avoid triggering symptoms, and allows the student to progress and learn. A 504 plan is often helpful for those with significant PTH, because these student athletes may also be dealing with cognitive changes related to the concussion in addition to the challenges with focus and attention that accompany severe headache. The Centers for Disease Control and Prevention has posted online resources that may be helpful for students, families, and schools (http://www.cdc.gov/headsup/providers/return_to_activities.html). Although each student's plan is different and depends on individual circumstances it may include the following:

- The ability to work and/or take tests in a quiet environment with limited distractions
- A syllabus or homework packet so that the student can complete missed assignments
- An arrangement at school to store books so the student does not have to carry a heavy backpack from class to class
- Providing a process for getting notes/assignments for missed classes
- Shorter or modified homework assignments during times of headache and/or missed class
- Extra time to make up assignments that were late or missed because of illness
- Time to make up missed examinations without penalty
- Excused absences for illness/severe headaches
- Provision of a quiet, dark place to rest in school to try to recover from a spike in headache while staying in school
- Ability to leave noisy or bright environments without penalty, with the provision that work missed can be made up at a later date
- Permission to carry a water bottle during class and have free access to the restroom
- Permission to pursue activities in physical education class that do not trigger headaches if/when strenuous physical activity exacerbates headaches
- Provision of a quiet place to eat lunch with a companion if/when the general cafeteria environment exacerbates headaches

OTHER HEADACHE EXACERBATED BY SPORT ACTIVITY
Chiari Malformation

Chiari type 1 malformation may be associated with headache that is exacerbated by physical effort; therefore, sports activities, such as those with frequent Valsalva maneuvers as seen in strength training, may bring this common anatomic variant to clinical attention. Chiari type 1 malformation is a craniocervical junction disorder with 5 mm of tonsillar ectopia (low-lying cerebellar tonsils) as a definition of an anatomically significant definition. Prevalence in the general population has varied from about 0.5% to 0.8% in MRI, surgical, and autopsy series.[68–70] The important element for clinical symptoms is a change in the flow of CSF at the level of the foramen magnum, which is frequently associated with syringomyelia (30%–70%). Onset of symptoms is frequently in teenage years or the 20s, and diagnosis may be delayed because of a variety of symptoms, which include headache, neck pain, dizziness, ataxia, limb weakness, or even bradycardia and syncope.

Headache is the most common symptom and the ICHD-3 criteria require at least one of three characteristics: precipitated by cough or other Valsalva maneuver, occipital or suboccipital location and lasts less than 5 minutes (ICHD-3;12). Although surgical repair is sometimes necessary, there is no correlation between amount of herniation and severity of headache, and many patients are symptomatic with minimal herniation, whereas others are asymptomatic with large herniations. Chiari type 1 malformation headache criteria and radiologic criteria need to be followed to make this association because other primary headache disorders can have similar clinical characteristics.[71,72]

Primary Exertional Headache

This primary headache type, also known as benign exertional headache, is a headache caused by any form of exercise in the absence of an intracranial disorder. It occurs only during or after strenuous physical exercise, although hot weather or altitude can decrease threshold for headache occurrence. Some name the headache according to the exercise that precipitates it, such as "weight-lifter's" headache. This headache is usually severe; has a sudden onset; lasts less than 48 hours, but usually seconds to a few hours; is throbbing, pulsating, or explosive in character; and bilateral in most cases.[73]

The mechanism of primary exertional headache is not known. Hypotheses center around vascular theories, such as venous or arterial dilation during exercise, and recent finding in patients with this headache type find that they have a significantly higher prevalence of internal jugular venous valve incompetence (70% compared with 20% of control subjects) suggesting venous distention as the precipitating mechanism of pain. Because serious intracranial pathology can present with similar headache characteristics, this is a headache type that needs evaluation. It is necessary to exclude such conditions as subarachnoid hemorrhage, arterial dissection, or herniation from intracranial mass.

Contact-Related Headache

Trauma-triggered headache is a specific, extremely rare migraine headache with aura that occurs mostly in children and adolescents or young adults. Some clinical descriptions labeled this type of headache as "footballer's migraine" and it differs from postconcussive headache because migraine symptoms are rapidly caused by minor blows or hits to the face or head, and the trauma triggers aura symptoms within minutes, usually visual or sensory symptoms, although in severe cases hemiplegia and aphasia have occurred.[74] Although the cause is not entirely clear, there have been cases of early seizures and cerebral edema after trivial head trauma associated with mutations of the CACNA1A gene. Other mutations in this and other genes have been reported.[75]

SUMMARY

PTH is the most common symptom after any TBI including sport-related concussion. PTH is frequent, with recent data from adult and pediatric populations reporting chronic and persistent symptoms. Most PTH is classified using primary headache disorder criteria to migraine-type or tension-type PTH. Whether or not phenotypically similar types of primary and secondary headaches respond similarly to the same treatment is unknown. Controlled, blinded clinical trials are needed to determine effective PTH management. Prevention of TBI and recurrent concussion remains the single most important management concern. Targeted efforts by government agencies (civilian and military), sports leagues, coaches and trainers, brain injury foundations, physicians, and parents are needed to prevent TBI.

REFERENCES

1. Lewis DW. Pediatric migraine. Pediatr Rev 2007;28:43–53.
2. Bompadre V, Jinguji TM, Yanez ND, et al. Washington State's Lystedt law in concussion documentation in Seattle Public High Schools. J Athl Train 2014;49: 486–92.
3. Lew HL, Lin PH, Fuh JL, et al. Characteristics and treatment of headache after traumatic brain injury: a focused review. Am J Phys Med Rehabil 2006;85:619–27.
4. Harmon KG, Drezner JA, Gammons M, et al. American Medical Society for Sports Medicine position statement: concussion in sport. Br J Sports Med 2013;47:15–26.
5. Echlin PS, Skopelja EN, Worsley R, et al. A prospective study of physician-observed concussion during a varsity university ice hockey season: incidence and neuropsychological changes. Part 2 of 4. Neurosurg Focus 2012;33:E2, 1–11.
6. Bazarian JJ, Veazie P, Mookerjee S, et al. Accuracy of mile traumatic brain injury case ascertainment using ICD-9 codes. Acad Emerg Med 2006;13:31–8.
7. Voss JD, Connolly J, Schwab KA, et al. Update on the epidemiology of concussion/mild traumatic brain injury. Curr Pain Headache Rep 2015;19:32–40.
8. Centers for Disease Control and Prevention (CDC). Traumatic brain injury statistics 2012. Available at: www.cdc.gov/traumaticbraininjury/statistics.html2012. Accessed December 30, 2016.
9. Evans RW. Post-traumatic headaches. Neurol Clin 2004;22(1):237–49, viii.
10. Linder S. Post-traumatic headache. Curr Pain Headache Rep 2007;11:396–400.
11. Hoffman J, Lucas S, Dikmen S, et al. Natural history of headache following traumatic brain injury. J Neurotrauma 2011;28:1–8.
12. Headache Classification Subcommittee of the International Headache Society. The international classification of headache disorders: 2nd edition. Cephalalgia 2004;24(Suppl 1):9–160.
13. Lucas S, Hoffman JM, Bell KR, et al. A prospective study of prevalence and characterization of headache following mild traumatic brain injury. Cephalalgia 2014; 34(2):93–102.
14. Uomoto JM, Esselman PC. Traumatic brain injury and chronic pain: differential types and rates by head injury severity. Arch Phys Med Rehabil 1993;74:61–4.
15. Eskridge SL, Macera CA, Galarneau MR, et al. Injuries from combat explosions in Iraq: injury type, location, and severity. Injury 2012;43:1678–82.
16. Couch JR, Bears C. Chronic daily headache in the posttrauma syndrome: relation to extent of head injury. Headache 2001;41:559–64.
17. Meehan WP 3rd, d'Hemecourt P, Comstock RD. High school concussions in the 2008-2009 academic year: mechanism, symptoms, and management. Am J Sports Med 2010;38:2405–9.
18. Chrisman SP, Rivara FP, Schiff MA, et al. Risk factors for concussive symptoms 1 week or longer in high school athletes. Brain Inj 2013;27:1–9.

19. Kontos AP, Elbin RJ, Lau B, et al. Posttraumatic migraine as a predictor of recovery and cognitive impairment after sport-related concussion. Am J Sports Med 2013;41(7):1497–504.

20. Mihalik JP, Register-Mihalik J, Kerr ZY, et al. Recovery of posttraumatic migraine characteristics in patients after mild traumatic brain injury. Am J Sports Med 2013;41(7):1490–6.

21. Barlow KM, Crawford S, Stevenson A, et al. Epidemiology of postconcussion syndrome in pediatric mild traumatic brain injury. Pediatrics 2010;126:e374–81.

22. Kuczynski A, Crawford S, Bodell L, et al. Characteristics of post-traumatic headaches in children following mild traumatic brain injury and their response to treatment: a prospective cohort. Dev Med Child Neurol 2013;55:636–41.

23. Kirk C, Nagiub G, Abu-Arafeh I. Chronic post-traumatic headache after head injury in children and adolescents. Dev Med Child Neurol 2008;50:422–5.

24. Eisenberg MA, Meehan WP 3rd, Mannix R. Duration and course of post-concussive symptoms. Pediatrics 2014;133:999–1006.

25. Blume HK, Vavilala MS, Jaffe KM, et al. Headache after pediatric traumatic brain injury: a cohort study. Pediatrics 2012;129:e31–9.

26. Lucas S, Hoffman JM, Bell KR, et al. Characterization of headache after traumatic brain injury. Cephalalgia 2012;32:600–6.

27. Victor TW, Hu X, Campbell JC, et al. Migraine prevalence by age and sex in the United States: a life-span study. Cephalalgia 2010;30:1065–72.

28. Martins H, Ribas V, Martins B, et al. Post-traumatic headache. Arq Neuropsiquiatr 2009;2009:43–5.

29. Lieba-Samal D, Platzer P, Seidel S, et al. Characteristics of acute post-traumatic headache following mild head injury. Cephalalgia 2011;31:1618–26.

30. Stovner LJ, Schrader H, Mickeviciene D, et al. Headache after concussion. Eur J Neurol 2009;16:112–20.

31. Haas DC. Chronic post-traumatic headaches classified and compared with natural headaches. Cephalalgia 1996;16:486–93.

32. Baandrup L, Jensen R. Chronic post-traumatic headache: a clinical analysis in relation to the International Headache Classification 2nd edition. Cephalalgia 2004;25:132–8.

33. Castillo J, Munoz P, Guitera V, et al. Kaplan Award 1998. Epidemiology of chronic daily headache in the general population. Headache 1999;39:190–6.

34. Couch J, Lipton R, Stewart W, et al. Head or neck injury increases the risk of chronic daily headache: a population-based study. Neurology 2007;69:1169–77.

35. Clark ME, Bair MJ, Buckenmaier CC, et al. Pain and combat injuries in soldiers returning from operations Enduring Freedom and Iraqi Freedom: implications for research and practice. J Rehabil Res Dev 2007;44:179–94.

36. Lay CL, Newman LC. Post-traumatic hemicrania continua. Headache 1999;39:275–9.

37. Matharu MJ, Goadsby PJ. Post-traumatic chronic paroxysmal hemicrania (CPH) with aura. Neurology 2001;56:273–5.

38. Piovesan EJ, Kowacs PA, Werneck LC. S.U.N.C.T. syndrome: report of a case preceded by ocular trauma. Arq Neuropsiquiatr 1996;54:494–7 [in Portuguese].

39. Gironda RJ, Clark ME, Ruff RL, et al. Traumatic brain injury, polytrauma, and pain: challenges and treatment strategies for the polytrauma rehabilitation. Rehabil Psychol 2009;54:247–58.

40. Lucas S, Devine J, Bell K, et al. Acute neuroimaging abnormalities associated with post-traumatic headache following traumatic brain injury (P04.020). Neurology 2013;80 (American Academy of Neurology meeting abstracts).

41. Choe MC, Blume HK. Pediatric posttraumatic headache: a review. J Child Neurol 2016;31:76–85.
42. Zemek R, Barrowman N, Freedman SB, et al. Clinical risk score for persistent postconcussion symptoms among children with acute concussion in the ED. JAMA 2016;315:1014–25.
43. Watanabe T, Bell K, Walker W, et al. Systematic review of interventions for post-traumatic headache. PM R 2012;4:129–40.
44. Jensen OK, Nielsen FF, Vosmar L. An open study comparing manual therapy with the use of cold packs in the treatment of post-traumatic headache. Cephalalgia 1990;10:241–50.
45. Dubrovsky AS, Friedman D, Kocilowicz H. Pediatric post-traumatic headaches and peripheral nerve blocks of the scalp: a case series and patient satisfaction survey. Headache 2014;54:878–87.
46. Packard RC. Treatment of chronic daily post-traumatic headache with divalproex sodium. Headache 2000;40:736–9.
47. Saran A. Antidepressants not effective in headache associated with minor closed head injury. Int J Psychiatry Med 1988;18:75–83.
48. Friedman MH, Peterson SJ, Frishman WH, et al. Intraoral topical nonsteroidal anti-inflammatory drug application for headache prevention. Heart Dis 2002;4(4): 212–5.
49. Gawel MJ, Rothbart P, Jacobs H. Subcutaneous sumatriptan in the treatment of acute episodes of post-traumatic headache. Headache 1993;33:96–7.
50. McBeath JG, Nanda A. Use of dihydroergotamine in patients with post-concussion syndrome. Headache 1994;34:148–51.
51. Erickson JC. Treatment outcomes of chronic post-traumatic headaches after mild head trauma in US soldiers: an observational study. Headache 2011;51:932–44.
52. DiTommaso C, Hoffman JM, Lucas S, et al. Medication usage patterns for head-ache treatment after mild traumatic brain injury. Headache 2014;54:511–9.
53. Lucas S. Headache management in concussion and mild traumatic brain injury. PMR 2011;3(10 Suppl 2):S406–12.
54. Evans RW. Expert opinion: post-traumatic headaches among United States sol-diers injured in Afghanistan and Iraq. Headache 2008;48:1216–25.
55. Seifert TD, Evans RW. Post-traumatic headache: a review. Curr Pain Headache Rep 2010;14:292–8.
56. McCrea M, Guskiewicz KM, Marshall SW, et al. Acute effects and recovery time following concussion in collegiate football players: the NCAA Concussion Study. JAMA 2003;290:2556–63.
57. Tfelt-Hansen PC. Evidence-based guideline update: pharmacologic treatment for episodic migraine prevention in adults: report of the quality standards subcom-mittee of the American academy of neurology and the American Headache Soci-ety. Neurology 2013;80:869–70.
58. Holland S, Silberstein SD, Freitag F, et al. Evidence-based guideline update: NSAIDs and other complementary treatments for episodic migraine prevention in adults: report of the quality standards subcommittee of the American Academy of Neurology and the American Headache Society. Neurology 2012;78:1346–53.
59. Lewis D, Ashwal S, Hershey A, et al. Practice parameter: pharmacological treat-ment of migraine headache in children and adolescents: report of the American Academy of Neurology quality standards subcommittee and the practice com-mittee of the Child Neurology Society. Neurology 2004;63:2215–24.

60. Wu A, Ying Z, Gomez-Pinilla F. Dietary strategy to repair plasma membrane after brain trauma: implications for plasticity and cognition. Neurorehabil Neural Repair 2014;28:75–84.

61. Wu A, Ying Z, Gomez-Pinilla F. Omega-3 fatty acids supplementation restores mechanisms that maintain brain homeostasis in traumatic brain injury. J Neurotrauma 2007;24:1587–95.

62. Wu A, Ying Z, Gomez-Pinilla F. Dietary omega-3 fatty acids normalize BDNF levels, reduce oxidative damage, and counteract learning disability after traumatic brain injury in rats. J Neurotrauma 2004;21:1457–67.

63. Oliver JM, Jones MT, Kirk KM, et al. Effect of docosahexaenoic acid on a biomarker of head trauma in American football. Med Sci Sports Exerc 2016; 48(6):974–82.

64. Ramsden CE, Faurot KR, Zamora D, et al. Targeted alteration of dietary n-3 and n-6 fatty acids for the treatment of chronic headaches: a randomized trial. Pain 2013;154(11):2441–51.

65. McCrory P, Heywood J, Ugoni A. Open label study of intranasal sumatriptan (Imigran) for footballer's headache. Br J Sports Med 2005;39:552–4.

66. Halstead ME, McAvoy K, Devore CD, et al. Returning to learning following a concussion. Pediatrics 2013;132:948–57.

67. Master CL, Gioia GA, Leddy JJ, et al. Importance of 'return-to-learn' in pediatric and adolescent concussion. Pediatr Ann 2012;41:1–6.

68. Alperin N, Loftus JR, Oliu CJ, et al. Imaging based features of headaches in Chiari malformation type I. Neurosurgery 2015;77:96–103.

69. Arnautovic A, Splavski B, Boop FA, et al. Pediatric and adult Chiari malformation type I surgical series 1965-2013: a review of demographics, operative treatment, and outcomes. J Neurosurg Pediatr 2015;15:161–77.

70. Speer MC, Enterline DS, Mehltretter L, et al. Chiari type I malformation with or without syringomyelia: prevalence and genetics. J Genet Couns 2003;12:297.

71. Stovner LJ. Headache associated with the Chiari type I malformation. Headache 1993;33:175–81.

72. Toldo I, Tangari M, Mardari R, et al. Headache in children with Chiari I malformation. Headache 2014;54:899–908.

73. Imperato J, Burstein J, Edlow JA. Benign exertional headache. Ann Emerg Med 2003;41:98–103.

74. Lansink JG, van Oosterhout WP, Borggreve AG, et al. Footballer's migraine instead of concussion. Ned Tijdschr Geneeskd 2014;158:A8434.

75. Stam AH, Luijckx GJ, Poll-The BT, et al. Early seizures and cerebral oedema after trivial head trauma associated with the CACNA1A S218L mutation. J Neurol Neurosurg Psychiatry 2009;80:1125–9.

76. Dikmen S, Machamer J, Fann JR, et al. Rates of symptom reporting following traumatic brain injury. J Int Neuropsychol Soc 2010;16:401–11.

77. Faux S, Sheedy J. A prospective controlled study in the prevalence of post-traumatic headache following mild traumatic brain injury. Pain Med 2008;9: 1001–11.

78. Marar M, McIlvain NM, Fields SK, et al. Epidemiology of concussions among United States high school athletes in 20 sports. Am J Sports Med 2012;40(4): 747–55.

79. Meehan WP 3rd, Mannix RC, Stracciolini A, et al. Symptom severity predicts prolonged recovery after sport-related concussion, but age and amnesia do not. J Pediatr 2013;163:721–5.

80. Eckner JT, Seifert T, Pescovitz A, et al. Is migraine headache associated with concussion in athletes? A case-control study. Clin J Sport Med 2017;27(3): 266–70.
81. Miller JH, Gill C, Kuhn EN, et al. Predictors of delayed recovery following pediatric sports-related concussion: a case-control study. J Neurosurg Pediatr 2016;17: 491–6.
82. Corbin-Berrigan LA, Gagnon I. Postconcussion symptoms as a marker of delayed recovery in children and youth who recently sustained a concussion: a brief report. Clin J Sport Med 2017;27(3):325–7.
83. Howell DR, O'Brien MJ, Beasley MA, et al. Initial somatic symptoms are associated with prolonged symptom duration following concussion in adolescents. Acta Paediatr 2016;105:e426–32.
84. Eisenberg MA, Andrea J, Meehan W, et al. Time interval between concussions and symptom duration. Pediatrics 2013;132(1):8–17.

Neurologic Health in Combat Sports

Tad Seifert, MD

KEYWORDS

- Combat sports • Neurologic injuries • Neurologic health • Combat sports clinicians

KEY POINTS

- Neurologic injuries of both an acute and chronic nature have been reported in the literature for various combat sport styles; however, reports of the incidence and prevalence of these injury types vary greatly.
- Combat sports clinicians must continue to strive for the development, implementation, and enforcement of uniform minimum requirements for brain safety.
- These health care providers must also seize on the honor to provide this oft-underserved population with the health care advocacy they very much deserve, but often do not receive.

INTRODUCTION

Because combat sports encourage deliberate blows to the head, much of the world's medical community has spoken out against this genre of sport, including the American Academy of Pediatrics and the American, Canadian, Australian, British and World medical associations.[1–6] Despite this opposition, mixed martial arts (MMA) continues to rapidly gain acceptance as a genuine combat sport, and is currently more popular than boxing, the National Hockey League (NHL), and the National Association for Stock Car Auto Racing (NASCAR) amongst males 18 to 34 years of age.[7] Boxing and MMA alike are both watched by millions of spectators annually in the United States and abroad. The May 2, 2015 "Fight of the Century" bout between Manny Pacquiao and Floyd Mayweather,Jr. generated 4.6 million pay-per-view purchases and generated a revenue of over $400 million; both figures remain all-time records within the world of combat sports. In the summer of 2016, the Ultimate Fighting Championship (UFC) was purchased by a group of outside investors for $4.2 billion, which was remarkable considering its original purchase for $2 million in 2000. Up to one-half of all fights in boxing, karate, and taekwondo result in injury, with a significant number of these injuries being to the head and neck region.[8–13] Despite this elevated public interest, chronic traumatic brain injury (CTBI) remains the most predominant safety

Norton Healthcare, 3991 Dutchmans Lane, Suite 310, Louisville, KY 40207, USA
E-mail address: Tad.Seifert@nortonhealthcare.org

Neurol Clin 35 (2017) 523–535
http://dx.doi.org/10.1016/j.ncl.2017.04.001
0733-8619/17/© 2017 Elsevier Inc. All rights reserved.
neurologic.theclinics.com

challenge in modern-day combat sports. With its inevitable association with central nervous system trauma, it is imperative that neurologists maintain an open line of communication and understanding with its combatants.

Boxing and other combat sports are different than other sporting pursuits due to the head being an intended and targeted place of contact. Despite the inherent goal of attempting to concuss an opponent, the current author suggests that calls to ban this genre of sport overlook the inherent benefit of active medical involvement in the context of combat sports. Sports medicine providers should emphasize the associated risks, insist on adequate safety precautions, and even prevent future participation due to disqualifying medical conditions. I stop short, however, of unwavering opposition due to other associated factors, such as socioeconomic considerations and the benefit of exercise, self-discipline, and familial structure. In a sports genre where a significant portion of participants arrive from humble socioeconomic backgrounds, the value of health care advocacy provided by sports medicine personnel cannot be underestimated.

Combat sports participation is associated with a risk of neurologic injury, both acute and chronic in nature. CTBI includes a number of disorders that are associated with long-term neurologic sequelae, including persistent post-traumatic headache, chronic postconcussion syndrome, post-traumatic Parkinsonism, post-traumatic dementia, dementia pugilistica, and chronic traumatic encephalopathy (CTE). Previous studies have estimated 20% to 50% of former boxers have symptoms of chronic brain injury.[14] Combat sport athletes are exposed to thousands of blows to the head over the course of their careers, with the cumulative endpoint often being that of chronic neurologic impairment. The complex mixture of applied force, induced head movement, and neurophysiological state at the time of injury contributes to the type & severity of brain injury incurred. Furthermore, there may be a time period of increased vulnerability after TBI where the brain is physiologically more susceptible to recurrent injury at a lower threshold. The early identification of high risk fighters is imperative to facilitate primary prevention efforts, such as decreasing the likelihood of reinjury (secondary prevention), and ensuring access to appropriate interventions that may reduce both personal and aggregate costs (tertiary prevention). The precise threshold of force necessary to induce both acute and chronic neuropathology remains unknown; therefore, the accurate and timely detection of neurologic injury in combat sports is of critical importance so that appropriate therapeutic management may be initiated.

ACUTE AND CHRONIC BRAIN INJURY

Issues regarding the neurologic health of fighters are generally divided into three categories: (1) pre-participation exams to assess baseline status (2) return to fight progression after concussion, and (3) serial assessments to evaluate the aptitude for continued sport participation. Most major professional sports leagues within the United States have formal concussion policies in place; however, return-to-fight management in combat sports participants remains much less standardized. Commonly used guidelines for return-to-sport progression after concussion are inconsistently applied, with significant variability being dependent upon the jurisdiction of medical suspension. In MMA and boxing, medical suspensions are generally issued after a technical knockout (TKO) or knockout (KO). During these restricted periods, fighters are prohibited from sparring and competition, but not from other activities, such non-contact risk conditioning. These suspensions range from 30 to 180 days, but vary greatly in criteria, uniformity, and regulation by the various athletic commissions.[15–18] The transient nature of fighters also provides a frequent barrier in delivering "best practice" medicine, as many competitors often travel to different jurisdictions or even internationally for training camps and competition; subsequently outpatient follow-up with these individuals is inconsistent at best, and nonexistent, at worst.

The frequency of acute traumatic brain injury (ATBI) in amateur boxing is low. The most common type of ATBI is concussion; however, more moderate to severe brain injuries such as diffuse axonal injury, cerebral contusion, subdural hematoma, intracranial hemorrhage, or epidural hematoma may uncommonly be experienced by participants.[19] A realistic aim in combat sports is ATBI risk reduction and minimization of injury, rather than elimination altogether. This goal is accomplished by performing prefight examinations to identify individuals predisposed to catastrophic brain injury. In Kentucky, for example, recent changes were instituted by the Kentucky Boxing and Wrestling Commission (KBWC) at the beginning of 2017 with the aim of improved fighter health & safety.[20] Combatants' comprehensive physicals are now required 15 days prior to licensure, so as to allow adequate time for the Commission's Medical Advisory Panel to review license applications.

Historically, most competitors in boxing, kickboxing, or MMA would be licensed on the day of the bout. A recurrent concern with this model, however, was that a pre-fight physical was not as in-depth as a physical conducted in a clinical setting, such as an outpatient physician's office. The doctors who attend these events must screen numerous contestants, so the time spent with each athlete is limited. Recognizing this concern, the KBWC now mandates that boxers, kickboxers, and mixed martial artists be required to have a comprehensive physical performed before the Commission issues a license. For the accuracy of medical history, this physical must be within the 90 days previous of an applicant seeking licensure. The KBWC also now mandates that an applicant for licensure apply for a license at least 15 days in advance of any scheduled bout, whether professional or amateur. This regulation is required to permit the KBWC's Medical Advisory Panel sufficient time to review an applicant's medical records to determine the applicant's fitness for licensure. Under the old model, such review was impossible, as a fighter was licensed and received a physical only hours before the fighter was set to compete. The accessibility of the Commission's Medical Advisory Panel also allows for the prompt review and subsequent approval of licensure applications in those rare, but unavoidable, situations that fight cards are altered within the 15 day pre-fight period.

The KBWC felt this approach was feasible for applicants, as virtually all health insurance plans cover 100% of the cost of a yearly physical. Combatants can, therefore, have their physician complete the Commission's required physical, and not require extensive out-of-pocket expense. Furthermore, pre-fight physicals, that all contestants must undergo, are provided free of charge. Finally, and most importantly, these changes were felt to be medically necessary to ensure the health and safety of all combatants, while drawing an appropriate balance against unnecessary restrictions.

The pathogenesis of fatal sport-related head injury in young athletes remains controversial. In Japan, judo-related fatalities due to brain injury are occurring at increased frequency and have become an issue of significant public concern[21]; however, validated epidemiologic data are less commonly reported. Deaths to boxing participants have been reported in a more comprehensive manner than judo-related fatalities, or any other combat sport type. The majority of deaths from boxing result from a subdural hematoma, and are often associated with an immediate loss of consciousness during a fight.[22,23] Although a small number of deaths in other combat sports have been the subject of a few case reports, rates of death in those sports cannot be accurately determined based upon the available literature.[24,25]

Neuroimaging applications extend far beyond their ability to rule out evidence of diffuse axonal injury or acute blood product formation following head trauma. Pre-participation radiographic screening can prove invaluable in the setting of preexisting intracranial pathology that may predispose to catastrophic outcomes. The primary objective with such imaging is to identify a structural lesion such as subdural or epidural hematoma, vascular malformation or aneurysm, or space-occupying arach-noid cyst, which could further elevate a fighter's morbidity and mortality during competition.[26] If detected, the significance of an abnormality is deferred to the respec-tive commission's chief medical officer or medical advisory panel. Subsequently, a fighter could conceivably be prohibited from obtaining licensure in one state due to intracranial pathology, while concurrently obtaining formal clearance to fight in another jurisdiction. Within the context of combat sports, there is no evidence-based data from which to derive guidelines for optimal frequency of MRI imaging; however, to reduce the likelihood of serious brain injury, serial monitoring of some type is warranted.

In addition to acute injury, chronic neurocognitive impairment is also a considerable concern in modern-day combat sports.[27,28] It has long been recognized that certain individuals exposed to cumulative head trauma may develop persistent, progressive, and even irreversible neurologic impairment despite the cessation of head trauma exposure (**Table 1**).[26] In the absence of reliable screening methods to consistently identify those fighters at high risk for CTBI, a vexing challenge for combat sports physicians and sanctioning bodies alike is determining when it is no longer safe for a participant to continue competitive involvement within the sport. It is possible that serial neuropsychological testing may help objectively identify those with chronic pro-gressive neurocognitive impairment, yet this is but one component of comprehensive neurologic monitoring. Regardless, baseline neuropsychological testing is recommen-ded so that an additional measure of recovery is available for the treating clinician to assist in return-to-fight decision making. Although inherent limitations exist, such testing can be useful in the assessment of cognitive and behavioral impairment following head trauma exposure.

Many states and jurisdictions require a more extensive neurologic evaluation for fighters considered to be "high risk." The determination of what comprises a high risk fighter is typically a confluence of factors; including age, number of rounds fought, or prolonged time period away from competition. Findings from the Professional Fighters Brain Health Study suggest that strictly using the criteria of age or number of rounds fought did not consistently correlate with decreased measures of cognitive function.[29] Instead, a Fight Exposure Index has been employed that combines several factors including age, number of professional fights, average fights per year, and num-ber of KOs. This formula, based on readily accessible information, correlates signifi-cantly with standard cognitive performance measures. Thus, the use of a risk index

Table 1 Chronic traumatic brain injury	
Long Term Consequences of Traumatic Brain Injury	
Chronic traumatic encephalopathy	Dementia pugilistica
Chronic post-concussion syndrome	Chronic neurocognitive impairment
Post-traumatic dementia	Post-traumatic cognitive impairment
Post-traumatic parkinsonism	Persistent post-traumatic headache

Data from Jordan BD. Brain injury in boxing. Clin Sports Med 2009;28:561–78.

to identify those fighters at highest risk of impairment can consistently be employed. For those fighters suspected of being higher risk, further evaluation with detailed neuroimaging, formal neuropsychological testing, and clinical neurologic evaluation is recommended. Further testing, such as PET imaging or specific MRI modalities (functional, diffusion tensor, or susceptibility weighted) may be indicated at the discretion of the treating neurologist or neurosurgeon.

HEADGEAR

The introduction of mandated headgear was introduced into Olympic boxing at the 1984 Los Angeles games due to an American Medical Association demand out of concern for long-term neurocognitive impairment in boxers. There was no scientific basis for this transition nor were the head guards designed to reduce the risk of head injury. The original use of headgear was designed to reduce the incidence of facial cuts; however, it is theorized that its use could potentially provide added protection due to energy absorption, and a displacement of peak impact to a greater surface area upon localized impact.[30] Since its inception, subsequent neurosurgical and neurotrauma literature specific to the topic has suggested that headgear efficacy is limited to moderate to severe head trauma, rather than mild traumatic brain injury (TBI) such as concussion.[31] More recent evidence also suggests that patients equipped with headgear do not have improved clinical outcome or protection against concussion when compared to an unhelmeted cohort.[32] Despite opportunistic marketing and a public perception otherwise, it remains unclear to what degree helmets are effective in concussion risk reduction.

The combat sports-specific literature within the context of headgear is quite sparse. In 2013, O'Sullivan and colleagues[33] showed that standard taekwondo headgear does not protect against low-energy (50 g) or high energy (150 g) head impacts thought to result in concussion. Two studies on amateur boxing revealed further evidence showing limited protection offered by headgear. A 2013 study by Bianco and colleagues[34] found that mandatory headgear use was associated with an overall increase in "referee stopped contest due to head injury," as well as "referee stopped contest" injuries overall. Bartsch, and colleagues[35] investigated the use of padded headgear and gloves in mixed martial artists. They found a reduction in linear impact dose, but no effect on rotational impact forces. The addition of headgear also led to increased weaponization of the head, as boxers developed a style of fighting with head placement more forward, resulting in an increase in head-to-head contact with their opponents. In 2013, the Amateur International Boxing Association (AIBA) ultimately mandated the banning of headgear in amateur male competition, citing internal data by chairman of the AIBA medical commission, Dr Charles Butler.[36] Dr Butler reported that removal of headgear was associated with reduced concussion rates among amateur boxers. Specifically, 7545 rounds without headgear use resulted in a concussion rate of 0.17%, while 7352 rounds with headgear resulted in an increased concussion rate of 0.38%. Of interesting note, this transition to headgear removal applied to adult-level amateur males only. It remains unclear why these rule changes were not extended to females and youth athletes also, as the mechanism of injury in those populations would be expected to be the same. To date, all female (any level) and all junior level male boxers are mandated to continue the usage of headgear in competition.

A number of other factors potentially increasing neurologic risk were considered during the evaluation of headgear efficacy. There is some concern that headgear decreases peripheral vision, allowing heavier kicks to be landed to the head, while concurrently slowing the fighter from taking any counter-defensive measure.[37] It is also important to note that increased cranial weight and bulk from headgear may contribute to greater magnitudes of injury via additional surface areas, which ultimately augment the force of contact.[38] In summary, there is little to no convincing evidence in the medical literature showing that mandatory use of headgear is necessary to either prevent head injury or to reduce concussion risk. A limitation of most pertinent published studies, however, is that headgear regulations have often coincided with other rule changes and implementation. For this reason, it is very difficult to definitively state the effects of mandatory headgear use alone.

WEIGHT-CUTTING

Combat sports medicine physicians remain gravely concerned over the increased occurrence and popularity of weight-cutting. There are overt dangers associated with dehydration, including electrolyte imbalance, hypoglycemia, and the danger of over-rehydration. To ensure a fair & competitive balance among participants, as well as guard against preventable injury, match-making for combat sport involves competition within specific weight classes. In attempt to obtain a competitive advantage within their respective weight class, many participants acutely reduce body mass & weight through a process known as "weight-cutting." This potentially provides an advantage by being the larger and stronger combatant while competing against lighter, weaker, and smaller opponents. Subsequently, many combat sports athletes compete in weight classes 5% to 10% below their normal body weight.[39,40] The prevalence of acute weight reduction is very high in certain combat sports, such as judo, wrestling, karate, boxing, jujitsu, and taekwondo.[41] Of significant concern is a population of younger athletes employing aggressive weight reduction measures. Artioli, and colleagues[39] found that approximately 60% of judo participants utilized rapid weight-cutting practices before competitions at very young ages (ie, 12–15 years). Another study found that 33% of high school wrestlers competed during season below minimum wrestling weight. Minimum wrestling weight was defined as a body fat measurement of 5% or less.[42] Evidence suggests that rapid weight cycling during adolescence can be problematic due to its negative impact upon development and growth.[43] Furthermore, it has been suggested that weight-cutting in youth athletes is associated with a higher risk of obesity after ceasing competitive sport participation.[43]

Despite objective evidence on the negative impact of acute dehydration upon various health-related parameters, combat sports have remained steeped in their own tradition and culture of weight-reducing measures. Although data concerning these practices are beginning to accumulate, the specific study of weight-cutting in combat sports is still a largely under-researched space. In instances of strict pre-bout weight monitoring of participants, weight losses of 3 to 4 kg are not uncommon in the week preceding competition.[39,44–47] A 2013 study evaluated thirty-two collegiate wrestlers who had initiated weight-cutting measures a day before pre-practice and post-practice testing.[48] The authors found pre-match decreased performance on both neuropsychometric measures as well as balance testing. A 2015 study of elite wrestlers found that 60.7% were found to be dehydrated (ie, plasma osmolarity of >290 mOsm/L) on the day of competition.[49] These practices of rapid weight loss invariably result in significant discrepancies among competitors. In sports such as wrestling and taekwondo, weight discrepancies of up to 10 kg may exist between weight divisions, whereas weight classes in professional and amateur boxing are separated by no more than 3 to 4 kg.[50] However, after weigh-in has been completed in competitive boxing or MMA, rehydration in excess of 9 kg by the time of actual competition has been reported.[51] This potentially allows for a significant mismatch within the ring/cage when a fighter rehydrates to 1, or even 2, weight-classes above his opponent by the time of actual competition.

In response to such situations and an overriding concern for fighter health & safety, the California State Athletic Commission in April of 2017 proposed an ambitious plan to address these ongoing concerns in a systematic manner.[52] Among the proposed revisions include: licensing fighters by weight class; the addition of new weight classes; making fighters move up a division if they miss weight more than once; dehydration checks; and 30-day and 10-day weight checks for high-level title fights. Arguably, the most substantial proposed change is a mandatory weight check on fight day to see if the athlete has gained back more than 10% of his or her body weight after weigh-ins. Per the proposal, if the fighter puts on more weight than the 10%, the fighter would be required to increase weight classification (ie, go up in weight) for his or her next bout.

Acute dehydration can also affect brain morphology, which has key implications, particularly in neurologic health. A study of regional brain changes found that rapid dehydration resulted in ventricular dilation, with the largest volume expansion occurring in the left lateral ventricle and an associated relative decrease in total brain volume.[53] Another study in adolescents observed a significant correlation between bodyweight loss and percentage change in ventricular volume, indicating that greater reductions in body mass were proportional with increases in lateral ventricular volumes.[54] The observed lateral ventricular enlargement is thought, in part, due to an osmotic gradient induced by acute dehydration. This gradient results in water leaving intracellular stores, causing a relative volume loss in astrocytes, which are key components of intracellular water & nutrient transport. The relatively subtle, but definite, degree of brain atrophy may manifest as a compensatory increase in ventricular volume.

Several studies have linked acute dehydration with an increased risk for musculoskeletal injuries during practice or competition.[55–57] The concern for acute and chronic brain injury is also heightened in the context of acute dehydration. Dehydration is accompanied by a number of adaptive hormonal responses that are aimed at the conservation of body fluids, including an increase in plasma vasopressin concentration. Vasopressin can substantially reduce blood flow to the choroid plexus, in turn, decreasing cerebrospinal fluid (CSF) formation.[58] CSF acts as a cushion, mitigating the effects of brain movement inside the skull after sudden jarring movements and/or impacts. Dehydration and concussion share a similar symptomatology, including dizziness, headache, and imbalance. It is critical for sports medicine personnel to understand how weight-cutting tactics affect clinical concussion measures in order to provide appropriate care to combat sport athletes. Unfortunately, negative effects of weight-cutting tactics can significantly skew the accuracy of clinical concussion assessments.[48] Furthermore, much like other realms of sports concussion research, there is a tremendous paucity of data investigating any potential link of acute dehydration and increased risk of neurologic injury. Clearly more information is needed to definitively establish an evidence-based association; however, until such data is available, clinicians should continue to utilize "best practices" medicine, and operate under the assumption of acute dehydration lowering the threshold for concussive injury.

Lastly, the psychological component of weight-cutting in combat sports athletes is often minimized or discounted altogether. For some competitors, strict weight regulation propagates the self-image of being, "a real athlete".[59] Weight-cutting in combat sports has also been intertwined as a long held tradition and culture of the sport;

however, few studies, however, have further explored the assumed mental and physical benefits or shortcomings of acute weight reduction among combat sport athletes. A 2013 study of Swiss Olympic combat sport athletes (wrestling, judo, and taekwondo) revealed the practice of weight-cutting to be a primary component of sport identity through both self-perception of one's standing as an athlete, as well how an athlete was perceived by others.[59] Consequently, the general practice of rapid weight cycling for the purpose of enhanced athletic performance and perceived competitive advantage was openly encouraged by coaches and teammates. Although recent efforts through entities such as the California State Athletic Commission (described previously) are commendable and long overdue, rule changes alone could potentially fail to address the deeply held beliefs and positive psychological effects associated with weight regulation. Psychological counseling provided for these athletes may be a viable adjunct to aid in the transition away from this longstanding practice and its closely held association with sport identity.[59]

PERFORMANCE ENHANCING DRUGS

The practice of performance enhancement via artificial means and/or compensatory substances is as old as competitive sport itself. As early as BC 776, Greek Olympians are rumored to have used substances such as mushrooms, dried figs, and strychnine to increase their athletic prowess.[60] The first death attributed to a performance enhancing drug (PED) occurred in 1896, when a Welsh cyclist, Andrew Linton, overdosed on a stimulant, trimethyl, although there is some dispute regarding the factual accuracy of the case.[61] The first report concerning the use of anabolic-androgenic steroids (AAS) by a competitive athlete dates back to 1954.[62] Reliable testing for anabolic steroids within Olympic sports was finally introduced in 1974. The International Olympic Committee formally added AAS to its list of prohibited substances in 1976.[63] AAS consistently remain the most commonly used PEDs in modern day Olympic competition. Their reach into the world of combat sports is undeniable despite their prohibition due to health concerns and the unfair competitive advantage provided. Their use also often violates federal laws within the United States regarding controlled substances; regardless, speculation suggests that PED use is more prevalent in combat sports today perhaps than ever before, in amateur and professional ranks alike.

Within the United States, drug testing via United States Anti-Doping Agency (USADA) guidelines has long been the ultimate standard for most professional and NCAA sport participants; however, mandatory Olympic-style drug testing in combat sports is present only at the highest levels of competition. Standard USADA testing can reportedly cost up to $50,000 per fighter for 8 weeks of random testing in the time surrounding a bout.[64] Low -level promoters and smaller state athletic commissions are often unable to ensure the testing of all fighters due to inherent financial constraints. Within the United States, state-to-state variations are commonplace, with some states requiring mandatory testing only for title bouts, while others have no formal testing policy whatsoever. Because of this, lower-level fighters can conceivably avoid detection if they were to continue to fight in venues outside certain jurisdictions or promotions. With no federal oversight or national governing body, such practice variations will almost certainly continue to persist, despite its detriment to the competitors in the ring and/or cage.

Boxers and MMA fighters indeed have unique sport-specific risks when stepping onto the stage of competition; however, fighters agree to face their opponents within a specific weight range, in accordance to the rules of their sport, including the working assumption that their opponent is void of PEDs. The consequences of PEDs extend far beyond what they may do to the offending party. It can be problematic for the unknowing opponent and decrease the threshold for catastrophic injury in this genre of sport where head trauma is routinely encountered. Due to the inherent risks of combat sports, having all fighters, professional or amateur, subjected to mandatory testing, is not unreasonable.

Testosterone remains a mainstay within the world of PED testing. This naturally occurring hormone plays a critical role in neuronal function; however, supratherapeutic levels can have harmful effects within the central nervous system. Estrada and colleagues[65] suggested that increased amounts of testosterone initiate the apoptotic cascade in otherwise healthy neurons. The authors found that elevated testosterone concentrations increased cell death, with these effects having longterm and potentially permanent effects on brain function. How AAS influence the brain's threshold of concussive injury remains largely unknown; however, a 2016 rodent study revealed that AAS exposure significantly exacerbates microgliosis and axonal injury after head trauma.[66] This suggests that AAS exposure likely alters the inherent neuronal response to mild traumatic brain injury (mTBI). An earlier study using a standard acceleration-deceleration model of mTBI, however, revealed no deleterious effect of AAS on the brain following head trauma.[67] Although approximately 20% of CTE cases report a history of substance use, including AAS, it remains uncertain whether a history of AAS use influences the behavioral and neuropathological responses seen with head trauma.[68] Well-designed prospective studies are necessary to better understand how AAS influence the long-term trajectory of post-TBI neurocognitive deficits.

A more recent structural study found negative correlations between AAS use and cortical thickness and brain volume.[69] Specifically AAS users, when compared to non-using controls, had thinner cortex measurements in multiple regions, as well as significantly smaller neuroanatomical volumes, including total gray matter, cerebral cortex, and putamen. Both thickness and volumetric measures remained relatively stable across different AAS subsets representing various degrees of AAS exposure. These findings raise concerns about possible deleterious effects of long-term AAS use on brain health. The cortical effects seem to persist after stopping AAS use. Large-scale longitudinal, and ideally prospective, studies are warranted to address the possible implication of accelerated cerebral atrophy caused by long-term AAS exposure.

SUMMARY

Neurologic injuries of both an acute and chronic nature have been reported in the literature for various combat sport styles; however reports of the incidence and prevalence of these injury types vary greatly. Large scale longitudinal, and ideally prospective, studies, such as the *Professional Fighters Brain Health Study* at the Lou Ruvo Center for Brain Health in Las Vegas, Nevada, are warranted to address the underlying neurologic implications of combat sport participation. Furthermore, newer areas of concern unrelated to direct head trauma exposure, such as the neurologic implications of weight-cutting and PEDs, also warrant systematic surveillance and diligent study by the combat sports medicine community. Concussion and lasting brain damage, however, remains the most significant risk for in this genre of sport, where the aim is, in fact, to deliver a concussive injury to the opponent. Combat sports clinicians must continue to strive for the development, implementation, and enforcement of uniform minimum requirements for neurologic safety. These health care providers must also seize upon the honor to provide this oft-underserved population with the health care advocacy they very much deserve, but often do not receive. As a whole, we can ensure both the long-term health of the athlete/patient within the ring of competition as well as the long-term viability of the sport itself.

REFERENCES

1. American Academy of Pediatrics, Council on Sports Medicine and Fitness, Canadian Paediatric Society, Healthy Active Living and Sports Medicine Committee. Policy statement–Boxing participation by children and adolescents. Pediatrics 2011;128:617–23.
2. Australian Medical Association. Boxing: 1997–reaffirmed. 2007. Available at: http://ama.com.au/node/444. Accessed April 06, 2017.
3. British Medical Association. Boxing: an update from the board of science. 2008. Available at: http://bmaopac.hosted.exlibrisgroup.com/exlibris/aleph/a21_1/apache_media/15BMGJ6PDYJ3HVSYNKPHV81SYB8ATR.pdf. Accessed April 06, 2017.
4. Lundberg GD. Boxing should be banned in civilized countries. JAMA 1983;249:250.
5. Dillner L. Boxing should be counted out, says BMA report. BMJ 1993;306:1561–2.
6. Cohen L. Should the sport of boxing be banned in Canada? Can Med Assoc J 1984;130:767–8.
7. Ross DJ, Hafner JW Jr, Yahuaca BI, et al. Injury patterns of mixed martial arts athletes in the United States. Ann Emerg Med 2013;62(4S):S108.
8. Zazryn T, Cameron P, McCrory P. A prospective cohort study of injury in amateur and professional boxing. Br J Sports Med 2006;40(8):670–4.
9. McLatchie G. Analysis of karate injuries sustained in 295 contests. Injury 1976;8(2):132–4.
10. Stricevic M, Patel M, Okazaki T, et al. Karate: historical perspective and injuries sustained in national and international tournament competitions. Am J Sports Med 1983;11(6):320–4.
11. Arriaza R, Leyes M. Injury profile in competitive karate: prospective analysis of three consecutive World Karate Championships. Knee Surg Sports Traumatol Arthrosc 2005;13:603–7.
12. Zemper E, Pieter W. Injury rates during the 1988 US Olympic team trials for taekwondo. Br J Sports Med 1989;23(3):161–4.
13. McLatchie G, Morris E. Prevention of karate injuries—a progress report. Br J Sports Med 1977;11:78–82.
14. Jordan BD. Chronic traumatic brain injury associated with boxing. Semin Neurol 2000;20:179–86.
15. Association of Boxing Commissions. Regulatory guidelines. Available at: http://abcboxing.com/documents/abcboxing_regulatory_guidelines.htm. Accessed April 06, 2017.
16. Medical Commission of the International Boxing Association. Medical handbook for boxing. Available at: http://www.aiba.org/documents/site1/docs/Medical%20Handbook%202013.pdf. Accessed April 06, 2017.
17. North Carolina Department of Public Safety. Boxing authority section of alcohol law enforcement division. Available at: https://www.ncdps.gov/div/boxing/documents/ncboxingrules.pdf. Accessed April 06, 2017.

18. World Medical Association. WMA statement on boxing. Available at: www.wma. net/en/30publications/10policies/b6/index.html. Accessed April 06, 2017.

19. Morris S, Jones WH, Proctor MR, et al. Emergent treatment of athletes with brain injury. Neurosurgery 2014;75:S96–105.

20. Kentucky Boxing and Wrestling Commission. Laws and Regulations. Available at: http://kbwa.ky.gov/Documents/Laws%20and%20Regulations.pdf. Accessed April 06, 2017.

21. Yokota H, Ida Y. Acute subdural hematoma in a judo player with repeated head injuries. World Neurosurg 2016;91(671):671.e1–3.

22. Unterharnscheidt F. A neurologist's reflection on boxing. 3:Vascular injuries. Rev Neurol 1995;23(122):847–55.

23. Cantu R. Head injuries in sport. Br J Sports Med 1996;30(4):289–96.

24. Oler M, Tomson W, Pepe H, et al. Morbidity and mortality in the martial arts: a warning. J Trauma 1991;31(2):251–3.

25. Jackson F, Earle K, Beamer Y, et al. Blunt head injuries incurred by marine recruits in hand-to-hand combat (judo training). Mil Med 1967;132(10):803–8.

26. Jordan BD. Brain injury in boxing. Clin Sports Med 2009;28:561–78.

27. McKee AC, Cantu RC, Nowinski CJ, et al. Chronic traumatic encephalopathy in athletes: progressive tauopathy after repetitive head injury. J Neuropathol Exp Neurol 2009;68:709–35.

28. Omalu B, Bailes J, Hamilton RL, et al. Emerging histomorphologic phenotypes of chronic traumatic encephalopathy in American athletes. Neurosurgery 2011;69: 173–83.

29. Bernick C, Banks S, Phillips M, et al. Professional fighters brain health study: rationale and methods. Am J Epidemiol 2013;178:280–6.

30. Medina M, Avila J. New perspectives on the role of tau in Alzheimer's disease. Implications for therapy. Biochem Pharmacol 2014;88:540–7.

31. Sone JY, Kondziolka D, Huang JH, et al. Helmet efficacy against concussion and traumatic brain injury: a review. J Neurosurg 2017;126(3):768–81.

32. Zuckerman SL, Lee YM, Odom MJ, et al. Sports-related concussion in helmeted vs. unhelmeted athletes: who fares worse? Int J Sports Med 2015;36:419–25.

33. O'Sullivan DM, Fife GP, Pieter W, et al. Safety performance evaluation of taekwondo headgear. Br J Sports Med 2013;47(7):447–51.

34. Bianco M, Loosemoore M, Daniele G, et al. Amateur boxing in the last 59 years. Impact of rules changes on the type of verdicts recorded and implications on boxers' health. Br J Sports Med 2013;47(7):452–7.

35. Bartsch AJ, Benzel EC, Miele VJ, et al. Boxing and mixed martial arts: preliminary traumatic neuromechanical injury risk analyses from laboratory impact dosage data. J Neurosurg 2012;116(5):1070–80.

36. Wang SS. Boxing group bans headgear to reduce concussions. The Wall Street Journal 2013.

37. McCrory P, Falvey E, Turner M. Returning to the golden age of boxing. Br J Sports Med 2012;46:459–60.

38. Timperley W. Banning boxing. Br Med J (Clin Res Ed) 1982;285:289.

39. Artioli GG, Gualano B, Franchini E, et al. Prevalence, magnitude, and methods of rapid weight loss among judo competitors. Med Sci Sports Exerc 2010;42(3): 436–42.

40. Filaire E, Sagnol M, Ferrand C, et al. Psychophysiological stress in judo athletes during competitions. J Sports Med Phys Fitness 2001;41(2):263–8.

41. Franchini E, Brito CJ, Artioli GG. Weight loss in combat sports: physiological, psychological and performance effects. J Int Soc Sports Nutr 2012;9(1):52.

42. Wroble RR, Moxley DP. Acute weight gain and its relationship to success in high school wrestlers. Med Sci Sports Exerc 1998;30(6):949–51.

43. Roemmich JN, Sinning WE. Weight loss and wrestling training: effects on growth-related hormones. J Appl Physiol 1997;82:1760–4.

44. Alderman BL, Landers DM, Carlson J, et al. Factors related to rapid weight loss practices among international-style wrestlers. Med Sci Sports Exerc 2004;36: 249–52.

45. Fleming S, Costarelli V. Eating behaviours and general practices used by Taekwondo players in order to make weight before competition. Nutr Food Sci 2009;39:16–23.

46. Hall CJ, Lane AM. Effects of rapid weight loss on mood and performance among amateur boxers. Br J Sports Med 2001;35:390–5.

47. Oppliger RA, Steen SA, Scott JR. Weight loss practices of college wrestlers. Int J Sport Nutr Exerc Metab 2003;13:29–46.

48. Weber AF, Mihalik JP, Register-Mihalik JK, et al. Dehydration and performance on clinical concussion measures in collegiate wrestlers. J Athl Train 2013;48(2): 153–60.

49. Irfan Y. Associations among dehydration, testosterone and stress hormones in terms of body weight loss before competition. Am J Med Sci 2015;350(2):103–8.

50. Langan-Evans C, Close GL, Morton JP. Making weight in combat sports. Strength Cond J 2011;33(6):25–39.

51. Jetton AM, Lawrence MM, Meucci M, et al. Dehydration and acute weight gain in mixed martial arts fighters before competition. J Strength Cond Res 2013;27(5): 1322–6.

52. Okamoto B. Ten-point plan intended to curb weight cutting coming to California. 2017. Available at: http://www.espn.com/mma/story/_/id/19023891/mma-ten-point-plan-intended-curb-weight-cutting-coming-california. Accessed April 07, 2017.

53. Kempton MJ, Ettinger U, Schmechtig A, et al. Effects of acute dehydration on brain morphology in healthy humans. Hum Brain Mapp 2009;30(1):291–8.

54. Kempton MJ, Ettinger U, Foster R, et al. Dehydration affects brain structure and function in healthy adolescents. Hum Brain Mapp 2011;32(1):71–9.

55. Agel J, Ransone J, Dick R, et al. Descriptive epidemiology of collegiate men's wrestling injuries: National Collegiate Athletic Association Injury Surveillance System, 1988–1989 through 2003–2004. J Athl Train 2007;42:303–10.

56. Oopik V, Paasuke M, Sikku T, et al. Effect of rapid weight loss on metabolism and isokinetic performance capacity. A case study of two well trained wrestlers. J Sports Med Phys Fitness 1996;36:127–31.

57. Green CM, Petrou MJ, Fogarty–Hover MLS, et al. Injuries among judokas during competition. Scand J Med Sci Sports 2007;17:205–10.

58. Faraci FM, Mayhan WG, Heistad DD. Effect of vasopressin on production of cerebrospinal fluid: possible role of vasopressin (V1)-receptors. Am J Physiol 1990; 258(1):R94–8.

59. Pettersson S, Ekstrom MP, Berg CM. Practices of weight regulation among elite athletes in combat sports: a matter of mental advantage? J Athl Train 2013; 48(1):99–108.

60. Grivetti LE, Applegate EA. From Olympia to Atlanta: a cultural historical perspective on diet and athletic training. J Nutr 1997;127(suppl):860–8.

61. Dimeo P. A history of drug use in sport 1876-1976: beyond good and evil. London: Routledge Publishing; 2007.

62. Yesalis CE, Courson SP, Wright J. History of anabolic steroid use in sport and exercise. In: Yesalis CE, editor. Anabolic steroids in sport and exercise. 2nd edition. Champaign (IL): Human Kinetics; 2000. p. 51–71.
63. Graf-Baumann T. Medicolegal aspects of doping in football. Br J Sports Med 2006;40(Suppl 1):i55–7.
64. Mazique B. PED use in combat sports should be a criminal offense. 2016. Available at: https://www.forbes.com/sites/brianmazique/2016/07/18/ped-use-in-combat-sports-should-be-a-criminal-offense/#365d42113c17l. Accessed April 07, 2017.
65. Estrada M, Varshney A, Ehrlich BE. Elevated testosterone induces apoptosis in neuronal cells. J Biol Chem 2006;281(35):25492–501.
66. Namjoshi DR, Cheng WH, Carr M, et al. Chronic exposure to androgenic-anabolic steroids exacerbates axonal injury and microgliosis in the CHIMERA mouse model of repetitive concussion. PLoS One 2016;11(1):e0146540.
67. Mills JD, Bailes JE, Turner RC, et al. Anabolic steroids and head injury. Neurosurgery 2012;70(1):205–9.
68. Maroon JC, Winkelman R, Bost J, et al. Chronic traumatic encephalopathy in contact sports: a systematic review of all reported pathological cases. PLoS One 2015;10(2):e0117338.
69. Bjomebekk A, Walhovd KB, Jorstad ML, et al. Structural brain imaging of long-term anabolic-androgenic steroid users and nonusing weightlifters. Biol Psychiatry 2016. http://dx.doi.org/10.1016/j.biopsych.2016.06.017.

Psychiatric Comorbidities in Sports

Claudia L. Reardon, MD[a,b],*

KEYWORDS

- Psychiatry • Sports • Sports psychiatry • Athletes • Mental health • Mental illness

KEY POINTS

- Depression and anxiety disorders may occur in athletes at least as commonly as they do in the general population.
- Eating disorders, attention-deficit/hyperactivity disorder, and substance use disorders may be even more common among athletes than in the general population.
- Psychiatric disorders may have unique presentations of symptoms and behaviors in athletes.
- Medical professionals across all specialties and disciplines should be able to screen for psychiatric disorders and treat or refer for appropriate treatment if disorders are suspected.

INTRODUCTION

Athletes are not immune to mental illness. Despite strong outward appearances, they suffer from a variety of psychiatric conditions ranging from depression and anxiety to eating disorders and bipolar disorder. The relationship between sport and mental illness in any given athlete may occur in one of three ways.[1]

First, the athlete's sport may somehow cause or worsen the mental illness. For example, an athlete on a women's lightweight rowing team may develop an eating disorder because of the pressures to maintain a low body weight and the culture she sees around her of athletes engaging in disordered eating behaviors.

Second, the athlete's psychiatric symptoms may somehow draw him or her to sport, perhaps as a way to cope with the symptoms or because the symptoms are somehow adaptive for the sport. For example, a soccer player with attention-deficit/hyperactivity disorder (ADHD) of the hyperactive/impulsive subtype may have enjoyed aerobic sports from a young age because they helped him dissipate energy, and

Dr C.L. Reardon has nothing to disclose.
[a] Department of Psychiatry, University of Wisconsin School of Medicine and Public Health, 6001 Research Park Boulevard, Madison, WI 53719, USA; [b] Counseling and Consultation Services, University Health Services, 333 East Campus Mall, Madison, WI 53715, USA
* Department of Psychiatry, University of Wisconsin School of Medicine and Public Health, 6001 Research Park Boulevard, Madison, WI 53719.
E-mail address: clreardon@wisc.edu

running around the playing field was much easier than sitting still to work on homework.

Finally, there may be no evident relationship between the sport and mental illness. For example, a diver may develop a major depressive episode in the middle of her career related to significant family stressors and underlying genetic predisposition that have nothing to do with diving.

This paper summarizes research and clinical experience on the presentation, epidemiology, and treatment principles of some of the most common psychiatric comorbidities in sports. Within these conditions, any of the previously mentioned three relationships between the sport and the mental illness may be seen.

MOOD DISORDERS
Major Depressive Disorder

Precipitants for depression in athletes may include the following[1]:

- Any of the same genetic or environmental factors that trigger depression in the general population
- Injury
- Competitive failure
- Retirement from sport, with predictors for postretirement depression including more psychological attachment to sport,[2] more devotion to sport to the exclusion of other activities,[2] less current physical activity,[3] and more physical pain[4]
- Overtraining (OT)
- Concussion[5]

The relationship between OT and depression is particularly complex, and OT is difficult to distinguish from primary major depressive disorder. Fatigue is a core overlap symptom between the two conditions, and a common source of referral to sports psychiatrists. A trial of rest from sport can help in distinguishing the two. Rest from sport should improve OT symptoms, whereas it would not be expected to do so, and in fact could even worsen symptoms, in primary depression.[1] Additionally, in OT, the primary realm of dysfunction caused by the symptoms is in the sport itself, whereas primary depression would also be expected to cause deterioration in work, social, and cognitive performance.[6]

Various reports have described rates of depression within different levels of athletes. At the high school level, at least one report has suggested that athletes have a decreased likelihood of depression and suicidal ideation compared with the general population.[7] At the college level, two studies of Division 1 athletes suggest similar frequencies of depression among college athletes compared with the general college population.[8,9] At the elite or professional level, there is a paucity of data comparing rates of depression in this cohort as compared with the general population. Within German elite athletes, 15% self-reported depression.[10] Within French elite athletes, 3.6% had diagnosable depression based on clinician interview.[11] However, neither of these studies reported comparison groups, so relative frequency of depression compared with the general population is unknown. Overall, rates of depression in athletes are suspected to be approximately similar to those in the general population based on available research.[1]

Bipolar Disorder

Bipolar disorder involves episodes of persistently and abnormally elevated, expansive, or irritable mood. Usually major depressive episodes also occur. Bipolar disorder in athletes has received minimal study, unfortunately.

It is possible to see substance-induced mood disorders, with either manic features or depressive features, in athletes who use anabolic steroids.[12] Another unique issue that has arisen in the literature is the possibility that vigorous exercise, as of course often occurs in athletes, may precipitate or worsen manic episodes in predisposed athletes.[13] Although this needs further study, the possibility is not necessarily surprising, because exercise is known to have antidepressant effects.[14] Many other interventions or behaviors that have antidepressant effects (eg, monotherapy with antidepressant medications, phototherapy, sleep deprivation) also may cause mania.

It is unknown how prevalent bipolar disorder is among athletes.

Treatment

Some principles apply when treating mood disorders in athletes. Individual psychotherapy alone may be sufficient treatment of mild cases of depression, or may be used in combination with medications. Athletes are good candidates for cognitive behavioral therapy (CBT), because they are accustomed to structure, direction, practice, goal setting, and self-reliance.[15]

Medications are often needed in bipolar disorder and in moderate to severe major depressive disorder. Choose medications that are more energizing, less sedating, and less likely to cause weight gain or cardiac toxicity. Fluoxetine has been better studied than have other antidepressants in athletes and may be a reasonable first choice for major depressive disorder.[1] Bupropion may also be a reasonable choice for this condition if comorbid anxiety is not present and the athlete is not vigorously exercising in extremely hot temperatures.[1]

Many mood stabilizers for bipolar disorder have side effects, such as tremor, weight gain, and sedation, which would be problematic for athletes. Antipsychotics, such as aripiprazole, that have fewer sedating and weight gain qualities are likely to be better tolerated. For less severe bipolar disorder, such as bipolar II disorder, lamotrigine may be a well-tolerated monotherapy option, although its antimanic effects are not as powerful as its antidepressant ones.[16]

ANXIETY DISORDERS
Sport-Related Performance Anxiety

Anxiety disorders have been less well-studied in athletes than depression has been. The data that exist suggest that of importance is distinguishing symptoms and behaviors in athletes that may resemble anxiety disorders, but are not pathologic, from the actual disorders, because there can be overlap. For example, athletes may become reasonably anxious before or during competition, and this is not pathologic if not extreme or detrimental to performance.[17] Such anxiety may even be facilitative, resulting in improved performance.[17] However, performance-associated anxiety can result in deterioration of performance to the point of causing a "slump" (an extended period of performance at a level less than demonstrated capabilities) or "choke" (debilitation to the point of acute inability to participate in sport).[17] Although sport-related performance anxiety per se does not always meet criteria for a specific anxiety disorder, it may warrant treatment if it is impacting functioning in sport, which is an area important to the athlete.[17]

Generalized Anxiety Disorder

Clinicians should evaluate for warning signs of actual anxiety disorders. For example, multiple worries extending beyond sport, causing significant distress and dysfunction, and present much of the time for at least 6 months suggest possible generalized anxiety disorder. This has not been uniquely studied in athletes.

Panic Disorder

Full-blown panic attacks may suggest panic disorder. Research generally shows that exercise has an overall anxiolytic effect, but some studies demonstrate that exercise can trigger heightened anxiety and acute panic attacks, with up to one-third of patients with panic disorder and/or agoraphobia reporting increased anxiety during acute exercise.[18] Consequently, people with panic disorder may avoid exercise.[19] The association between exercise and panic may relate to the physical sensations of exercise, such as shortness of breath, mimicking those of panic, and thus the panic disorder–suffering exerciser worries he or she indeed is going to have a panic attack, which exacerbates further symptoms of panic.[20] Although the association of panic attacks with exercise in the athlete population per se has not been studied, clinicians should be aware that athletes are not immune from this condition. If an athlete presents with panic attacks, and concomitant with development of that condition is discussing dropping out of sport, the clinician should evaluate if the athlete's panic seems worse when exercising. In such a situation, treating the panic disorder, and not encouraging phobic avoidance of sport and exercise, is the recommended intervention.

Social Anxiety Disorder

A pattern of fear of social evaluation, especially if extending to other social venues outside of sport, merits evaluation for social anxiety disorder. One study of 180 students showed a correlation between social anxiety and avoidance of individual sports but not team sports.[21] It is important to distinguish social anxiety disorder from sport-related performance anxiety. In true social anxiety disorder, the focus of fears is interaction with and scrutiny by others, whereas in sport-related performance anxiety, the symptoms are limited to sport participation, with fear of scrutiny by others not a primary factor.[17]

Obsessive Compulsive Disorder

Rituals and superstition are prevalent among athletes, who often face significant unpredictability, such as in what their opponent does, the weather, the spectators, and whether they catch an illness before competition. Rituals help athletes feel more in control. Such rituals must be distinguished from obsessive compulsive disorder (OCD).[22] Although most rituals and superstitions are harmless and may even be helpful, they can evolve into OCD. In the latter case, the rituals become increasingly rigid, take up more and more of the athlete's time, and extend outside of the athletic realm. Athletes feel distraught and anxious if the rituals cannot be performed. By definition, OCD usually involves at least an hour per day of obsessions or compulsions in a way that significantly interferes with daily functioning.

Posttraumatic Stress Disorder

Athletes may also suffer from posttraumatic stress disorder (PTSD). Traumas leading to symptoms of PTSD in this population include the usual traumas that lead to the condition in the general population, but also catastrophic injuries and catastrophic losses to self-esteem and social expectations, such as with the loss of a crucial game or public recognition as a doper.[23] If injury led to PTSD, consequences of the condition in athletes may include interference with rehabilitation and return to sport. This can happen via avoidance of challenging aspects of the sport, nightmares or flashbacks after return to the setting where the injury occurred or when watching the sport in the media, and hypervigilance leading to premature action within the sport.[23]

Medical Conditions

It is particularly important to consider medical conditions that are especially likely to present as anxiety symptoms in athletes. Asthma and vocal cord dysfunction are among the most common in the athlete population.[17]

Prevalence

Anxiety disorder prevalence among athletes has not been well studied. However, a study of Australian elite athletes asked to self-report symptoms demonstrated 14.7% met criteria for social anxiety, 7.1% for generalized anxiety disorder, and 4.5% for panic disorder.[24] The authors concluded that these numbers are similar to those observed in general populations.

Treatment

CBT without medication for sport-related performance anxiety is recommended for this condition.[17] Psychotherapy (including CBT, exposure therapy, and others) with or without selective serotonin reuptake inhibitors, such as fluoxetine, are good options for generalized anxiety disorder, panic disorder, social anxiety disorder, OCD, and PTSD. As with treatment of mood disorders, medication selection should be made with an effort to minimize impact on physical performance and to minimize likelihood of side effects that are dangerous in vigorously exercising athletes.[1]

Avoid benzodiazepines, because side effects are likely to impede sport-related performance.[1,17] β-Blockers, such as propranolol, are also generally avoided because of negative performance effects in some sports (eg, endurance sports), and unfair performance advantage in others (eg, archery).[1]

EATING DISORDERS

Eating disorders in athletes are probably the best studied psychiatric disorders in this population. The disorders include anorexia nervosa, bulimia nervosa, binge eating disorder, and other specified/unspecified eating disorder. The latter grouping may include, for example, athletes who otherwise meet the criteria for anorexia nervosa but who are within the normal weight range. Risk factors for athlete development of eating disorders include the following:

- Participation in "leanness" sports in which there are weight classes or in which lean physique is regarded as physically or aesthetically advantageous, such as lightweight rowing, distance running, figure skating, gymnastics, and diving[1]
- Female sex, although males are also at risk, especially within leanness sports; male athletes have higher rates of eating disorders than male nonathletes[25]
- Early start of sport-specific training[26]
- Perfectionism and overcompliance with coaches' recommendations[26]
- Injury[26]

Presenting symptoms and behaviors of eating disorders that are especially seen in athletes include:

- Stress fractures and other injuries
- Declining athletic performance
- Chest pain, palpitations, and dizziness when practicing or competing
- Exercising more than expected by the coach

- Sweat runs and avoidance of fluid intake before weigh-ins in weight-class sports
- Body weight that may not be significantly low, caused by significant muscle mass
- Amenorrhea even if body weight is not significantly low
- Denial of symptoms in an effort to continue participation[25] or because of a tendency toward intellectualization among perfectionistic athletes

Prevalence

Although many psychiatric conditions have not been studied in athletes such that prevalence compared with the general population is unknown, numerous studies demonstrate that eating disorders are more prevalent in athletes than in other groups.[1,25] Among elite female athletes, two well-regarded, large studies demonstrated an overall eating disorder prevalence of 18% to 20%.[27,28] Rates were found to be twice as high in leanness sports compared with other sports.[28] The same authors recently reported that up to 70% of elite athletes in weight class sports diet or exhibit abnormal eating behaviors to reduce weight before competition.[29]

Studies on the prevalence of eating disorders in high school and college athletes have been more variable, complicated by the use of self-report measures in several of these studies.[26] One study demonstrated that 32% of women collegiate varsity respondents to an anonymous survey had engaged in at least one weight-control behavior (self-induced emesis or use of laxatives, diuretics, or diet pills) daily for at least 1 month.[30] Disordered eating behaviors may be far more common than diagnosable eating disorders in the college athlete population.[31]

Assessment and Treatment

Laboratory evaluation and diagnostic testing depends on the severity of malnourishment and symptoms. All patients with eating disorders, at a minimum, should have their electrolytes, renal function, liver function, thyroid function, and blood counts checked, and assessment beyond this, such as electrocardiograms and bone density testing, may be needed in some athletes.[25]

Incorporate an experienced multidisciplinary team approach to treatment. This includes a general medical physician, dietician, psychiatrist, and psychologist. Eating disorders should be treated as injuries, with use of evidence-based return-to-play guidelines.[25,32]

Fluoxetine is a medication option that is approved by the US Food and Drug Administration for bulimia nervosa, but other antidepressants are often used off-label, for the core eating disorder symptoms and for the commonly comorbid depression and anxiety. Bupropion is contraindicated in patients with eating disorders because of seizure risk.

ATTENTION-DEFICIT/HYPERACTIVITY DISORDER

Athletes with ADHD may initially have been drawn to sport because of a general inclination toward physical activity,[33] especially when fast-paced.[34] For example, higher rates of ADHD may be seen in football, with lower rates in sports requiring extended concentration.[35] Even though athletes with ADHD may be drawn to sport, the condition can interfere with practice and competition. For example, athletes may be easily distracted and intolerant of boring or repetitive drills and may have low frustration tolerance when things are not going well.[35] They may also be at higher risk of sustaining concussion.[36]

Treatment

Behavioral interventions, such as skill-based psychotherapy, should be undertaken for all athletes with ADHD.[37]

Stimulants are performance enhancing,[1,37] and accordingly, are tightly regulated at collegiate and professional/elite levels of sport. If stimulants are needed at the US collegiate level, then clinicians must maintain appropriate documentation to be submitted to the National Collegiate Athletic Association if an athlete tests positive for this class of medications.[38] If believed necessary at the professional/elite level, then therapeutic use exemption paperwork must be completed before prescribing the medication.[39]

Nonstimulant options, such as atomoxetine and bupropion (the latter especially if depression is comorbid), are reasonable first-line approaches especially within higher levels of competition in which stimulants confer greater concerns about unfair performance enhancement.[37]

SUBSTANCE USE DISORDERS

Substance use disorders in athletes may develop for several reasons, including use of substances for the purpose of performance enhancement, or they may involve use of substances for other reasons, such as recreation, pleasure, and coping with stressors.[40] Stressors that may lead athletes to turn to substances include performance pressure, pressure from teammates, injuries, physical pain, and retirement from sport.[41] Athletes may also use substances to self-treat undiagnosed mental health disorders. Finally, the culture of certain sports, in which victories may be celebrated and losses consoled with substances, may contribute.[41]

Epidemiology

As in the general population, alcohol is the most commonly overused substance among athletes.[42] Alcohol, cannabis, and smokeless tobacco are the top three most commonly used substances, in that order, by college athletes.[43] Substances that athletes across all levels commonly use for performance-enhancement effects include anabolic steroids, stimulants, smokeless tobacco, growth hormone and growth factors, β-agonists, β-blockers, and opioids.[40] Overall, athletes seem to use substances of abuse more often than does the general population.[1]

The relationship between concussion and substance use is important. Substance use by athletes who have suffered concussion may lead to worsened cognitive impairment, more prominent disinhibition, and more prolonged intoxicating effects.[41]

Treatment

Refer for evidence-based psychotherapeutic interventions, including motivational enhancement, CBT/relapse prevention, and network therapy.[41]

Twelve-step groups, such as Alcoholics Anonymous, are helpful but athletes are often concerned about confidentiality in group settings.[41]

In cases of severe substance use disorders, medication treatment with naltrexone, acamprosate, or disulfiram for alcohol use disorder, buprenorphine for opioid use disorder, and other appropriate agents should be considered.[41]

Comorbid psychiatric illness, such as depression and anxiety, is common and should simultaneously be treated.[40]

SUMMARY

Athletes suffer from psychiatric disorders. Some such conditions, such as depression and anxiety disorders, are probably just as common in athletes as in the general population. Others, such as eating disorders, ADHD, and substance use disorders, may be even more common. Clinicians across all specialties who are working with athletes should keep in mind the following principles of evaluation and treatment, regardless of specific psychiatric condition:

- Screen athletes for mental health disorders, especially if they are presenting with conditions that are commonly comorbid with mental illness or symptoms that could be caused by mental illness.
- If necessary, refer to experienced sports medicine physicians, mental health clinicians, and other multidisciplinary team members to help in management of the suspected disorder.
- Medication choices when prescribing for athletes should be made in an effort to minimize performance-limiting side effects and safety concerns, and in accordance with antidoping rules of national and international regulatory bodies.
- Referral for psychotherapy, especially CBT, is an important part of treatment of most conditions.

REFERENCES

1. Reardon CL, Factor RM. Sport psychiatry: a systematic review of diagnosis and medical treatment of mental illness in athletes. Sports Med 2010;40(11):961–80.
2. Parham WD. The intercollegiate athlete: a 1990s profile. Couns Psychol 1993;21:411–29.
3. Backmand H, Kaprio J, Kujala U, et al. Influence of physical activity on depression and anxiety of former elite athletes. Int J Sports Med 2003;24:609–16.
4. Schwenk TL, Gorenflo DW, Dopp RR, et al. Depression and pain in retired professional football players. Med Sci Sports Exerc 2007;39(4):599–605.
5. Wolanin A, Gross M, Hong E. Depression in athletes: prevalence and risk factors. Curr Sports Med Rep 2015;14(1):56–60.
6. Schwenk TL. The stigmatization and denial of mental illness in athletes. Br J Sports Med 2000;34(1):4–5.
7. Oler MJ, Mainous AG, Martin CA, et al. Depression, suicidal ideation, and substance use among adolescents: are athletes at less risk? Arch Fam Med 1994;3:781–3.
8. Yang J, Peek-Asa C, Corlette JD, et al. Prevalence of and risk factors associated with symptoms of depression in competitive collegiate student athletes. Clin J Sport Med 2007;17(6):481–7.
9. Wolanin A, Hong E, Marks D. Prevalence of clinically elevated depressive symptoms in college athletes and differences by gender and sport. Br J Sports Med 2016;50:167–71.
10. Nixdorf I, Hautzinger M, Beckmann J. Prevalence of depressive symptoms and correlating variables among German elite athletes. J Clin Sport Psychol 2013;7(4):313–26.
11. Schael K, Tafflet M, Nassif H, et al. Psychological balance in high level athletes: gender-based differences and sport-specific patterns. PLoS One 2011;6(5):e19007.
12. Pope H, Katz D. Affective and psychotic symptoms associated with anabolic steroid use. Am J Psychiatry 1988;145(4):487–90.
13. Melo MC, Daher EF, Albuquerque SG, et al. Exercise in bipolar patients: a systematic review. J Affect Disord 2016;198:32–8.
14. Schuch FB, Vancampfort D, Richards J, et al. Exercise as a treatment for depression: a meta-analysis adjusting for publication bias. J Psychiatr Res 2016;77:42–51.

15. Stillman MA, Ritvo EC, Glick ID. Psychotherapeutic treatment of athletes and their significant others. In: Baron DA, Reardon CL, Baron SH, editors. Clinical sports psychiatry: an international perspective. Oxford (United Kingdom): Wiley-Blackwell; 2013. p. 117–23.
16. Ng F, Hallam K, Lucas N, et al. The role of lamotrigine in the management of bipolar disorder. Neuropsychiatr Dis Treat 2007;3(4):463–74.
17. Patel DR, Omar H, Terry M. Sport-related performance anxiety in young female athletes. J Pediatr Adolesc Gynecol 2010;23:325–35.
18. Cameron OG, Hudson CJ. Influence of exercise on anxiety level in patients with anxiety disorders. Psychosomatics 1986;27:720–3.
19. Broocks A, Meyer TF, Bandelow B, et al. Exercise avoidance and impaired endurance capacity in patients with panic disorder. Neuropsychobiology 1997;36: 182–7.
20. Strohle A, Graetz B, Scheel M, et al. The acute antipanic and anxiolytic activity of aerobic exercise in patients with panic disorder and healthy control subjects. J Psychiatr Res 2009;43:1013–7.
21. Northon PJ, Burns JA, Hope DA. Generalization of social anxiety to sporting and athletic situations: gender, sports involvement, and parental pressure. Depress Anxiety 2000;12:193–202.
22. Kamm RL. Interviewing principles for the psychiatrically aware sports medicine physician. Clin Sports Med 2005;24(4):745–69.
23. Wenzel T, Zhu LJ. Posttraumatic stress in athletes. In: Baron DA, Reardon CL, Baron SH, editors. Clinical sports psychiatry: an international perspective. Oxford (United Kingdom): Wiley-Blackwell; 2013. p. 102–14.
24. Gulliver A, Griffiths K, Mackinnon A, et al. The mental health of Australian elite athletes. J Sci Med Sport 2015;18(3):255–61.
25. Joy E, Kussman A, Nattiv A. 2016 update on eating disorders in athletes: a comprehensive narrative review with a focus on clinical assessment and management. Br J Sports Med 2016;50:154–62.
26. Bratland-Sanda S, Sundgot-Borgen J. Eating disorders in athletes: overview of prevalence, risk factors and recommendations for prevention and treatment. Eur J Sport Sci 2013;13(5):499–508.
27. Sundgot-Borgen J, Torstveit MK. Prevalence of eating disorders in elite athletes is higher than in the general population. Clin J Sport Med 2004;14:25–32.
28. Sundgot-Borgen J. Prevalence of eating disorders in elite female athletes. Int J Sport Nutr 1993;3:29–40.
29. Sundgot-Borgen J, Torstveit MK. Aspects of disordered eating continuum in elite high intensity sports. Scand J Med Sci Sports 2010;20(Suppl 2):112–21.
30. Burckes-Miller ME, Black DR. Behaviors and attitudes associated with eating disorders: perceptions of college athletes about food and weight. Health Educ Res 1988;3:203–8.
31. Greenleaf C, Petrie TA, Carter J, et al. Female collegiate athletes: prevalence of eating disorders and disordered eating behaviors. J Am Coll Health 2009;57(5): 489–95.
32. De Souza MJ, Nattiv A, Joy E, et al. 2014 female athlete triad coalition consensus statement on treatment and return to play of the female athlete triad: 1st International Conference held in San Francisco, California, May 2012 and 2nd International Conference held in Indianapolis, Indiana, May 2013. Br J Sports Med 2014;48:289.
33. Burton RW. Mental illness in athletes. In: Begel D, Burton RW, editors. Sport psychiatry: theory and practice. New York: WW Norton; 2000. p. 61–81.

34. Barkley RA. Attention-deficit hyperactivity disorder; a handbook for diagnosis and treatment. 2nd edition. New York: Guilford; 1998.

35. Esfandiari A, Broshek D. Psychiatric and neuropsychological issues in sports medicine. Clin Sports Med 2011;30:611–27.

36. Nelson LD, Guskiewicz KM, Marshall SW, et al. Multiple self-reported concussions are more prevalent in athletes with ADHD and learning disability. Clin J Sport Med 2016;2:120–7.

37. Reardon CL, Factor RM. Considerations in the use of stimulants in sport. Sports Med 2015;46:611–7.

38. Drug-testing exceptions procedures. NCAA Health and Safety; 2016. Available at: http://www.ncaa.org/health-and-safety/sport-science-institute/2015-16-drug-testing-exceptions-procedures-medical-exceptions. Accessed April 22, 2017.

39. Therapeutic use exemptions. World Anti-Doping Agency; 2017. Available at: https://www.wada-ama.org/en/what-we-do/science-medical/therapeutic-use-exemptions. Accessed April 22, 2017.

40. Reardon CL, Creado S. Drug abuse in athletes. Sub Abuse Rehab 2014;5:95–105.

41. Morse ED. Substance use in athletes. In: Baron DA, Reardon CL, Baron SH, editors. Clinical sports psychiatry: an international perspective. Oxford (United Kingdom): Wiley-Blackwell; 2013. p. 3–12.

42. Johnson LD, O'Malley PM, Bachman JG, et al. Monitoring the future national survey on drug use, 1975–2003, volume II. College students and adults ages 19-25. NIH publication no. 04-5508. Bethesda (MD): National Institute on Drug Abuse; 2004.

43. Green GA, Uryasz FD, Petr TA, et al. NCAA study of substance abuse habits of college student-athletes. Clin J Sport Med 2001;11(I):51–6.

Sleep, Recovery, and Performance in Sports

Raman K. Malhotra, MD

KEYWORDS

- Sleep deprivation • Sleep apnea • Insomnia • Jet lag • Circadian rhythm disorder
- Recovery • Hypersomnia • Concussion

KEY POINTS

- Poor duration, quality, and timing of sleep can lead to poor performance, slower recovery, and higher risk of injury in athletes.
- Although the exact prevalence is unknown, athletes commonly suffer from many sleep disorders, such as insomnia, insufficient sleep, jet lag, and obstructive sleep apnea.
- Improving sleep in athletes has been shown in some studies to improve performance on the field.
- Sleep symptoms are commonly seen after concussion and should be managed appropriately, as poor sleep can exacerbate or prolong any concussion symptoms.

Over the past several years, an increasing number of athletes and their medical teams have come to recognize the importance of adequate sleep duration and quality on athletic performance and recovery. Many professional sports teams have consulted sleep specialists to help their athletes who suffer from widespread sleep issues, such as sleep deprivation, insomnia, and jet lag. As sleep researchers and clinicians continue to learn more about the impact of sleep duration, timing, and quality on human performance and recovery, it is not surprising that athletes are quickly adopting these principles to attempt to gain an advantage over their opponents. Poor sleep not only puts athletes at risk for injury, but plays a vital role in recovery from injuries and procedures. Adequate sleep and sleep extension appear to improve on field performance. Sleep plays a prominent role in concussion management given that sleep complaints are commonly noted after mild traumatic brain injury, and may play a role in exacerbating other concussion symptoms and slowing recovery.

SLEEP DURATION

Recently, evidence-based consensus recommendations have been published stating that adults need at least 7 hours of sleep for optimal health.[1] Even more sleep is

The author has nothing to disclose.
Department of Neurology, Saint Louis University School of Medicine, Monteleone Hall, 1438 South Grand Boulevard, St Louis, MO 63104, USA
E-mail address: Rmalhot1@slu.edu

Neurol Clin 35 (2017) 547–557
http://dx.doi.org/10.1016/j.ncl.2017.03.002
neurologic.theclinics.com

required for adolescents and children.[2] Insufficient sleep is prevalent in our society, with more than a third of the adult US population reporting sleep durations of less than the recommended 7 hours of sleep, and about 15% reporting sleep durations of less than 6 hours.[3] This is also true of athletes, who many times have even more responsibilities and distractions to reduce the amount of time dedicated for sleep. Early morning practices, frequent travel, and in the case of student athletes, classes and studying, many times leave it impossible for athletes to obtain adequate sleep. One study of high school athletes demonstrated poor sleep quality in more than 80% of respondents using the Pittsburgh Sleep Quality Index, a validated self-reported questionnaire regarding sleep quality.[4] Another study of professional rugby and cricket players showed poor sleep quality in 50% of respondents.[5]

Effects of Sleep Deprivation

Inadequate sleep affects overall human function and performance, ranging from neurocognitive function to immune function to life expectancy[6] (**Box 1**). Sleep deprivation is associated with higher risks of motor vehicle crashes, work place accidents, and poor work performance. Sleep is needed to help with memory consolidation and learning, and sleep disruption may be associated with decreased ability to learn and improve skills necessary for team performance.[7] There appears to be a dose-response relationship between hours of sleep deprivation and cognitive function. Human performance starts to decrease after even 17 hours of wakefulness. One group has shown that 17 to 19 hours of wakefulness was equivalent to reaction time and attention in a person with a blood alcohol concentration of 0.05%.[8]

Specifically with regard to athletes, important skills, such as decision making, reaction time, fine motor coordination, and imprinting memories and skills that were practiced, can be affected by inadequate amounts of sleep. There are only a few studies that have attempted to demonstrate decrements in function and performance with sleep deprivation in athletes. Interestingly, many of these studies have not consistently shown decrements with acute sleep deprivation when evaluating strength or endurance specifically. One explanation for the absence of an effect from sleep deprivation is that elite athletes react differently, and are "protected" from sleep deprivation. Individual variation is known to occur, as some individuals may be more or less likely to be affected by sleep deprivation. Another possible explanation is that other factors such as motivation or the adrenaline rush of performance can blunt the effects of sleep

---

Box 1
Effects of sleep deprivation

Decreased reaction time

Decreased alertness

Impaired concentration

Impaired memory and learning

Higher motor vehicle crash rate

Higher risk of depression and anxiety

Decreased immune function

Impaired glucose control

Weight gain

deprivation and thus not affect eventual performance.[9,10] Increased heart rate and increased oxygen consumption have been noted in athletes who are acutely sleep deprived, suggesting that they may be compensating to maintain their performance.[11] However, chronic, partial sleep deprivation, which is more likely the case with athletes, does seem to cause decrease in performance. Two major skills that can deteriorate with chronic, partial sleep deprivation are reaction time and sustained attention, both of which are crucial for many athletes. One study in major league baseball players demonstrated that plate discipline (how often a player swings and makes contact with a pitch) deteriorated over the course of the season, most likely due to progressive sleep deprivation. One would expect timing and hitting to improve with repetition of the season.[12] Another study demonstrated worse serve accuracy in tennis players who were sleep deprived.[13]

Sleep Extension

Some studies have shown improvement in athletic performance with sleep extension. Sleep extension is allowing athletes more time in bed, resting or sleeping, to presumably make up sleep debt that has accrued over a period of time. This additional sleep also may be necessary in athletes, as some have suggested that athletes may require more sleep than the general population to assist in recovery due to the increased mental and physical demand on their bodies. This recovery sleep or extra napping can be completed prophylactically before a predicted period of sleep deprivation. Studies have shown that it typically takes several nights of recovery sleep to return back to baseline functioning after sleep deprivation.[14] Studies have evaluated whether sleep extension (allowing subjects to sleep as much as possible, including naps) can improve athletic performance. College basketball players were prescribed sleep extension for 5 to 7 weeks. Baseline and follow-up measurements were taken of parameters, such as sprint time, free throw percentage, and 3-point field goal percentage. As total sleep time was reported higher during the sleep extension period, improvements in sprint time, free throw percentage (9% increase), and 3-point field goal percentage (9% increase) were also noted.[15] Similar studies demonstrated improvements in serve accuracy in tennis players.[16]

POOR SLEEP QUALITY AND SLEEP DISORDERS IN ATHLETES

Even if athletes are able to get adequate amounts of sleep, many of them suffer from primary sleep disorders that can affect the quality of their sleep. Sleep disorders in athletes many times remain undiagnosed, just as they go unnoticed in the general population (**Table 1**). Disorders such as obstructive sleep apnea (OSA), insomnia, restless legs syndrome, and circadian rhythm disorders can affect athletic performance if left untreated. Although we have a clear understanding of prevalence and risk factors of these conditions in the general population, very little research exists in athletes.

Table 1
Common sleep disorders found in athletes

Sleep Disorder	Risk Factors (That May Be Seen in Athletes)
Obstructive sleep apnea	Large body mass index, enlarged neck circumference, male
Insomnia	High-stress situations (anxiety), frequent travel, pain, sleeping in unfamiliar environments
Circadian rhythm disorders	Frequent travel, varying practice times
Insufficient sleep	Poor sleep hygiene, busy schedules

Obstructive Sleep Apnea

OSA is characterized by repetitive episodes of complete (apnea) or partial (hypopnea) upper airway obstruction occurring during sleep. It occurs when the muscles relax during sleep, causing soft tissue in the back of the throat to collapse and block the upper airway. This leads to sleep fragmentation, hypoxia, and/or abnormal sympathetic activation. Symptoms include snoring, apneas, unrefreshing sleep, excessive daytime sleepiness, fatigue, and neurocognitive dysfunction. Long-term health consequences, such as hypertension, cardiovascular disease, and diabetes, are also associated with this condition if left untreated. Prevalence in the general population is estimated at 5% to 7%.

Some athletes, such as football players, have large body mass indices and neck circumferences, which can put them at risk for OSA. A recent study demonstrated prevalence of 8% in college football players.[17] Thirty-eight percent of professional rugby and cricket players reported snoring, with 8% reporting apneas.[5] In professional football players, one study demonstrated sleep apnea in 27% (14/52) of participants confirmed by sleep study[18] and 19% in a more recent study.[19] This risk seems to be related to position, as defensive and offensive lineman, along with linebackers, had higher rates of OSA as compared with other positions. Retired professional football players were found to have a higher rate of cardiovascular disease and mortality, some of which may be attributed to sleep apnea.[20] Untreated OSA may lead to problems with attention and concentration during team meetings and games, higher risk of injury, and longer recovery time. In addition, snoring itself can be disruptive to other teammates if players share rooms on the road or in college.

Diagnosis is typically made by asking patients and their bedpartners about risk factors and performing a detailed upper airway, pulmonary, and cardiac examination. If suspicion is high for OSA based on these findings, either home sleep apnea testing or in-lab, attended polysomnography is necessary to confirm the diagnosis (**Table 2**). Treatment for OSA in adults typically involves continuous positive airway pressure (CPAP) in conjunction with conservative measures, such as weight loss and avoiding supine sleep. However, some patients may be treated with mandibular advancement devices or surgery. There are anecdotal cases of athletes having improved performance after being treated for OSA, but formal studies in this population are lacking. One study showed golfers with sleep apnea had improvement in sleep measures and golf scores with use of CPAP.[21]

Insomnia

Insomnia is a common sleep complaint in both, the general population, as well as athletes. Per the International Classifications of Sleep Disorders-3rd Edition, insomnia is defined as a persistent difficulty with sleep initiation, duration, consolidation, or quality that occurs despite adequate opportunity and circumstances for sleep, and results in

Table 2
Obstructive sleep apnea risk factors and diagnostic evaluation

Risk Factors (History)	Risk Factors (Physical Examination Findings)	Diagnostic Testing
• Snoring	• Obesity	• Home sleep apnea testing
• Apneas	• Enlarged neck circumference	• In-lab polysomnography
• Daytime sleepiness/fatigue	• Age	
• Morning headaches	• Male gender	
• History of hypertension	• Crowded oropharynx	

some form of daytime impairment. Elite athletes are at high risk for this condition due to the high stress related to their occupation, especially anxiety or worry before or after a game. One survey reported more than 60% of athletes had difficulties with insomnia the night before a competition.[22] Frequent travel and pain may also lead to insomnia in the athlete. Athletes may also have insomnia for the same reasons as the general population, secondary to anxiety, depression, restless legs syndrome, jet lag, or poor sleep hygiene.

The first step in management of insomnia is a focused history and physical examination on possible causes of insomnia, ruling out conditions that can cause difficulty falling asleep or awakenings at night, such as restless legs syndrome, circadian rhythm disorders, mood disorders, and sleep apnea. Many times, sleep logs, diaries, or sleep trackers (consumer wearables) can be helpful. If the insomnia seems more related to stress or anxiety, cognitive-behavioral therapy for insomnia (CBT-I) is the most effective and safest long-term therapy. CBT-I is typically performed by a psychologist, but alternative methods such as online CBT-I are available and can be effective.[23] Although there are cases in which hypnotics and sleep aids should be used, clinicians should be aware of abuse potential and possible side effects, such as early morning grogginess or fogginess, which may affect athletic performance the following day (**Table 3**). Clinicians should also educate athletes regarding appropriate sleep hygiene and advise against the use of recreational drugs like alcohol for treatment of their insomnia.

Circadian Rhythm Disorders

There is variation in performance throughout the 24-hour day due to the circadian rhythm. The circadian rhythm is the body's internal clock that helps regulate processes that differ based on time of day. It controls functions such as body temperature, release of certain hormones (ie, melatonin, cortisol, and growth hormone), and cardiovascular function. There is circadian control of functions that are important to athletes, such as alertness, concentration, strength, and coordination. These skills seem to peak in the early evening time, which not coincidentally, is when most world records in running and swimming are set.[24] These skills tend to function less optimally in the early afternoon and the period before or after bedtime. Depending on the time of the competition or practice, this may have an effect on the athlete's ability to function optimally (**Fig. 1**).

Specific skills in sports have been evaluated throughout the day and evening to determine if there are peaks and valleys in performance. Highest functioning is typically expected in the early evening during circadian peaks. This has been noted in

Table 3	
Commonly used pharmacologic treatments for insomnia	
Medication	**Comments**
Zolpidem and Zolpidem ER	Possible side effect: sleep-driving or other sleep-related behaviors
Eszopiclone	Possible side effect: metallic taste
Doxepin	Start with low dose (3 or 6 mg)
Trazodone	Consider with comorbid depression
Melatonin	Not regulated in the United States
Ramelteon	Melatonin receptor agonist
Suvorexant	Orexin antagonist

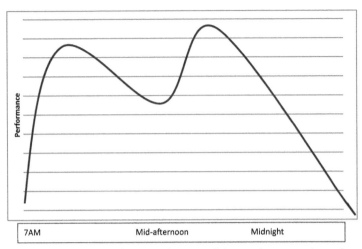

Fig. 1. Circadian rhythm and performance by time of day. Performance throughout the day fluctuates based on the circadian rhythm with peaks of performance in the mid-morning and late evening. Decreases in performance are noted late at night and in the mid-afternoon.

activities such as badminton serving,[25] tennis serves,[26] and swimming.[27] Overall strength and endurance also have been shown to fluctuate based on circadian rhythm, with peak performance in the late afternoon or early evening.

Besides looking at specific skills of athletes, evaluation on whether there was an effect of the circadian rhythm on the field regarding wins and losses has also been performed. Frequent travel by professional teams, many times across multiple time zones, contributes to what many teams already recognize as a negative effect on performance. It has been noted that baseball teams in major league baseball do worse if they have to travel across time zones and play a game, even if it means traveling across those time zones to play at home.[28] A circadian advantage was also found in professional football as it relates to Monday Night Football. West coast football teams seem to have an advantage (even after taking into consideration the point spread in Las Vegas) over east coast teams, as games may end as late as after midnight Eastern Standard Time, which is later than most east coast players' habitual bedtimes.[29]

Some athletes may be "morning" types or "evening" types, which may affect timing of optimal performance. It is not surprising for certain athletes who are night owls who have difficulties with practice or remaining alert during team meetings in the early morning. This decrement in function may also be seen in "morning larks" at the end of games that go late into the evening when their brain is trying to transition to sleep. This was seen in major league baseball players regarding to batting average. Players who were found to be more morning types had better hitting statistics (batting average) during day games versus night games. The opposite was true of players who were evening types.[28]

Management of circadian rhythm disorders in athletes first involves correct identification of the circadian rhythm disorder. Properly timed light therapy and melatonin may be effective in advancing or delaying an athlete's circadian rhythm to fit their desired schedule. For example, if an athlete is typically a night owl and having difficulties waking up early for practice, light therapy would be given immediately on awakening to phase advance his rhythm and melatonin would be administered in the evening time after dinner. For athletes or teams struggling with travel across time zones and jet lag, it may be necessary for travel plans to include time to adjust to the new schedule or adjusting to the destination schedule before travel. If travel to another time zone will be for a short time, one strategy may include keeping sleep schedules on the "home" time zone. Careful use of hypnotics may be considered short term in some cases, but care must be taken with regard to abuse potential and league rules regarding to banned substances.

Narcolepsy/Hypersomnia from Traumatic Brain Injury

Although narcolepsy and other central nervous system hypersomnias are much less common than sleep apnea and insomnia described previously, it is important to mention these conditions in athletes, as they are more commonly seen in patients with traumatic brain injury and concussion. In patients who have suffered traumatic brain injury, they are 10 times more likely to have narcolepsy than the general population. Even more have hypersomnia or excessive daytime sleepiness in relation to their head injury.[30] In patients with hypersomnia, treatments are available, such as wake-promoting medications (modafinil) and traditional stimulants (methylphenidate, dextroamphetamines). Clinicians should be careful with use of these medications in athletes, as they may be prohibited or banned without proper clearance due to abuse of these types of medication as performance enhancers.

SLEEP AND RISK OF INJURY

There is minimal available evidence that poor sleep leads to injury in athletes. However, there are substantial data linking poor sleep to fatigue-related accidents and injury in other populations, such as transportation workers and in the military. Insufficient sleep and primary sleep disorders, such as OSA, put people at higher risks of motor vehicle crashes and work-related accidents. This is likely the case with athletes as well. One study demonstrated that sleeping fewer than 6 hours or having inadequate rest was associated with injury in young athletes.[31] Another found that adolescents sleeping more than 8 hours were less likely to be injured.[32] This gives further reason for teams to ensure their athletes are obtaining adequate duration, timing, and quality of sleep.

SLEEP AND RECOVERY

Sleep has been known to help the body with recovery from injury or physical and mental exertion during wakefulness. Sleep plays a role in cellular homeostasis and maintenance of function.[33] Sleep is also important for normal endocrine and immune function, vital to recovery. Several athletes report poor quality and less sleep immediately after games.[34] This decrease in sleep may affect recovery of the athlete, although large studies in this population are lacking. Small studies have demonstrated that recovery is impaired by sleep restriction and sleep deprivation in professional athletes.[35]

SLEEP AND CONCUSSION

Sleep symptoms and complaints are common after concussion. These symptoms can be excessive daytime sleepiness, fatigue, disrupted sleep, or insomnia. It is not surprising that these symptoms can develop after a concussion, as many of the parts of the brain important for control of sleep and wake are susceptible to traumatic injury. It is possible that patients with persistent sleep complaints, such as insomnia may

---

Box 2
Good sleep habits and hygiene

Keep a consistent bedtime and wake time

Avoid light 1 to 2 hours before bedtime (including electronic devices)

Find a quiet and comfortable place to sleep

Avoid alcohol and caffeine after dinner

Use bed for sleep and sex only. Do not do other activities in bed, such as eating or watching television

Avoid long naps (>30 minutes) during the day, as this can make it more difficult to fall asleep at night

Avoid heavy meals immediately before bed

---

have prolonged recovery times. This has led some clinicians to aggressively treat insomnia at the onset of concussion to hopefully reduce severity and length of concussion symptoms. Melatonin levels have been shown to be decreased in some patients with traumatic brain injury; thus, melatonin may be a reasonable first choice in treatment of insomnia in this population.[36]

Before concussion, as mentioned previously, many athletes may have predisposing sleep disorders. These sleep disorders, if left untreated, may put athletes at risk for concussion or other injury. Sleep symptoms and poor sleep should be screened for before baseline computerized concussion testing, as this may affect scores.[37]

MANAGEMENT STRATEGIES TO ADDRESS SLEEP ISSUES IN ATHLETES

Given the growing evidence mentioned in this article regarding sleep and athletic performance and recovery, there are also several management strategies to address sleep issues in athletes. Education regarding the importance of sleep and how improved sleep will benefit athletes in performance on the field and in their personal health is key. Discussing good sleep habits and good sleep hygiene can be helpful, as this group may lack education on these principles. Additionally, many aspects of athletes' schedules place them at risk for breaking good sleep habits (**Box 2**).

Medical staff should screen for common sleep disorders, such as sleep apnea, insomnia, and restless legs syndrome, during yearly physicals. Numerous questionnaires are available to assist in this screening process (**Table 4**).

Another high-yield intervention would be to review travel plans ahead of time to help minimize the effects of jet lag on the athletes. The effects of jet lag can be reduced slowly by adapting to the destination time zone several days leading up to the game

---

Table 4
Screening tools for common sleep disorders in athletes

Sleep Disorder	Screening Questionnaire(s)
Obstructive sleep apnea	STOP-BANG, Berlin Questionnaire
Restless legs syndrome	International Restless Legs Syndrome Study Group Criteria
Insomnia	Insomnia Severity Index
Circadian rhythm disorder	Horne-Ostberg Questionnaire, Morningness-Eveningness Questionnaire

or by traveling to the destination with plenty of time to allow the body to adjust to the new time zone. It has been suggested that it can take 1 day per time zone crossed to acclimate. Careful use of melatonin and proper timing of light therapy also can be used to help synchronize the clock. Prioritizing and ensuring athletes have the opportunity to get adequate sleep, and making sure the timing of team meetings and other team activities coincide with the times of greatest alertness (per the circadian rhythm) also may be helpful.

SUMMARY

Poor sleep can lead to decreases in performance and recovery for athletes. Sleep disorders and symptoms are commonly seen in athletes, and may be unrecognized. It is important to educate athletes on getting adequate duration, quality, and timing of sleep. Interventions may include changes to practice times or careful planning for travel to games in different time zones. In addition, it is important to screen and treat sleep disorders, such as sleep apnea and insomnia, that are seen in some athletes. In patients who suffer concussion, it is important to address their sleep issues, as poor sleep can prolong or exacerbate other concussion symptoms.

REFERENCES

1. Watson NF, Badr MS, Belenky G, et al. Recommended amount of sleep for a healthy adult: a joint consensus statement of the American Academy of Sleep Medicine and Sleep Research Society. Sleep 2015;38(6):843–4.
2. Paruthi S, Brooks LJ, D'Ambrosio C, et al. Recommended amount of sleep for pediatric populations: a consensus statement of the American Academy of Sleep Medicine. J Clin Sleep Med 2016;12(6):785–6.
3. Centers for Disease Control and Prevention. Effect of short sleep duration on daily activities—United States, 2005-2008. MMWR Morb Mortal Wkly Rep 2011;60: 239–42.
4. Samuels C. Sleep, recovery, and performance: the new frontier in high-performance athletics. Neurol Clin 2008;26(1):169–80.
5. Swinbourne R, Gill N, Vaile J, et al. Prevalence of poor sleep quality, sleepiness and obstructive sleep apnoea risk factors in athletes. Eur J Sport Sci 2016;16(7): 850–8.
6. Kripke DF, Garfinkel L, Wingard DL, et al. Mortality associated with sleep duration and insomnia. Arch Gen Psychiatry 2002;59:131–6.
7. Walker M, Stickgold R. It's practice, with sleep, that makes perfect: implications of sleep-dependent learning and plasticity for skill performance. Clin Sports Med 2005;24:301–17.
8. Dawson D, Reid K. Fatigue, alcohol and performance impairment [letter]. Nature 1997;388:235.
9. Blumert PA, Crum AJ, Ernsting M, et al. The acute effects of twenty-four hours of sleep loss on the performance of national-caliber male collegiate weightlifters. J Strength Cond Res 2007;21(4):1146–54.
10. Reilly T, Piercy M. The effect of partial sleep deprivation on weight-lifting performance. Ergonomics 1994;37(1):107–15.
11. Mougin F, Simon-Rigaud ML, Davenne D, et al. Influence of partial sleep deprivation on athletic performance. Sci Sports 1990;5:83–90.
12. Kutscher SJ, Song Y, Wang L, et al. Validation of a statistical model predicting possible fatigue effect in major league baseball. Sleep 2013;36(Abstract Suppl):A408.

13. Reyner LA, Horne JA. Sleep restriction and serving accuracy in performance tennis players, and effects of caffeine. Physiol Behav 2013;120:93–6.

14. Belenky G, Wesensten NJ, Thorne DR, et al. Patterns of performance degradation and restoration during sleep restriction and subsequent recovery: a sleep dose-response study. J Sleep Res 2003;12:1–12.

15. Mah CD, Mah KE, Kezirian EJ, et al. The effects of sleep extension on the athletic performance of collegiate basketball players. Sleep 2011;34:943–50.

16. Schwartz J, Simon RD. Sleep extension improves serving accuracy: a study with college varsity tennis players. Physiol Behav 2015;151:541–4.

17. Dobrosielski DA, Nichols D, Ford J, et al. Estimating the prevalence of sleep-disordered breathing among collegiate football players. Respir Care 2016; 61(9):1144–50.

18. George CF, Kab V, Kab P, et al. Sleep and breathing in professional football players. Sleep Med 2003;4(4):317–25.

19. Rice TB, Dunn RE, Lincoln AE, et al, National Football League Subcommittee on Cardiovascular Health. Sleep-disordered breathing in the National Football League. Sleep 2010;33(6):819–24.

20. Albuquerque FN, Kuniyoshi FH, Calvin AD, et al. Sleep-disordered breathing, hypertension, and obesity in retired National Football League players. J Am Coll Cardiol 2010;56(17):1432–3.

21. Benton ML, Friedman NS. Treatment of obstructive sleep apnea syndrome with nasal positive airway pressure improves golf performance. J Clin Sleep Med 2013;9(12):1237–42.

22. Juliff LE, Halson SL, Peiffer JJ. Understanding sleep disturbance in athletes prior to important competitions. J Sci Med Sport 2015;18(1):13–8.

23. Lancee J, Van Straten A, Morina N, et al. Guided online or face-to-face cognitive behavioral treatment for insomnia: a randomized wait-list controlled trial. Sleep 2016;39(1):183–91.

24. Atkinson G, Reilly T. Circadian variation in sports performance. Sports Med 1996; 21(4):292–312.

25. Edwards BJ, Lindsay K, Waterhouse J. Effect of time of day on the accuracy and consistency of the badminton serve. Ergonomics 2005;48:1488.

26. Atkinson G, Speirs L. Diurnal variation in tennis service. Percept Mot Skills 1998; 86:1335–8.

27. Deschodt VJ, Arsac LM. Morning vs. evening maximal cycle power and technical swimming ability. J Strength Cond Res 2004;18:149–54.

28. Winter WC, Potenziano BJ, Zhang Z, et al. Chronotype as a predictor of performance in major league baseball batters. Sleep 2011;34:A167–8.

29. Smith RS, Efron B, Mah CD, et al. The impact of circadian misalignment on athletic performance in professional football players. Sleep 2013;36(12):1999–2001.

30. Castriotta RJ, Wilde MC, Lai JM, et al. Prevalence and consequences of sleep disorders in traumatic brain injury. J Clin Sleep Med 2007;3(4):349–56.

31. Luke A, Lazaro RM, Bergeron MF, et al. Sports-related injuries in youth athletes: is overscheduling a risk factor? Clin J Sport Med 2011;21(4):307–14.

32. Von Rosen P, Frohm A, Kottorp A, et al. Too little sleep and an unhealthy diet could increase the risk of sustaining a new injury in adolescent elite athletes. Scand J Med Sci Sports 2016. [Epub ahead of print].

33. Vyazovskiy VV, Delogu A. NREM and REM sleep: complementary roles in recovery after wakefulness. Neuroscientist 2014;20(3):203–19.

34. Eagles A, Mclellan C, Hing W, et al. Changes in sleep quantity and efficiency in professional rugby union players during home based training and match-play. J Sports Med Phys Fitness 2004. [Epub ahead of print].
35. Skein M, Duffield R, Minett G, et al. The effect of overnight sleep deprivation after competitive rugby league matches on postmatch physiological and perceptual recovery. Int J Sports Physiol Perform 2013;8:556–64.
36. Grima NA, Ponsford JL, St Hilaire MA, et al. Circadian melatonin rhythm following traumatic brain injury. Neurorehabil Neural Repair 2016;30(10):972–7.
37. McClure DJ, Zuckerman SL, Kutscher SJ, et al. Baseline neurocognitive testing in sports-related concussions: the importance of a prior night's sleep. Am J Sports Med 2014;42(2):472–8.

Peripheral Nerve Injuries in Sport

Ricardo Olivo, MD, Bryan Tsao, MD*

KEYWORDS

- Peripheral nerve • Nerve injury • Sports related

KEY POINTS

- Sport-related peripheral nerve injuries (SNRIs) can be acute or chronic and often related to the specific mechanics of individual sports.
- The diagnosis of SNRIs includes identifying its pathophysiology and severity in order to initiate appropriate treatment.
- The diagnosis of SRNIs requires a detailed clinical history and examination, the use of imaging and electrodiagnostic techniques, and awareness of other conditions that affect peripheral nerves.
- Treatment includes medications, rest, physical and occupational therapy, injection therapy, and modification (if possible) of sporting mechanics. Surgical treatment is indicated when these measures fail but can be successful when candidates are appropriately selected.

INTRODUCTION

Sport-related peripheral nerve injury (SRNI) can affect any level of the peripheral axis, including the nerve root, plexus, and peripheral nerves. Nerve injuries that occur during a specific sport account for less than 0.5% of all traumatic peripheral nerve injuries, but recent studies suggest a higher rate in the United States.[1-5] The risk and type of SRNIs varies by sport and can be generally classified by their onset, that is, acute or chronic, or whether they occur in full-contact or noncontact sports. Most acute SRNIs occur in full-contact sports whereby high-velocity impacts cause acute nerve traction or compression, for example, stingers with football tackles. In contrast, chronic SRNIs tend to occur in the setting of high-frequency repetitive movements, for example, ulnar neuropathy in baseball pitchers and suprascapular neuropathy in swimmers and volleyball players.[6]

The diagnosis of SRNI requires a detailed clinical history, examination, and the appropriate use of diagnostic modalities (eg, high-frequency ultrasound, MRI,

Author Disclosures: None.
Department of Neurology, Loma Linda University School of Medicine, 11175 Campus Street, Coleman Pavilion 11112, Loma Linda, CA 92354, USA
* Corresponding author.
E-mail address: btsao@llu.edu

computed tomography [CT], and electrodiagnostic [EDX] studies). Moreover, SRNIs often occur in the setting of musculoskeletal symptoms. This can make a clinical diagnosis more challenging, especially when symptoms are nonspecific in nature and distribution, that is, vague shoulder pain, scattered numbness or paresthesias not confined to a single dermatome, or intermittent pain without weakness.[7] This article reviews the diagnosis and treatment of SRNIs and further addresses some of the more common and complicated SRNIs seen in competitive and noncompetitive sports.

FACTORS

Factors that predispose athletes to injury include improper technique, age, overtraining, the number of repetitive stresses, and protective equipment.[8,9] Any disruption along the nerve pathway, such as a ganglionic cyst, increases the risk for nerve injury.

MECHANISM AND PATHOPHYSIOLOGY

There are many mechanisms whereby peripheral nerves can be injured during sports participation, including compression, stretch, traction, laceration, and crush.[7] The severity and duration of these different mechanisms result in varying degrees of axon loss, demyelination, or a combination of both. Axon loss is the most common form of pathophysiology with SRNIs followed by demyelination. Prognosis with axon loss lesions varies depending on the severity and location of injury, whereas the prognosis with focal demyelinating lesions is good assuming that further compression is avoided. Confirming pathophysiology often requires use of the EDX examination that includes nerve conduction studies and needle electromyography in addition serial clinical evaluations.

The decision to return to play after sustaining a potential SRNI is less distinct than the evolving guidelines for field concussion assessments. Defining the mechanism and severity of an SRNI requires a detailed description of how the injury occurred and an examination that incorporates both musculoskeletal and neurological components. The use of a grading scale for peripheral nerve injuries, that is, the Sunderland grades I to V, ranging from I or neurapraxia/focal demyelination to V or complete nerve transection or loss of function, allows for more accurate prognosis but can at times only be determined by serial examinations and imaging and electrophysiological tests[7] (**Table 1**).

Table 1
Sunderland classification and expected recovery

Injured Structure	Seddon	Sunderland	Spontaneous Recovery
Myelin	Neurapraxia	Grade 1	Excellent
Myelin, axon	Axonotmesis	Grade 2	Good
Myelin, axon, endoneurium		Grade 3	Variable
Myelin, axon, endoneurium, perineurium		Grade 4	Poor
Myelin, axon, endoneurium, perineurium, epineurium	Neurotmesis	Grade 5	None

From Tsao B, Bethoux F, Murray B. Peripheral nerve trauma. In: Bradley WG, Daroff RB, Fenichel GM, et al. editors. Neurology in clinical practice. 6th edition. Philadelphia: Butterworth Heinemann; 2012. p. 986; with permission.

Acute nerve traction or compressive injuries are most often composed of axon loss lesions of varying degrees with the notable exception of burners/stingers which are primarily composed of neurapraxic lesions.[5,10,11] Chronic compressive injuries are most likely to cause focal demyelination or neurapraxia (eg, as with carpal tunnel syndrome); but if the degree and duration of compression is sufficient, then axon loss occurs.[12]

TYPES OF SPORT-RELATED PERIPHERAL NERVE INJURIES

SRNIs classified by full-contact, limited-contact, and noncontact sports are presented with the presumed onset and the associated pathophysiology in **Tables 2–4**.[1,11,13–49] Inadvertent contact and injury that occurs in sports traditionally classified as limited or noncontact is not addressed.

DISCUSSION ON SPECIFIC SPORT-RELATED PERIPHERAL NERVE INJURIES
Burners and Stingers

Burners (also known as burners and stingers) are common in contact sports and frequently reported in American and Canadian nation football leagues. They result from high-velocity impacts that cause rapid inferior displacement of the shoulder from the neck, that is, when making a football tackle or hockey check with resultant compression or stretching of the C5-6 nerve roots and upper brachial plexus.[5,10,11,39,50,51] There is typically rapid onset of pain, tingling, numbness, and at times weakness in the distribution of the affected dermatomes and myotomes. Most burners are composed of neurapractic lesions (Sunderland grade I with focal demyelination); therefore, symptoms resolve within minutes to a few hours.[5] Players often do not seek medical attention because of the rapid spontaneous recovery and the lack of prominent weakness.[5]

The unilaterality of symptoms and mechanism of injury, if identifiable, separate this diagnosis from more concerning cervical spinal cord injury. In the former, the presence of bilateral symptoms and weakness should immediately tip the examiner to the possibility of a central lesion.[52]

Ulnar Neuropathy

Ulnar neuropathy at the elbow can occur in many different sports but is most commonly seen with baseball pitchers. The degree of ulnar nerve mobility and the extreme biomechanics that occur during both overhead and underhanded pitching contribute to the high frequency of nerve injury.[45,53]

The pathway the ulnar nerve travels is along the elbow between the medical epicondyle and the olecranon. The nerve passes by the 2 heads of flexor carpi ulnaris under the humeral-ulnar aponeurotic arcade forming the cubital tunnel along the ligaments. At the wrist, the ulnar nerve enters the hand via the Guyon canal. The ulnar nerve then divides to superficial and deep branches.

The significant rapid acceleration, forces, and precision in the throwing motion in baseball pitchers cause increased tension in regions on the throwing arm. The throwing motion, when the arm is cocked back and then rapidly accelerated forward, causes the shoulder to externally rotate with forces generated across the anterior shoulder. The flexion of the elbow is between 90° and 120° with pronation of the forearm. During the motion forward, the shoulder internally rotates rapidly to 7000°/s with the elbows accelerating up to 3000°/s with increased valgus stress in the medial aspect of the elbow up to 64 N.[6,24,45,54–57] This stretching produces pressure on the ulnar nerve within its surrounding ligaments and aponeurotic arcade. This repetitive

Table 2
Peripheral nerve injuries in full-contact sports

Sport	Onset	Most Common Pathophysiology
Basketball		
Suprascapular neuropathy	Chronic	Axon loss
Median neuropathy (wheelchair basketball player)	Chronic	Demyelinating/axonal
Ulnar neuropathy (wheelchair basketball player)	Chronic	Axon loss
Boxing		
Stingers	Acute	Demyelinating > axon loss (for Stinger)
Football tackle		
Brachial plexus	Acute	Axon loss
Stinger	Acute	Demyelinating > axon loss
Thoracic outlet syndrome: quarterback	Acute	Axon loss
Axillary neuropathy	Acute	Axon loss
Suprascapular neuropathy	Acute/chronic	Axon loss
Ulnar neuropathy	Chronic	Axon loss
Median neuropathy (distal or proximal)	Acute/chronic	Demyelinating > axon loss
Long thoracic neuropathy	Acute	Axon loss
Radial neuropathy	Acute/chronic	Axon loss
Iliohypogastric neuropathy	Acute	Axon loss
Fibular neuropathy	Acute	Axon loss
Sciatic nerve (hamstring syndrome)	Chronic	Axon loss
Ice hockey		
Axillary neuropathy	Acute	Axon loss
Stinger	Acute	Demyelinating > axon loss
Long thoracic neuropathy	Acute	Axon loss
Peroneal neuropathy	Acute	Axon loss
Martial arts		
Spinal accessory neuropathy	Acute	Axon loss
Long thoracic neuropathy	Acute	Axon loss
Axially neuropathy	Acute	Axon loss
Ulnar neuropathy	Acute	Axon loss
Peroneal neuropathy	Acute	Axon loss
Plantar neuropathy	Acute?	Axon loss
Motor cross		
Median neuropathy (distal)	Chronic	Demyelinating > axon loss
Axillary neuropathy	Acute	Axon loss
Spinal accessory neuropathy	Acute	Axon loss
Peroneal neuropathy	Acute	Axon loss
Rodeo		
Ulnar	Acute	Axon loss
Axillary neuropathy	Acute	Axon loss

(continued on next page)

Table 2 (continued)		
Sport	**Onset**	**Most Common Pathophysiology**
Rugby		
Stinger	Acute	Demyelinating/axon loss
Axillary neuropathy	Acute	Axon loss
Obturator neuropathy	Acute	Axon loss
Soccer		
Peroneal	Acute	Axon loss
Water polo		
Ulnar	Chronic	Axon loss
Wrestling		
Stinger	Acute	Demyelinating/axon loss
Brachial plexopathy	Acute	Axon loss
Axillary neuropathy	Acute	Axon loss
Ulnar neuropathy	Acute/chronic	Axon loss
Median neuropathy (distal)	Chronic	Demyelinating > axon loss
Long thoracic neuropathy	Acute	Axon loss
Suprascapular neuropathy	Acute	Axon loss

motion leads to trauma of the nerve as well as hypertrophy and further compression by the ulnar collateral ligament.[6,24,45,54–57]

Ulnar neuropathy present with sensory (pain, numbness, and paresthesias in digit 5 and half of digit 4) and motor (finger flexion or grip weakness) symptoms or any combination of both. The clinical diagnosis is often complicated by the presence of combined musculoskeletal pain in the elbow region.

Distal ulnar neuropathy in the hand is divided into 4 different types based on location and symptoms (pure sensory, pure motor to all intrinsic hand muscles, pure motor to abductor digiti minimi (ADM), and mixed).[25] These distal ulnar neuropathies most commonly result from repetitive compression in the hand or wrist, for example, in wheelchair athletes, cyclists, and skiers.[15,25,58]

DIAGNOSIS

The clinical evaluation should include a detailed history with the precise date, location, and description of the mechanism of injury; the presence of sensorimotor symptoms; the degree of functional loss; and pain. The neuromuscular examination should include signs of trauma, a detailed sensory and motor examination, an estimated nerve-muscle distance, and correlative reflexes. The use of incorporating grading scales for pain, motor, and sensory helps to quantify and verify recovery.[7]

The EDX examination can define the pathophysiology of injury and the location and severity of the injured segments and ideally provide prognostic information.[12] In general, nerve conduction studies (NCS) should be performed at least 10 days after the onset of symptoms so that motor and sensory nerve conduction results can differentiate subacute axon loss (axon failure or axon discontinuity conduction block) from demyelinating conduction block. The needle electromyogram (EMG) should be performed at least 3 weeks after the injury to allow the development of fibrillation

Table 3
Peripheral nerve injuries in limited-contact sports

Sport	Onset	Most Common Pathophysiology
Backpacking/mountain climbing		
Brachial plexopathy	Acute	Axon loss
Suprascapular neuropathy	Acute	Axon loss
Thoracic outlet syndrome	Acute	Axon loss
Baseball		
Thoracic outlet syndrome	Acute	Axon loss
Suprascapular neuropathy	Acute/chronic	Axon loss
Axillary neuropathy	Acute	Axon loss
Musculocutaneous neuropathy	Acute	Axon loss
Radial neuropathy	Chronic	Axon loss
Ulnar neuropathy	Chronic	Axon loss > demyelinating
Anterior interosseous nerve	Chronic	Axon loss
Digital neuropathy	Chronic	Axon loss
Bicycling		
Ulnar neuropathy	Chronic	Axon loss
Median neuropathy (distal)	Chronic	Demyelinating > axon loss
Pudendal neuropathy	Chronic	Axon loss
Posterior cutaneous nerve of the thigh	Acute	Axon loss
Sciatic neuropathy	Chronic?	Axon loss
Cheerleading		
Digital neuropathy	Chronic	Axon loss
Median neuropathy (distal)	Chronic	Demyelinating > axon loss
Gymnastics		
Lateral femoral cutaneous neuropathy	Chronic	Axon loss
Femoral neuropathy	Acute?	Axon loss
Racquetball/tennis (noncontact)		
Posterior interosseous neuropathy	Chronic	Axon loss
Suprascapular neuropathy	Acute/chronic	Axon loss
Long thoracic neuropathy	Acute	Axon loss
Radial neuropathy	Acute	Axon loss
Skating (ice, in-line roller skating)		
Peroneal neuropathy	Acute	Axon loss
Skiing (cross-country)		
Femoral neuropathy	Acute	Axon loss
Ulnar neuropathy	Chronic	Axon loss > demyelinating
Softball, squash		
Radial neuropathy	Chronic	Axon loss > demyelinating
Ulnar neuropathy	Chronic	Axon loss > demyelinating
Ultimate Frisbee		
Posterior interosseous neuropathy	Chronic	Axon loss
Volleyball		
Suprascapular neuropathy	Acute/chronic	Axon loss

(continued on next page)

Table 3 (continued)		
Sport	**Onset**	**Most Common Pathophysiology**
Long thoracic neuropathy	Acute	Axon loss
Axillary neuropathy	Acute	Axon loss
Windsurfing or surfing		
Common peroneal neuropathy	Acute	Axon loss
Saphenous neuropathy	Acute	Axon loss

potentials. The timing for serial EDX examinations depends on the nature of the lesion but can be repeated in 3 to 5 months if symptoms progress or surgical repair is being considered. In relation to SRNIs, the EDX study has its highest value in the assessment of cervical radiculopathy, mononeuropathy (ie, ulnar or median nerves), or plexopathy.

It is important to note that the routine EDX examination primarily assesses the mid-plexus to lower plexus (C6/7–T1 myotomes) and that the assessment of complicated peripheral nerve lesions requires additional sensory and motor NCSs and extra muscles on needle EMG.[59] In the lower limb, the routine EDX examination primarily assesses the L5 to S1 dermatomes and myotomes.

Imaging plays an important role in helping diagnosis peripheral nerve injuries. Proximal lesions seen in posttraumatic plexopathy are complicated and may require imaging to exclude other injuries, such as acute cord injury and nerve root avulsions. Cervical CT myelogram and MRI with gadolinium are relatively comparable methods for detecting suspected nerve root avulsion.[7] MRI neurography uses diffusion-weighted, T2-weighted, and short T1 inversion recovery images. In the hands of experienced musculoskeletal radiologists and a 3.0-T scanner, this can demonstrate various signal changes in correlative peripheral nerves and muscle.[60] Diffusion tensor imaging and high-frequency sonography of the peripheral nerves can provide additional information on localization and, to some degree, severity of peripheral nerve lesions. High-frequency ultrasound of peripheral nerve and muscle has the advantage of being relatively inexpensive, quickly accessible, and allows for dynamic observation of in vivo nerve segments and their surrounding structures.

DIFFERENTIAL DIAGNOSIS

Parsonage-Turner syndrome (PTS) or neuralgic amyotrophy is an uncommon sporadic or hereditary condition that has been associated with a variety of triggers, including strenuous exercise, trauma, viral disease, recent surgery, immunizations, and autoimmune disease.[61] The association with heavy exercise can mimic shoulder girdle and brachial plexus neuropathies. PTS typically presents with severe and intractable pain in the neck or shoulder girdle region that can radiate into the upper limb. This pain, often nocturnal in initial onset, usually lasts 1 to 2 weeks and then subsides and is followed by weakness, muscle atrophy, and at times sensory loss.[61] Although unilateral in most cases, up to one-half of patients have EDX changes in the contralateral or asymptomatic side. Although PTS can be clinically indistinguishable from cervical radiculopathy, the presence of marked muscle atrophy supports PTS over the latter condition, whereby atrophy is uncommon.

The EDX examination differentiates PTS from cervical radiculopathy, upper brachial plexopathies, or other musculoskeletal mimickers. PTS has a predilection

Table 4
Nerve injuries in noncontact sports

Sport	Onset	Most Common Pathophysiology
Archery		
Digital neuropathies	Chronic	Axon loss
Median neuropathy (distal and proximal)	Chronic	Demyelinating > axon loss
Long thoracic nerve palsy	Acute/chronic	Axon loss
Bowling		
Digital neuropathy of the thumb	Acute/chronic	Axon loss
Crew		
Axillary	Acute	Axon loss
Dancing: ballet, modern, jazz		
Suprascapular neuropathy	Acute?	Axon loss
Femoral neuropathy	Acute?	Axon loss
Peroneal neuropathy	Chronic?	Axon loss
Sural neuropathy	Chronic	Axon loss
Dorsal cutaneous neuropathy	Chronic	Axon loss
Morton neuroma	Chronic	Axon loss
Golf		
Median neuropathy (distal)	Chronic	Demyelinating > axon loss
Ulnar neuropathy	Chronic	Axon loss/demyelinating
Riflery		
Long thoracic neuropathy	Acute	Axon loss
Running		
Lateral femoral cutaneous neuropathy	Chronic	Axon loss
Peroneal neuropathy	Chronic	Axon loss
Tibial neuropathy	Chronic	Axon loss
Plantar neuropathies	Chronic	Axon loss
Calcaneal neuropathy	Chronic	Axon loss
Sural neuropathy	Chronic	Axon loss
Superficial peroneal neuropathy	Chronic	Axon loss
Saphenous neuropathy	Chronic	Axon loss
Scuba diving		
Lateral femoral cutaneous neuropathy	Chronic	Axon loss
Sky jumping, skiing, snowboarding		
Brachial plexopathy	Acute	Axon loss
Femoral neuropathy	Acute	Axon loss
Ulnar neuropathy wrist	Acute	Axon loss
Swimming		
Thoracic outlet syndrome	Chronic	Axon loss
Suprascapular neuropathy	Chronic	Axon loss
Lateral antebrachial cutaneous	Chronic	Axon loss
Tennis		Axon loss
Posterior interosseous neuropathy	Chronic	Axon loss
Radial neuropathy	Chronic	Axon loss
Suprascapular neuropathy	Acute	Axon loss
Long thoracic neuropathy	Acute	Axon loss

for motor branches and is less often a true brachial plexopathy. The motor branches involved usually include the anterior interosseous, posterior interosseous, suprascapular, long thoracic, phrenic, and cranial (IX and XII) nerves. The prognosis for PTS is favorable with significant recovery of weakness within 6 month to 3 years.[62]

TREATMENT

Peripheral nerve recovery depends on the severity and location of nerve injury. Sunderland classification of grade 1 nerve injury with focal demyelination or neurapraxia has the most favorable prognosis. If there is continuous compression in a grade 1 lesion, imaging studies should be considered, for example, baseball players' ulnar neuropathy.

The management in most sports nerve injury requires clinical and, at times, diagnostic surveillance. Most SRNIs recover with conservative management, such as medication, rest, and physical therapy; however, there are instances that surgery is needed. In the acute setting, the first step is to remove the player from repetitive nerve injury. In many circumstances in contact sports, other serious central nerve injuries need to be rapidly differentiated.

Acute neuropathic and musculoskeletal pain can have a large impact in preventing optimal physical therapy and to help prevent chronic pain syndromes.[63] The choice of pain management medications varies depending on if there is a large musculoskeletal component of pain. A combination of nonsteroidal antiinflammatory drugs and neuropathic pain medication are sometimes needed depending on the severity and the type of pain. There is a diversity of neuropathic pain medications, which are classified as tricyclic antidepressants, serotonin-norepinephrine reuptake inhibitors, calcium channel alpha 2 delta ligands, tropical agents, antiepileptic drugs, and opioids. The preference of medication depends on the side effects, potential dual benefits, and efficacy. A combination of pain medications may be needed for acute severe pain, for example, a short course of opioids with another neuropathic pain medication for potential long-term usage. There are instances when braces, slings, or splints are needed to provide optimal limb position for nerve recovery. Optimizing pain management strategies will help initiate physical therapy early to maintain passive range of motion in the affected joints and to maintain strength in noneffected muscles.

Injection therapy is used frequently in nerve injuries to help decrease the swelling and discomfort provisionally. In many instances, a combination of steroid injection with local anesthesia is used for acute pain and inflammation or with local anesthesia alone for nerve blocks, for example, lidocaine. There is growing concern for the use and overuse of steroid injection in structural areas. Local injection of steroid can cause muscle atrophy and weaken tendons, which may increase the risk of more collateral damage.[64,65] For example, the use of steroids is admonitory because of the importance for sound structure in the elbow area to avert more injuries. Injection therapy is currently used as an additional tool for acute pain reduction with the combination of other long-term treatment strategies discussed previously. Other injection treatments, such as platelet-rich plasma (PRP), is showing promise in tissue regeneration; however, there are limited data in nerve injuries outcomes.[66,67]

Working with a qualified sports physical therapist for specific stretching, range of motion, and exercises is vital and helps provide clinical feedback to the physician.[68] The guidance of a sports therapist will help tailor treatment, optimize nerve recovery, and guide a safe return to sport.[69] If associated with an entrapment neuropathy early, surgical intervention should be considered. The decision for operative exploration should be determined by about 5 months for severe nerve injuries, regardless of the level, so that surgical repair can ideally occur within 6 months of the injury.[7,70]

In terms of surgical treatment, the guiding principle is to optimize preventive and nonsurgical treatment modalities, including injection therapy. Surgical management of chronic SRNIs, for example, distal median neuropathy or carpal tunnel syndrome, involves decompressive surgery for the ulnar neuropathy intermuscular transposition in addition to local decompression.[71] For ulnar nerve at the elbow in baseball pitchers, the Tommy John surgery has allowed many players to continue their pitching careers.[56,57]

PREVENTIVE THERAPY

Sport-specific stretching programs and general warm-up seem to have an impact on preventing injury. However, nonsport stretching has little or no effect on the reduction of injury incidence.[72] Prevention of peripheral nerve entrapments may involve special equipment, for example, in wheelchair athletes the use of padded gloves to protect the volar surface of the wrist.[58] There are prevention guidelines in youth baseball to limit the number of pitches and require rest between games.[9,73] Many professional athletes have an athletic trainer that helps tailor stretching, reduction of repetitive injury, and recovery.[11,36,69,74–79]

SUMMARY

SRNIs are still seen despite advances in equipment and training and are often difficult to diagnose if they are mild and seen with concomitant musculoskeletal symptoms. Early recognition is important to obtain the best outcome and prevent further injury. The pressure to perform and win in any level of competitive sports should not outweigh the health of the individual athlete.[80] Diagnosis of SRNIs requires an adequate history of the injury, understanding of its mechanism, and using diagnostic imaging and other modalities as indicated. Nonsurgical treatment of SRNIs includes alternation of mechanics, physical therapy/occupational therapy, other new therapy (PRP), and pain management. Surgical management of SRNIs is less common and is indicated when there is a noncontinuity nerve lesion of an acute SRNI or for chronic SRNIs that have failed conservative therapy.

REFERENCES

1. Hirasawa Y, Sakakida K. Sports and peripheral nerve injury. Am J Sports Med 1983;11:420–6.
2. Krivickas LS, Wilbourn AJ. Sports and peripheral nerve injuries: report of 190 injuries evaluated in a single electromyography laboratory. Muscle Nerve 1998;21: 1092–4.
3. Krivickas LS, Wilbourn AJ. Peripheral nerve injuries in athletes: a case series of over 200 injuries. Semin Neurol 2000;20:225–32.
4. Charbonneau RM, McVeigh SA, Thompson K. Brachial neuropraxia in Canadian Atlantic University sport football players: what is the incidence of "stingers"? Clin J Sport Med 2012;22:472–7.
5. Feinberg JH. Burners and stingers. Phys Med Rehabil Clin N Am 2000;11: 771–84.
6. Anderson MW, Alford BA. Overhead throwing injuries of the shoulder and elbow. Radiol Clin North Am 2010;48:1137–54.

7. Tsao B, Bethoux F, Murray B. Peripheral nerve trauma. In: Bradley WG, Daroff RB, Fenichel GM, et al, editors. Neurology in clinical practice. 6th edition. Philadelphia: Butterworth Heinemann; 2012. p. 984–1002.

8. Andrews JR, Fleisig GS. Preventing throwing injuries. J Orthop Sports Phys Ther 1998;27:187–8.

9. Hawkins D, Metheny J. Overuse injuries in youth sports: biomechanical considerations. Med Sci Sports Exerc 2001;33:1701–7.

10. Levitz CL, Reilly PJ, Torg JS. The pathomechanics of chronic, recurrent cervical nerve root neurapraxia. The chronic burner syndrome. Am J Sports Med 1997;25: 73–6.

11. Weinberg J, Rokito S, Silber JS. Etiology, treatment, and prevention of athletic "stingers". Clin Sports Med 2003;22:493–500.

12. Wilbourn AJ. Electrodiagnostic testing of neurologic injuries in athletes. Clin Sports Med 1990;9:229–45.

13. Bohu Y, Klouche S, Lefevre N, et al. The epidemiology of 1345 shoulder dislocations and subluxations in French rugby union players: a five-season prospective study from 2008 to 2013. Br J Sports Med 2015;49:1535–40.

14. Brooks JH, Fuller CW, Kemp SP, et al. Epidemiology of injuries in English professional rugby union: part 2 training injuries. Br J Sports Med 2005;39:767–75.

15. Burnham RS, Steadward RD. Upper extremity peripheral nerve entrapments among wheelchair athletes: prevalence, location, and risk factors. Arch Phys Med Rehabil 1994;75:519–24.

16. Cho D, Saetia K, Lee S, et al. Peroneal nerve injury associated with sports-related knee injury. Neurosurg Focus 2011;31:E11.

17. Clancy WG, Brand RL, Bergfield JA. Upper trunk brachial plexus injuries in contact sports. Am J Sports Med 1977;5:209–16.

18. Colburn NT, Meyer RD. Sports injury or trauma? Injuries of the competition off-road motorcyclist. Injury 2003;34:207–14.

19. Collins K, Storey M, Peterson K, et al. Nerve injuries in athletes. Phys Sportsmed 1988;16:92–100.

20. Cordova CB, Owens BD. Infraspinatus muscle atrophy from suprascapular nerve compression. JAAPA 2014;27:33–5.

21. Cummins CA, Schneider DS. Peripheral nerve injuries in baseball players. Phys Med Rehabil Clin N Am 2009;20:175–93.

22. Dawson DM. Entrapment neuropathies of the upper extremities. N Engl J Med 1993;329:2013–8.

23. Feinberg JH, Nadler SF, Krivickas LS. Peripheral nerve injuries in the athlete. Sports Med 1997;24:385–408.

24. Field LD, Altchek DW. Elbow injuries. Clin Sports Med 1995;14:59–78.

25. Jackson DL, Hynninen BC, Caborn DN, et al. Electrodiagnostic study of carpal tunnel syndrome in wheelchair basketball players. Clin J Sport Med 1996;6: 27–31.

26. Kaplan PE. Posterior interosseous neuropathies: natural history. Arch Phys Med Rehabil 1984;65:399–400.

27. Kawasaki T, Ota C, Yoneda T, et al. Incidence of stingers in young rugby players. Am J Sports Med 2015;43:2809–15.

28. Kelly BT, Barnes RP, Powell JW, et al. Shoulder injuries to quarterbacks in the national football league. Am J Sports Med 2004;32:328–31.

29. Lee S, Saetia K, Saha S, et al. Axillary nerve injury associated with sports. Neurosurg Focus 2011;31:E10.

30. Lotem M, Fried A, Levy M, et al. Radial palsy following muscular effort. A nerve compression syndrome possibly related to a fibrous arch of the lateral head of the triceps. J Bone Joint Surg Br 1971;53:500–6.
31. Manske PR. Compression of the radial nerve by the triceps muscle: a case report. J Bone Joint Surg Am 1977;59:835–6.
32. Meyers MC, Laurent CM. The rodeo athlete: injuries - part II. Sports Med 2010;40:817–39.
33. Meyers MC, Laurent CM. The rodeo athlete: sport science: part I. Sports Med 2010;40:417–31.
34. Mitsunaga MM, Nakano K. High radial nerve palsy following strenuous muscular activity. A case report. Clin Orthop Relat Res 1988;(234):39–42.
35. Nieman EA, Swann PG. Karate injuries. Br Med J 1971;1:233.
36. Olson DE, Sikka RS, Hamilton A, et al. Football injuries: current concepts. Curr Sports Med Rep 2011;10:290–8.
37. Rayan GM. Archery-related injuries of the hand, forearm, and elbow. South Med J 1992;85:961–4.
38. Safran MR. Nerve injury about the shoulder in athletes, part 1: suprascapular nerve and axillary nerve. Am J Sports Med 2004;32:803–19.
39. Safran MR. Nerve injury about the shoulder in athletes, part 2: long thoracic nerve, spinal accessory nerve, burners/stingers, thoracic outlet syndrome. Am J Sports Med 2004;32:1063–76.
40. Seckler MM, DiStefano V. Peroneal nerve palsy in the athlete: a result of indirect trauma. Orthopedics 1996;19:345–8.
41. Sinson G, Zager EL, Kline DG. Windmill pitcher's radial neuropathy. Neurosurgery 1994;34:1087–90.
42. Terzis JK, Kostas I. Suprascapular nerve reconstruction in 118 cases of adult posttraumatic brachial plexus. Plast Reconstr Surg 2006;117:613–29.
43. Toth C, McNeil S, Feasby T. Peripheral nervous system injuries in sport and recreation: a systematic review. Sports Med 2005;35:717–38.
44. Toth C. Peripheral nerve injuries attributable to sport and recreation. Phys Med Rehabil Clin N Am 2009;20:77–100.
45. Treihaft MM. Neurologic injuries in baseball players. Semin Neurol 2000;20:187–93.
46. Visser CP, Coene LN, Brand R, et al. The incidence of nerve injury in anterior dislocation of the shoulder and its influence on functional recovery. A prospective clinical and EMG study. J Bone Joint Surg Br 1999;81:679–85.
47. Visser CP, Coene LN, Brand R, et al. Nerve lesions in proximal humeral fractures. J Shoulder Elbow Surg 2001;10:421–7.
48. Weiss AP, Idler RS. Radial nerve rupture after a traction injury: a case report. J Hand Surg Am 1992;17:69–70.
49. Zanette G, Lauriola MF, Picelli A, et al. Isolated musculocutaneous nerve injury in a kickboxer. Muscle Nerve 2015;52:1137–9.
50. Kelly JD, Aliquo D, Sitler MR, et al. Association of burners with cervical canal and foraminal stenosis. Am J Sports Med 2000;28:214–7.
51. Shannon B, Klimkiewicz JJ. Cervical burners in the athlete. Clin Sports Med 2002;21:29–35.
52. Rihn JA, Anderson DT, Lamb K, et al. Cervical spine injuries in American football. Sports Med 2009;39:697–708.
53. Post EG, Laudner KG, McLoda TA, et al. Correlation of shoulder and elbow kinetics with ball velocity in collegiate baseball pitchers. J Athl Train 2015;50:629–33.

54. Andrews JR, Timmerman LA. Outcome of elbow surgery in professional baseball players. Am J Sports Med 1995;23:407–13.
55. Erickson BJ, Harris JD, Chalmers PN, et al. Ulnar collateral ligament reconstruction: anatomy, indications, techniques, and outcomes. Sports Health 2015;7: 511–7.
56. Jobe FW, Stark H, Lombardo SJ. Reconstruction of the ulnar collateral ligament in athletes. J Bone Joint Surg Am 1986;68:1158–63.
57. Vitale MA, Ahmad CS. The outcome of elbow ulnar collateral ligament reconstruction in overhead athletes: a systematic review. Am J Sports Med 2008;36: 1193–205.
58. Klenck C, Gebke K. Practical management: common medical problems in disabled athletes. Clin J Sport Med 2007;17:55–60.
59. Di Benedetto M, Markey K. Electrodiagnostic localization of traumatic upper trunk brachial plexopathy. Arch Phys Med Rehabil 1984;65:15–7.
60. Grant GA, Britz GW, Goodkin R, et al. The utility of magnetic resonance imaging in evaluating peripheral nerve disorders. Muscle Nerve 2002;25:314–31.
61. Ferrante MA, Wilbourn AJ. Lesion distribution among 281 patients with sporadic neuralgic amyotrophy. Muscle Nerve 2016. [Epub ahead of print].
62. Tsairis P, Dyck PJ, Mulder DW. Natural history of brachial plexus neuropathy. Report on 99 patients. Arch Neurol 1972;27:109–17.
63. Kujala U, Orava S, Parkkari J, et al. Sports career-related musculoskeletal injuries: long-term health effects on former athletes. Sports Med 2003;33:869–75.
64. Babwah T. Common peroneal neuropathy related to cryotherapy and compression in a footballer. Res Sports Med 2011;19:66–71.
65. Drez D, Faust DC, Evans JP. Cryotherapy and nerve palsy. Am J Sports Med 1981;9:256–7.
66. Foster TE, Puskas BL, Mandelbaum BR, et al. Platelet-rich plasma: from basic science to clinical applications. Am J Sports Med 2009;37:2259–72.
67. Mishra A, Harmon K, Woodall J, et al. Sports medicine applications of platelet rich plasma. Curr Pharm Biotechnol 2012;13:1185–95.
68. Saliba S, Saliba EN, Pugh KF, et al. Rehabilitation considerations of a brachial plexus injury with complete avulsion of c5 and c6 nerve roots in a college football player: a case study. Sports Health 2009;1:370–5.
69. Lorei MP, Hershman EB. Peripheral nerve injuries in athletes. Treatment and prevention. Sports Med 1993;16:130–47.
70. Isaacs J. Major peripheral nerve injuries. Hand Clin 2013;29:371–82.
71. Biundo JJ, Harris MA. Peripheral nerve entrapment, occupation-related syndromes and sports injuries, and bursitis. Curr Opin Rheumatol 1993;5:224–9.
72. Lewis J. A systematic literature review of the relationship between stretching and athletic injury prevention. Orthop Nurs 2014;33:312–20.
73. Harada M, Takahara M, Mura N, et al. Risk factors for elbow injuries among young baseball players. J Shoulder Elbow Surg 2010;19:502–7.
74. Bahr R, Krosshaug T. Understanding injury mechanisms: a key component of preventing injuries in sport. Br J Sports Med 2005;39:324–9.
75. Faude O, Rößler R, Junge A. Football injuries in children and adolescent players: are there clues for prevention? Sports Med 2013;43:819–37.
76. Mazur LJ, Yetman RJ, Risser WL. Weight-training injuries. Common injuries and preventative methods. Sports Med 1993;16:57–63.
77. Meister K. Injuries to the shoulder in the throwing athlete. Part one: biomechanics/ pathophysiology/classification of injury. Am J Sports Med 2000;28:265–75.

78. Nissen SJ, Laskowski ER, Rizzo TD. Burner syndrome: recognition and rehabilitation. Phys Sportsmed 1996;24:57–64.
79. Whiteside JA, Andrews JR, Fleisig GS. Elbow injuries in young baseball players. Phys Sportsmed 1999;27:87–102.
80. Vaccaro AR, Klein GR, Ciccoti M, et al. Return to play criteria for the athlete with cervical spine injuries resulting in stinger and transient quadriplegia/paresis. Spine J 2002;2:351–6.

Neurologic Injuries in Noncontact Sports

Robert J. Marquardt, DO, Andrew Blake Buletko, MD, Andrew Neil Russman, DO*

KEYWORDS

- Noncontact sports • Muscle injury • Cervicocephalic dissection • Concussion
- Return to play • Spinal cord injury

KEY POINTS

- Concussion among noncontact sport participants requires similar assessment and management, but may differ most in aspects related to return to play.
- Cerebrovascular disease may affect athletes who participates in noncontact sports, and presents clinical challenges related to return to exercise and play.
- Muscle and spine disorders may occur with some frequency in noncontact sport participants, and raise knowledge gaps in clinical management, recovery, and return to sport.

NONCONTACT SPORT CONCUSSION

Concussion may be a consequence of unintended falls, head impact, and acceleration or deceleration injury in noncontact sports. The overall evaluation and management of sports concussion are discussed elsewhere. This article focuses on some of the unique aspects of concussion in noncontact sports.

Incident Reporting

The Cleveland Clinic's Concussion Center provides evaluation and management to student-athletes throughout the greater Cleveland, Ohio, area with concussion. In an effort to optimize community-based sports concussion care, the Concussion Center developed and implemented standardized methods of reporting, evaluating, and managing concussion injury in youth and high school athletes.

The collection and reporting of head injury details (eg, symptoms, date, time, location of injury, and action taken) facilitates the collaboration of care between athletic trainers on the sideline and physicians in the hospital or office. The development and deployment of the Concussion Incident Report (IR) module to a mobile tablet device or smartphone allows athletic trainers, who are typically the first medical

Disclosure Statement: The authors have nothing to disclose.
Department of Neurology, Cleveland Clinic, 9500 Euclid Avenue, Cleveland, OH 44195, USA
* Corresponding author.
E-mail address: russmaa@ccf.org

personnel to evaluate an injured athlete, to track head injury details. Additional assessment modules are used to objectively characterize aspects of cognitive and motor status.

Tables 1–3 illustrate the tracking of incidents of concussion among student-athletes at schools with athletic trainers employed by the Cleveland Clinic. From August 2014 through July 2016, Cleveland Clinic athletic trainers completed IR on 1778 student-athletes with concussion, 1071 of which occurred during competition and 707 of which occurred during practice. The use of an IR tool provides data that will guide process improvement, facilitate patient hand-offs, and allow calculation of injury rates for communication to community partners.

Concussion IR were substantially higher in contact sports (n = 1313; 73.8%) and semicontact sports (n = 413; 23.2%), than in noncontact sports (n = 52; 2.9%). Boys football and girls soccer had the highest overall rates of sports concussion (see **Table 1**). Rates of concussion were higher in competition, than in practice, for all contact and semicontact sports, except boys football, and boys wrestling (see **Tables 1** and **2**). Among noncontact sports, concussion IR was most common in girls swimming and diving and girls track and field (see **Table 3**). Rates of noncontact sports concussion, especially girls swimming and diving, were higher when compared with a national sample (see **Table 3**).[1] A greater number of noncontact sport concussion occurred in practice than in competition in the Cleveland Clinic patient population (see **Table 3**). Also, higher rates of observed contact and semicontact sport concussions were reported among girls soccer, basketball, and volleyball when compared with a national sample (see **Tables 1** and **2**).[1] The presence of Cleveland Clinic high school athletic trainers at soccer, basketball, and volleyball practices and competitions likely improved detection. The increased popularity of soccer, as well as community education and awareness of concussion signs and symptoms, may contribute to greater incidence among these athletes.

Exertional Recovery

Guidelines from the American Academy of Neurology[2] and the National Athletic Trainers' Association,[3] which are based on the 2012 International Consensus

Table 1
Frequency of concussion among contact sport athletes, 2014 to 2016

Contact Sport	Game/Event, n (%)	Practice, n (%)	Total, n (%)
Boys football	332 (31.0)	365 (51.6)	697 (39.2)
Girls soccer	183 (17.1)	35 (5.0)	218 (12.3)
Boys soccer	99 (9.2)	22 (3.1)	121 (6.8)
Boys wrestling	42 (3.9)	55 (7.8)	97 (5.5)
Boys lacrosse	44 (4.1)	14 (2.0)	58 (3.3)
Boys hockey	39 (3.6)	6 (0.8)	45 (2.5)
Girls lacrosse	21 (2.0)	11 (1.6)	32 (1.8)
Boys rugby	17 (1.6)	4 (0.6)	21 (1.2)
Girls rugby	11 (1.0)	1 (0.1)	12 (0.7)
Girls hockey	4 (0.4)	2 (0.3)	6 (0.3)
Girls field hockey	3 (0.3)	1 (0.1)	4 (0.2)
Boys boxing	2 (0.2)	0 (0.0)	2 (0.1)
Totals	797 (74.4)	516 (73.0)	1313 (73.8)

Table 2
Frequency of concussion among semicontact sport athletes, 2014 to 2016

Semicontact Sport	Game/Event, n (%)	Practice, n (%)	Total, n (%)
Girls basketball	96 (9.0)	35 (5.0)	131 (7.4)
Girls volleyball	51 (4.8)	30 (4.2)	81 (4.6)
Boys basketball	51 (4.8)	23 (3.3)	74 (4.2)
Girls softball	27 (2.5)	22 (3.1)	49 (2.8)
Boys baseball	19 (1.8)	13 (1.8)	32 (1.8)
Girls cheerleading	3 (0.3)	16 (2.3)	19 (1.1)
Boys cheerleading	0 (0.0)	2 (0.3)	2 (0.1)
Boys volleyball	3 (0.3)	2 (0.3)	5 (0.3)
Boys softball	3 (0.3)	1 (0.1)	4 (0.2)
Boys other	6 (0.6)	2 (0.3)	8 (0.4)
Girls other	1 (0.1)	7 (1.0)	8 (0.4)
Totals	260 (24.3)	153 (21.6)	413 (23.2)

Conference on Concussion in Sport,[4] recommend a graduated program of exertional recovery after sports concussion toward return to play. Controversy exists as to the optimal duration and content of rest after sports concussion.[5] The American Academy of Neurology 2013 guideline recommends that athletes not return to "contact-risk activity" until their concussion symptoms have resolved.[2] For athletes participating in noncontact sports, the risk of recurrent concussion is very low and reduction in physical activity may be more harmful, than return to participation. Beginning a program of exertional recovery in a noncontact sport should strive to exercise within the

Table 3
Frequency of concussion among noncontact sport athletes, 2014 to 2016

Noncontact Sport	Game/Event, n (%)	Practice, n (%)	Total, n (%)
Girls swimming	2 (0.2)	16 (2.3)	18 (1.0)
Girls track and field	2 (0.2)	6 (0.8)	8 (0.4)
Girls equestrian	1 (0.1)	4 (0.6)	5 (0.3)
Boys cycling	1 (0.1)	1 (0.1)	2 (0.1)
Boys swimming	0 (0.0)	2 (0.3)	2 (0.1)
Boys track and field	2 (0.2)	0 (0.0)	2 (0.1)
Boys weightlifting	1 (0.1)	1 (0.1)	2 (0.1)
Girls cross country	1 (0.1)	1 (0.1)	2 (0.1)
Girls diving	0 (0.0)	2 (0.3)	2 (0.1)
Girls gymnastics	1 (0.1)	1 (0.1)	2 (0.1)
Girls tennis	2 (0.2)	0 (0.0)	2 (0.1)
Girls weightlifting	0 (0.0)	1 (0.1)	1 (0.1)
Girls cycling	0 (0.0)	1 (0.1)	1 (0.1)
Girls figure skating	0 (0.0)	1 (0.1)	1 (0.1)
Girls nonsport other	1 (0.1)	0 (0.0)	1 (0.1)
Boys nonsport other	0 (0.0)	1 (0.1)	1 (0.1)
Totals	14 (1.3)	38 (5.4)	52 (2.9)

submaximal symptom exacerbation threshold, to limit significant symptomatic worsening.[5] We rarely restrict athletes in noncontact sports with mild ongoing concussion symptoms, from return to noncontact activity. However, we must remain mindful of the need to manage concussion symptoms, and avoid specific exercises that may significantly aggravate symptoms, especially for an athlete with posttraumatic neck muscle weakness, cervicalgia, and cervicogenic headache.

STROKE AMONG ATHLETES IN NONCONTACT SPORTS

Stroke is the second leading cause of mortality and the third most common cause of disability worldwide.[6] Stroke can be divided into 2 broad categories, ischemic and hemorrhagic, with ischemic strokes accounting for about 80% of all strokes. There have been no large studies looking specifically at the epidemiology of stroke in athletes. In this section, we highlight the most common causes of stroke in noncontact sports, along with some diagnostic and management practices.

Cervicocephalic Arterial Dissection

Arterial dissection occurs when there is a small tear in the innermost lining of the arterial wall known as the tunica intima. This allows blood to enter the space between the inner and outer layers leading to either narrowing or occlusion of the vessel. Strokes may then occur owing to occlusion of the vessel involved and poor collateral circulation or from thromboemoli occluding distal vessels. In noncontact sports, dissection of the cervical arteries (carotids and vertebrals) have been described in softball, cycling, skating, weightlifting, diving, and golf.[7]

Carotid artery dissection can occur extracranially or intracranially, and usually is a result of forceful head turning or Valsalva maneuvers in about 40% of people with spontaneous carotid artery dissections.[8] Some common risk factors for carotid artery dissection include connective tissue disorders, family history of dissection, spondylotic bone spurs, anatomic anomalies, and atherosclerotic plaque.[9] Specific to athletes, carotid dissections are usually the result of a direct blow to the artery (eg, baseball or softball strike to the neck). Other causes more specific to noncontact sports include stretch injuries such as cervical hyperextension, rotation, or traction, which can be seen in tennis, cycling, weightlifting, and less often golf (usually a vertebral artery injury; see below).[7] Carotid artery dissection typically presents with cervical pain and headache, although in most cases, there will be focal neurologic symptoms depending on the location of dissection and whether ischemia ensues.

Vertebral artery dissections usually occur between C1 and C2 or as the artery enters the C6 transverse foramen. This has been best described in golfers, and is commonly referred to as "golfer's stroke." Rapid head rotation through the golfer's swing leads to asymmetric forward and downward displacement of the contralateral atlantoaxial joint, leading to contralateral vertebral artery dissection given its fixed position between C1 and C2. A similar mechanism exists at C6 owing to contraction of a fibrous anchoring band leading to contusion of the artery in the transverse foramen.[9] Symptoms occur within seconds to days and include occipital headaches or neck pain (radiating to the ipsilateral frontotemporal areas), dysarthria, dysmetria, ataxia, diplopia, dysphagia, vertigo, nystagmus, ipsilateral Horner syndrome, hearing loss, and crossed sensory deficits.

The diagnosis of cervical artery dissection is most commonly made with imaging modalities such as MRI, MR angiography, or computed tomography angiography. Luminal irregularities, intimal flaps, pseudoaneurysms, complete vessel occlusion, or a tapered appearance of the vessel either as a "flame sign" or "string sign" are characteristics seen on angiography.[9] Carotid Doppler imaging is also useful for identifying carotid artery dissections, but is less sensitive.

The treatment and prognosis of cervical artery dissections varies and depends on many factors such as location (carotid vs vertebral, extracranial vs intracranial), presenting symptoms, acuity, and severity. If presenting symptoms include transient ischemic attack or stroke, patients should be treated with intravenous thrombolysis with alteplase (intravenous recombinant tissue plasminogen activator) if eligible.[10] There is evidence to support the use of aspirin over anticoagulation for patients who are presenting in the postacute setting with either extracranial (grade 2B) or intracranial (grade 2C) dissection, although some expert opinions differ on this.[11,12] There are no well-established guidelines on duration of treatment, although repeat imaging between 3 and 6 months to reevaluate the affected vessel and assess for recanalization/healing can often help to guide treatment duration. Endovascular options such as stenting are also available and usually reserved for dissections causing recurrent ischemic events despite antithrombotic therapy or for those who present with concurrent dissection and subarachnoid hemorrhage. Headaches and cervicalgia owing to dissection can usually be managed with common analgesics or preventive medications.

Complete or near complete recovery occurs in 70% to 85% of patients with extracranial dissection, although 10% to 25% will have disabling deficits, and the overall morbidity and mortality rates for extracranial dissection is 5% to 10% (higher with intracranial dissection). Carotid artery dissections more often present with ischemic strokes compared with vertebral artery dissections and, therefore, usually have a more unfavorable outcome at 3 months.[13] Most dissections undergo recanalization within the first several months. The rate of recurrence varies from study to study, and has not been well-established at this time. There are no generalized guidelines for return to play after a cervical artery dissection at this time and should be assessed at an individual level. For athletes with complete recanalization of a cervicocephalic dissection, return to play noncontact sports may be reasonable as long as blood pressure can be controlled, and avoidance of hyperflexion, hyperextension, or hyperrotation can be attained with sport performance. Consideration should be given to an exercise physiology evaluation to determine a safe threshold for exercise-associated increases in blood pressure and heart rate.

Patent Foramen Ovale as a Cause of Stroke

About 40% of ischemic strokes do not have an identifiable cause and are therefore classified as cryptogenic. Some cryptogenic strokes have been attributed to a "paradoxic embolism" crossing from the venous system into the arterial circulation through a patent foramen ovale (PFO; a connection between the right and left atria of the heart). For this to occur, there must initially be clot formation in the venous system (usually the deep veins of the pelvis or lower extremities). Deep vein thrombosis is a result of either vascular endothelial damage, stasis of blood flow, or hypercoagulability of blood as first described in 1856 by Rudolph Virchow.[14] More specifically, the most common risk factors associated with deep vein thrombosis, and specifically in young adults/athletes include hip or leg fractures, any major orthopedic or general surgeries, spinal cord injury, trauma, genetic predispositions, malignancy, oral contraceptive therapy, pregnancy, prolonged travel, and obesity.[15]

There are a few case reports and series describing athletes with acute strokes who were found to have PFOs with either a known deep vein thrombosis or negative stroke workup otherwise, thus attributing the stroke to a paradoxic embolus. Risk factors described in these cases included oral contraceptives, surgeries, genetic pre-disposition to clotting disorders, and long periods of travel.

The management of these athletes who may suffer a stroke with PFO is not well-established. Prospective, randomized trials concluded that there is no benefit of PFO closure to prevent recurrent strokes or transient ischemic attacks.[16,17] We recommend a multidisciplinary vascular neurology and interventional cardiology eval-uation to develop an individualized treatment approach for stroke risk reduction, re-covery, and consideration of return to play.

Heat Stroke

Heat stroke, which is a misnomer, is presented despite its lack of a vascular etiology, but rather to review the neurologic signs and symptoms which may present in noncon-tact athletes with excessive heat exposure. The definition of heat stroke is a core body temperature above 104°F (40°C) accompanied by hot, dry skin and central nervous system abnormalities such as delirium, convulsions, or coma. Heat stroke can be a manifestation of environmental high temperatures, strenuous exercise, or a combina-tion of both, as often seen with training athletes.[18] In the United States, the incidence of heat stroke is very low, with cases reported between 17.6 and 26.5 per 100,000 population.[19] Runners have the highest reported incidence of heat stroke for noncon-tact sports (football being the highest reported for contact sports).[18] Also, heat stroke is more commonly seen in people taking medications such as diuretics (which alter the salt and water content of the body), anticholinergic agents, amphetamines, cocaine, or medications that may impair sweating. The pathogenesis of heat stroke seems to be a combination of thermal dysregulation, acute phase response, heat shock proteins, and the systemic and cellular response to this heat stress on the body.[20]

When discussing heat stroke, it should be noted that it is the most severe form of a constellation of progressive symptoms in a general condition known as heat illness. The spectrum of heat illness (from least to most severe) includes heat edema, heat rash, heat cramps, heat syncope, heat exhaustion, and heat stroke.[21] These condi-tions are characterized in **Table 4**.

The most common signs and symptoms of athletes suffering from heat stroke are hyperthermia, tachycardia, tachypnea, and central nervous system dysfunction, such as confusion, impaired judgment, delirium, or coma. In most athletes, exertional heat stroke presents as a combination of respiratory alkalosis and lactic acidosis with severe cases presenting with multi-system organ failure. The cornerstone of treating patients suffering from heat stroke is immediate cooling. The use of pharmacologic agents to accelerate the cooling process, such as dantrolene, have been shown to be ineffective in heat stroke.[22] If not recognized, heat stroke can be fatal. Rapid iden-tification of the signs and symptoms of heat stroke followed by fanning, applying cold water to the skin, ice packs, and cooling blankets are effective methods of cooling and can be life saving. With proper recognition and cooling, most athletes fully recover and should be advised to rest and avoid any heat stress for a minimum of 48 hours before returning to activity, although data on return to play are limited.[23]

Knowledge of heat illnesses, especially in training athletes, may greatly lower the incidence through prevention. To best prevent heat stroke in athletes, practices and training should be scheduled during cooler times of the day when able, athletes should be provided frequent breaks, emphasis on adequate water and salty foods should be made, and training should be moved inside when environmental conditions are too extreme. Of these preventative measures, hydration may be the most important. For every 1% of body weight lost to dehydration, it has been shown that core body tem-perature rises 0.15°C to 0.2°C.[21]

Table 4
Heat illness

	Core Temperature	Signs and Symptoms	Treatment
Heat edema	Normal	Dependent edema (ankles, feet, hands)	Rest
Heat rash	Normal	Pruritic rash usually over clothed areas	Rest
Heat cramps	Normal or elevated <104°F (40°C)	Painful muscle contractions (calf, quadriceps, abdominal)	Stretch, ice, massage, oral fluid replacement
Heat syncope	Normal or elevated <104°F (40°C)	Loss of consciousness, rapid mental status recovery	Rest supine with feet up; monitor vital signs
Exertional heat exhaustion	98.6°F–104°F (37°C–40°C)	Dizziness, fatigue, nausea, vomiting, headache, hypotension, flushing, diaphoresis, normal mental status	ABCs, cooling, rest, monitor temperature and vital signs, oral fluids
Exertional Heat stroke	>104°F (40°C)	Mental status change, ataxia, nausea, vomiting, headache, hypotension, tachycardia, tachypnea, anhydrosis, coma, DIC, ARF	ABCs, rapid cooling, call EMS, monitor temperature and vital signs, IVFs if available

Abbreviations: ABS, airway, breathing, circulating; ARF, acute respiratory failure; DIC, disseminated intravascular coagulation; EMS, emergency medical services; IVFs, intravenous fluids.
Data from Howe AS, Boden BP. Heat-related illness in athletes. Am J Sports Med 2007;35(8): 1384–95; and Coris EE, Ramirez AM, Van Durme DJ. Heat illness in athletes: the dangerous combination of heat, humidity and exercise. Sports Med 2004;34(1):9–16.

MUSCLE AND NERVE DISORDERS AFTER NONCONTACT SPORTS INJURY
Complex Regional Pain Syndrome

Complex regional pain syndrome (CRPS) is a disorder classically characterized by pain, swelling, erythema, vasomotor changes, and bone demineralization that can lead to significant disability. The incidence varies, but a recent population-based study suggested 26.2 cases per 100,000 person-years.[24] There is usually an inciting event with the most common being fracture, followed by trauma causing soft tissue injury (eg, sprain), and then surgery. Up to 10% of patients will not have an identifiable cause.[25] Symptoms completely resolve within 5 years in 75% of patients, with a recurrence of 10%.[26] The pathophysiology is not well understood, but bone microvascular changes, increase in proinflammatory cytokines (interleukin [IL]-1β, IL-2, IL-6, tumor necrosis factor-alpha), central sensitization, sympathetic hyperactivity with catecholamine hypersensitivity, and autoimmune mechanisms have been suggested.[27–29] Neurology consultation is frequently requested because of the weakness associated with CRPS, or the development of other movement disorders including contractures, tremor, and dystonia,[30] which is seen less commonly.

The diagnosis of CRPS is clinical and should be suspected in anyone presenting with signs and symptoms and evidence of an inciting event. Diagnostic criteria have been developed and we recommend use of the Budapest Consensus Criteria[31] (https://www.ncbi.nlm.nih.gov/pubmed/20493633).

The best treatment for CRPS is prevention. Several small, randomized, controlled trials have evaluated vitamin C (>500 mg/d) immediately after a fracture or surgery for a duration of 50 days with some studies showing a significant reduction in development of CRPS, although others showed no benefit.[32,33] Given its relative safety, vitamin C should be considered in any patient undergoing limb surgery or who suffers a distal limb fracture. Once CRPS develops, nonsteroidal antiinflammatory drugs are first-line therapies, with typical neuropathic pain agents such as anticonvulsants (gabapentin and pregabalin) and tricyclic antidepressants (amitriptyline and nortriptyline) being second-line therapies. A single, small, placebo-controlled trial of 58 patients investigating gabapentin was completed and showed no benefit.[34] Other therapies may include bisphosphonates, topical lidocaine, or capsaicin creams. A final option to consider is oral glucocorticoids. Given their side effect profile and limited evidence of efficacy, oral glucocorticoids should be reserved for patients with symptoms refractory to other agents.[34]

Concurrent medical therapy along with multidisciplinary treatments including physical, occupational, and psychosocial therapy may be beneficial as well. If these fail, then referral to a pain specialist should be provided for consideration of other, more invasive approaches, such as nerve blocks, trigger point injections, spinal cord stimulators, sympathectomy,[35] and epidural clonidine injection or infusion.[36]

Rhabdomyolysis

Rhabdomyolysis is a syndrome of muscle breakdown and necrosis with resultant release of its intracellular components into systemic circulation. Recurrent episodes after seemingly insufficient exertion, a family history of rhabdomyolysis, or a history of exercise intolerance with muscle cramps going back to childhood, should prompt consideration of a metabolic myopathy.

Rhabdomyolysis can be owing to trauma, overexertion, or other nonexertional, nontraumatic causes (eg, amphetamines, cocaine, medications like statins, certain viruses). This can lead to a triad of symptoms including severe muscle pain characteristically described as diffuse myalgias, weakness, and dark urine. Multiorgan system involvement can be life threatening, with a mortality rate of up to 8%.[37] The overall incidence of exertional (nontraumatic) rhabdomyolysis is likely underreported and estimated at 26,000 cases per year.[38]

In athletes with rhabdomyolysis, the serum creatinine kinase (CK) level will be increased to at least 5 times the upper limit of normal and can be more than 100,000 IU/L. CK begins to increase within several hours of the inciting activity and peaks within 1 to 5 days. Marked electrolyte abnormalities occur, including hyperkalemia and hyperphosphatemia, owing to release from muscle cell breakdown. Hypocalcemia results from calcium deposition in the damaged muscle tissue. These abnormalities can lead to a variety of issues, including cardiac arrhythmias and diffuse weakness. Acute kidney injury is a common complication that may lead to renal failure in up to 4% of cases.[37] This can be owing to marked volume depletion causing renal ischemia or heme pigment casts causing renal tubular obstruction. The most extreme cases include reports of compartment syndrome and disseminated intravascular coagulation, although these are rare.

Diagnosis is based on a typical presentation; elevation of the CK levels in the blood, and myoglobinuria on urinalysis. Further diagnostic workup usually is not necessary and prompt supportive care should ensue. Treatment involves aggressive volume resuscitation with crystalloid intravenous fluids and correction of electrolyte abnormalities.

With noncontact sports, it often results from overexertion in the setting of sudden alteration in a training regimen, improper hydration, or lack of appropriate training for a particular event. Sports that have reported exertional rhabdomyolysis include swimming, weightlifting, and running.[39] Supplements have also been linked as potential contributors, with at least 1 case of a weightlifter who developed rhabdomyolysis with compartment syndrome while on creatine monophosphate.[40] High-protein and caffeine supplements, as well as the use of nonsteroidal antiinflammatory drugs, have been linked to rhabdomyolysis.[41]

There are no evidence-based guidelines for return to play. For adolescents and adults a Consortium for Health and Military Performance[42] consensus guideline recommends a conservative return to play model (http://journals.lww.com/acsm-csmr/fulltext/2008/11000/Return_to_Physical_Activity_After_Exertional.8.aspx). Other authors have suggested that patients who are deemed low risk (rapid CK correction, no major organ involvement, no personal or family history of rhabdomyolysis) may be able to return more quickly to regular activity once symptom free.[39]

Dystonia

Dystonia is a hyperkinetic movement disorder defined as sustained or intermittent muscle contraction causing abnormal, often repetitive movements, postures, or both. It is often initiated or worsened by movement and the muscles involved in the action are typically the ones involved in the dystonia. It can be classified by age of onset, affected body region (focal, segmental, generalized), its temporal pattern (static, progressive, task specific), and by any associated features like other movement disorders (tremor, myoclonus, parkinsonism).[43] In sports, dystonia usually presents as a task-specific problem with 2 well-described disorders.

The first is known as runner's dystonia. There are multiple case series describing this disorder,[44,45] which involves the onset of dystonia in the lower limb, not necessarily just in runners, but any athlete undergoing repetitive lower limb exercise. Sports reported as causative factors include running and cycling.[46] Athlete's dystonia usually starts in one leg and is task specific. Athletes may notice relief with a "sensory trick," which involves touching a specific area in the affected limb that provides relief of the dystonia or pain. In most patients, symptoms may progress to involve walking. Often the diagnosis is delayed, perhaps because of underrecognition, which can lead to unnecessary and unsuccessful invasive procedures.[47] Diagnosis is primarily clinical, but electromyography can be helpful. Unfortunately, this disorder tends to be refractory to treatment leading to much frustration, because it limits the athlete's ability to exercise. Treatments most commonly used are presented in **Table 5**.

The second disorder is another task-specific movement disorder called "yips." It is described as an involuntary motor phenomenon in the wrist and forearm muscles that occurs while putting during golf. Yips are exacerbated by high-stress situations and symptoms typically include jerks (most common), tremors, or "freezing" of the hands and forearms, resulting in poor putting performance. Owing to the high-stress circumstance, it has been suggested that yips could reflect performance anxiety.[7] However electromyography, electroencephalogram with somatosensory evoked potentials, and video analysis have been used to investigate this disorder. Cocontraction of the wrist flexors and extensors was found in 50% of yips-affected golfers immediately before putting, with all affected golfers having visible twisting and jerking movements of the wrists and forearms during putting.[48] This led to the conclusion that yips are a task-specific dystonia. The prevalence of this disorder is not well known, but is estimated it to be between 16.7% and 22.4%.[49] The average yips-affected golfer plays 75 rounds per year.[50] Treatment is symptomatic and, as with other types of dystonia, sensory tricks are useful (such as altering grip). Medications used for treatment of yips are also listed in **Table 5**.

Table 5
Treatment options for dystonia

Name of Agent	Typical Daily Dosage (Usually Divided into 2–3 Doses)	Common Adverse Effects
First line		
Botulinum toxin	Site and toxin type specific, injected approximately every 3 mo.	Weakness, Bruising, Pain
Second line		
Dopamine agents		
Carbidopa/levodopa	75/300–500/2000 mg	Orthostasis, nausea
Tetrabenazine	12.5–100 mg	Akithisia, anxiety, suicidality, parkinsonism
Benzodiazepines		
Clonazepam	1–4 mg	Drowsiness, fatigue, transaminitis
Anticholinergics		
Trihexyphenidyl	6–40 mg	Blurry vision, confusion, urinary retention, constipation
GABA-B agonist		
Baclofen	40–120 mg	Drowsiness, fatigue, nausea, muscle weakness
Anticonvulsants		
Carbamazepine	300–600 mg	Dizziness, nausea, constipation, ataxia, blurry vision
Gabapentin	900–3600 mg	Leg edema, drowsiness, dizziness

SPINAL CORD INJURIES AMONG NONCONTACT ATHLETES
Cauda Equina and Conus Medullaris Syndromes

Lumbosacral radiculopathy is a common disorder with an overall prevalence of 3% to 5% among adults.[51] Usually, this is in the setting of lumbar neural foramen degeneration seen with aging, but in relationship to sports, it can be the result of a traumatic disk herniation compressing multiple nerve roots within the central canal. When this occurs below the level of L2 it causes cauda equina syndrome, whereas if it is at L2 where the spinal cord typically ends it causes conus medullaris syndrome.

Cauda equina syndrome is a neurologic emergency resulting from compression, or infiltration, of multiple lumbosacral nerve roots within the central spinal canal.[52] The overall incidence is reported to be one case per 50,000 to 100,000 people, with up to 70% of these caused by disk herniation.[53] Presentation typically begins with intense low back pain, including a radicular component, that is worse when lying flat and accompanied by asymmetric saddle anesthesia, decreased rectal tone, micturition dysfunction, defecation dysfunction, and asymmetric weakness. On examination there will be asymmetric weakness in muscles innervated by the impinged nerve roots with radicular distribution of sensory loss. Reflexes are reduced and sphincter function on digital rectal examination will disclose decreased tone.

Conus medullaris syndrome is similar, but results from compression or infiltration of the terminal conus portion of the spinal cord. Comparatively, in conus medullaris syndrome there is often earlier prominent urinary retention and constipation, as well as sexual dysfunction. The sensory loss is often more symmetric and motor loss is much less than that seen in cauda equina syndrome. Pain is also reported less commonly.[54]

Diagnosis of either condition is made based on history and physical examination, followed by emergent MRI of the lumbosacral spine. Contrast should only be given if traumatic compression is not suspected and metastatic, infectious, or infiltrative disease is thought to be the cause.

Management for both syndromes includes immediate surgical evaluation and decompression with or without discectomy within 48 hours of symptom onset.[55,56] Return to play has been evaluated for symptomatic disc herniation (without resultant cauda equina or conus medullaris syndromes), with studies indicating that conservatively managed athletes can return in less than 5 months but if surgical management is required, patients will be out for closer to 6 months.[57] Because these syndromes are more severe, resulting in surgery almost as a rule, it is likely these athletes would miss substantially more time and require more physical therapy for recovery.

To our knowledge, there have been no studies to date regarding the incidence of these syndromes in noncontact sports. Weightlifting is commonly associated with injury to the lower back. General weightlifting resulted in low back injury in 20% of athletes in 1 study, and this increased to 30% to 50% with powerlifting.[58] Low back injury was associated with deadlifts and squat lifts.

Cervical Cord Neurapraxia

Cervical cord neurapraxia is a sports-related injury defined by a transient neurologic deficit after trauma to the cervical spinal cord. It was initially described by Torg and colleagues[59] as transient quadriplegia after trauma to the cervical spine. Neurologic deficits are recognized as ranging from limb paresthesias to flaccid quadriplegia, depending on the region of the cord affected and the severity. Typically, deficits can last several minutes to 48 hours. The mechanism of injury is typically cervical hyperextension, hyperflexion or excessive axial load where the spine is temporarily "pinched."[60] In adults, preexisting cervical spine stenosis has a strong causal relationship[61,62] and in the pediatric and adolescent population, the relative immaturity of the cervical spine may be a risk factor.[62]

Management primarily consists of rest and physical therapy, but neuropathic pain agents can be used, if needed. Return to play may be considered after anterior cervical discectomy and fusion, if the athlete was asymptomatic from cervical radiculopathy symptoms,[62–64] although the recurrence rate is suggested to be as high as 56%.[60] Owing to the risk of recurrence, several authors have suggested that even a single episode of cervical cord neurapraxia should preclude return to sport participation.[65]

Surfer's Myelopathy

Surfer's myelopathy is rare, but may occur in beginner surfers who develop an acute paraparesis while surfing for the first time. It was first described in 2004 and subsequently there have been more than 60 reported cases in the literature.[7] It begins with the surfer feeling a "crack" or "pop" sensation followed by back pain and lower limb weakness. Myelopathy symptoms progress to mimic acute spinal infarction with paraplegia, urinary retention, and spinal level on sensory examination. Diagnosis may be confirmed with MRI revealing restricted diffusion usually at the level of the artery of Adamkiewicz around T8 to T12. Unfortunately, the prognosis is poor with many patients having significant residual deficits; no therapy has proven effective for this condition.

REFERENCES

1. Marar M, McIlvain NM, Fields SK, Comstock RD. Epidemiology of concussions among United States high school athletes in 20 sports. Am J Sports Med 2012; 40(4):747–55.
2. Giza CC, Kutcher JS, Ashwal S, et al. Summary of evidence-based guideline update: evaluation and management of concussion in sports: report of the Guideline Development Subcommittee of the American Academy of Neurology. Neurology 2013;80(24):2250–7.
3. Broglio SP, Cantu RC, Gioia GA, et al. National Athletic Trainers' Association position statement: management of sport concussion. J Athl Train 2014;49(2): 245–65.
4. McCrory P, Meeuwisse WH, Aubry M, et al. Consensus statement on concussion in sport: the 4th International Conference on Concussion in Sport held in Zurich, November 2012. Br J Sports Med 2013;47(5):250–8.
5. Leddy J, Hinds A, Sirica D, et al. The role of controlled exercise in concussion management. PM R 2016;8(3 Suppl):S91–100.
6. Lozano R, Naghavi M, Foreman K, et al. Global and regional mortality from 235 causes of death for 20 age groups in 1990 and 2010: a systematic analysis for the Global Burden of Disease Study 2010. Lancet 2012;380(9859):2095–128.
7. Conidi F. Some unusual sports-related neurologic conditions. Continuum (Minneap Minn) 2014;20(6 Sports Neurology):1645–56.
8. Dharmasaroja P, Dharmasaroja P. Sports-related internal carotid artery dissection: pathogenesis and therapeutic point of view. Neurologist 2008;14(5):307–11.
9. Maroon JC, Gardner P, Abla AA, et al. "Golfer's stroke": golf-induced stroke from vertebral artery dissection. Surg Neurol 2007;67(2):163–8 [discussion: 168].
10. Engelter ST, Rutgers MP, Hatz F, et al. Intravenous thrombolysis in stroke attributable to cervical artery dissection. Stroke 2009;40(12):3772–6.
11. Kennedy F, Lanfranconi S, Hicks C, et al. Antiplatelets vs anticoagulation for dissection: CADISS nonrandomized arm and meta-analysis. Neurology 2012; 79(7):686–9.
12. Chowdhury MM, Sabbagh CN, Jackson D, et al. Antithrombotic treatment for acute extracranial carotid artery dissections: a meta-analysis. Eur J Vasc Endovasc Surg 2015;50(2):148–56.
13. Debette S, Grond-Ginsbach C, Bodenant M, et al. Differential features of carotid and vertebral artery dissections: the CADISP study. Neurology 2011;77(12): 1174–81.
14. Bagot CN, Arya R. Virchow and his triad: a question of attribution. Br J Haematol 2008;143(2):180–90.
15. Anderson FA Jr, Spencer FA. Risk factors for venous thromboembolism. Circulation 2003;107(23 Suppl 1):I9–16.
16. Furlan AJ, Reisman M, Massaro J, et al. Closure or medical therapy for cryptogenic stroke with patent foramen ovale. N Engl J Med 2012;366(11):991–9.
17. Carroll JD, Saver JL, Thaler DE, et al. Closure of patent foramen ovale versus medical therapy after cryptogenic stroke. N Engl J Med 2013;368(12):1092–100.
18. Knochel JP, Reed G. Disorders of heat regulation. In: Narins RG, editor. Maxwell & Kleeman's clinical disorders of fluid and electrolyte metabolism, vol. 5. New York: McGraw-Hill; 1994. p. 1549–90.
19. Jones TS, Liang AP, Kilbourne EM, et al. Morbidity and mortality associated with the July 1980 heat wave in St Louis and Kansas City, Mo. JAMA 1982;247(24): 3327–31.

20. Bouchama A, Knochel JP. Heat stroke. N Engl J Med 2002;346(25):1978–88.
21. Coris EE, Ramirez AM, Van Durme DJ. Heat illness in athletes: the dangerous combination of heat, humidity and exercise. Sports Med 2004;34(1):9–16.
22. Bouchama A, Cafege A, Devol EB, et al. Ineffectiveness of dantrolene sodium in the treatment of heatstroke. Crit Care Med 1991;19(2):176–80.
23. Pryor RR, Roth RN, Suyama J, et al. Exertional heat illness: emerging concepts and advances in prehospital care. Prehosp Disaster Med 2015;30(3):297–305.
24. Winston P. Early treatment of acute complex regional pain syndrome after fracture or injury with prednisone: why is there a failure to treat? a case series. Pain Res Manag 2016;2016:7019196.
25. de Mos M, de Bruijn AG, Huygen FJ, et al. The incidence of complex regional pain syndrome: a population-based study. Pain 2007;129(1–2):12–20.
26. Sandroni P, Benrud-Larson LM, McClelland RL, et al. Complex regional pain syndrome type I: incidence and prevalence in Olmsted county, a population-based study. Pain 2003;103(1–2):199–207.
27. Corradini C, Bosizio C, Moretti A. Algodystrophy (CRPS) in minor orthopedic surgery. Clin Cases Miner Bone Metab 2015;12(Suppl 1):21–5.
28. Bussa M, Guttilla D, Lucia M, et al. Complex regional pain syndrome type I: a comprehensive review. Acta Anaesthesiol Scand 2015;59(6):685–97.
29. Wasner G, Schattschneider J, Heckmann K, et al. Vascular abnormalities in reflex sympathetic dystrophy (CRPS I): mechanisms and diagnostic value. Brain 2001; 124(Pt 3):587–99.
30. Birklein F, Riedl B, Sieweke N, et al. Neurological findings in complex regional pain syndromes–analysis of 145 cases. Acta Neurol Scand 2000;101(4):262–9.
31. Harden RN, Bruehl S, Perez RS, et al. Validation of proposed diagnostic criteria (the "Budapest criteria") for complex regional pain syndrome. Pain 2010;150(2): 268–74.
32. Meena S, Sharma P, Gangary SK, et al. Role of vitamin C in prevention of complex regional pain syndrome after distal radius fractures: a meta-analysis. Eur J Orthop Surg Traumatol 2015;25(4):637–41.
33. Ekrol I, Duckworth AD, Ralston SH, et al. The influence of vitamin C on the outcome of distal radial fractures: a double-blind, randomized controlled trial. J Bone Joint Surg Am 2014;96(17):1451–9.
34. Abdi Salahadin MDP. Complex regional pain syndrome in adults: prevention and management. Vol 20162016.
35. O'Connell NE, Wand BM, Gibson W, et al. Local anaesthetic sympathetic blockade for complex regional pain syndrome. Cochrane Database Syst Rev 2016;(7):CD004598.
36. Kingery WS. A critical review of controlled clinical trials for peripheral neuropathic pain and complex regional pain syndromes. Pain 1997;73(2):123–39.
37. Bagley WH, Yang H, Shah KH. Rhabdomyolysis. Intern Emerg Med 2007;2(3): 210–8.
38. DeFilippis EM, Kleiman DA, Derman PB, et al. Spinning-induced rhabdomyolysis and the risk of compartment syndrome and acute kidney injury: two cases and a review of the literature. Sports Health 2014;6(4):333–5.
39. Tietze DC, Borchers J. Exertional rhabdomyolysis in the athlete: a clinical review. Sports Health 2014;6(4):336–9.
40. Do KD, Bellabarba C, Bhananker SM. Exertional rhabdomyolysis in a bodybuilder following overexertion: a possible link to creatine overconsumption. Clin J Sport Med 2007;17(1):78–9.

41. Hummel K, Gregory A, Desai N, et al. Rhabdomyolysis in adolescent athletes: review of cases. Phys Sportsmed 2016;44(2):195–9.
42. O'Connor FG, Brennan FH Jr, Campbell W, et al. Return to physical activity after exertional rhabdomyolysis. Curr Sports Med Rep 2008;7(6):328–31.
43. Shanker V, Bressman SB. Diagnosis and management of dystonia. Continuum (Minneap Minn) 2016;22(4 Movement Disorders):1227–45.
44. Cutsforth-Gregory JK, Ahlskog JE, McKeon A, et al. Repetitive exercise dystonia: a difficult to treat hazard of runner and non-runner athletes. Parkinsonism Relat Disord 2016;27:74–80.
45. Wu LJ, Jankovic J. Runner's dystonia. J Neurol Sci 2006;251(1–2):73–6.
46. Katz M, Byl NN, San Luciano M, et al. Focal task-specific lower extremity dystonia associated with intense repetitive exercise: a case series. Parkinsonism Relat Disord 2013;19(11):1033–8.
47. McClinton S, Heiderscheit BC. Diagnosis of primary task-specific lower extremity dystonia in a runner. J Orthop Sports Phys Ther 2012;42(8):688–97.
48. Adler CH, Crews D, Hentz JG, et al. Abnormal co-contraction in yips-affected but not unaffected golfers: evidence for focal dystonia. Neurology 2005;64(10):1813–4.
49. Klampfl MK, Philippen PB, Lobinger BH. Self-report vs. kinematic screening test: prevalence, demographics, and sports biography of yips-affected golfers. J Sports Sci 2015;33(7):655–64.
50. Smith AM, Adler CH, Crews D, et al. The 'yips' in golf: a continuum between a focal dystonia and choking. Sports Med 2003;33(1):13–31.
51. Tarulli AW, Raynor EM. Lumbosacral radiculopathy. Neurol Clin 2007;25(2):387–405.
52. Tarulli AW. Disorders of the cauda equina. Continuum (Minneap Minn) 2015;21(1 Spinal Cord Disorders):146–58.
53. Fuso FA, Dias AL, Letaif OB, et al. Epidemiological study of cauda equina syndrome. Acta Ortop Bras 2013;21(3):159–62.
54. Salardini A, Biller J. The hospital neurology book. Chapter 39. Columbus (OH): McGraw-Hill Education; 2016.
55. Shapiro S. Medical realities of cauda equina syndrome secondary to lumbar disc herniation. Spine 2000;25(3):348–51 [discussion: 352].
56. Todd NV. Cauda equina syndrome: the timing of surgery probably does influence outcome. Br J Neurosurg 2005;19(4):301–6 [discussion: 307–8].
57. Iwamoto J, Sato Y, Takeda T, et al. Return to play after conservative treatment in athletes with symptomatic lumbar disc herniation: a practice-based observational study. Open Access J Sports Med 2011;2:25–31.
58. Keogh JW, Winwood PW. The epidemiology of injuries across the weight-training sports. Sports Med 2016;47(3):479–501.
59. Torg JS, Naranja RJ Jr, Pavlov H, et al. The relationship of developmental narrowing of the cervical spinal canal to reversible and irreversible injury of the cervical spinal cord in football players. J Bone Joint Surg Am 1996;78(9):1308–14.
60. Page S, Guy JA. Neurapraxia, "stingers," and spinal stenosis in athletes. South Med J 2004;97(8):766–9.
61. Clark AJ, Auguste KI, Sun PP. Cervical spinal stenosis and sports-related cervical cord neurapraxia. Neurosurg Focus 2011;31(5):E7.
62. Herman MJ. Cervical spine injuries in the pediatric and adolescent athlete. Instr Course Lect 2006;55:641–6.
63. Joaquim AF, Hsu WK, Patel AA. Cervical spine surgery in professional athletes: a systematic review. Neurosurg Focus 2016;40(4):E10.

64. Maroon JC, El-Kadi H, Abla AA, et al. Cervical neurapraxia in elite athletes: evaluation and surgical treatment. Report of five cases. J Neurosurg Spine 2007;6(4): 356–63.
65. Castro FP Jr. Stingers, cervical cord neurapraxia, and stenosis. Clin Sports Med 2003;22(3):483–92.

Index

Note: Page numbers of article titles are in **boldface** type.

A

Abortive therapies
    in PTH management, 515
Acute brain injury
    in combat sports, 524–527
Acute postinjury assessment
    in neuropsychological screening of SRCs, 494–495
ADHD. *See* Attention-deficit/hyperactivity disorder (ADHD)
Anxiety
    sport-related performance, 539
Anxiety disorders
    in sports, 539–541
        medical conditions, 541
        prevalence of, 541
        treatment of, 541
Athlete(s)
    sleep quality and sleep disorders in, **547–557** *See also* Sleep; Sleep disorders; Sleep
        issues
Attention-deficit/hyperactivity disorder (ADHD)
    in sports, 542–543

B

Baseline neurocognitive testing
    Benign exertional headache, 516
Biomarker(s)
    blood-based
        in SRC identification, **473–485** *See also* Blood-based biomarkers, in SRC
            identification
Bipolar disorder
    in sports, 538–539
Blood-based biomarkers
    in SRC identification, **473–485**
        overview of, 476–480
Brain injury
    acute and chronic
        in combat sports, 524–527
    traumatic *See* Traumatic brain injury (TBI)
Burners and stingers, 561

Neurol Clin 35 (2017) 589–599
http://dx.doi.org/10.1016/S0733-8619(17)30053-1
0733-8619/17

neurologic.theclinics.com

Moving?

Make sure your subscription moves with you!

To notify us of your new address, find your **Clinics Account Number** (located on your mailing label above your name), and contact customer service at:

Email: journalscustomerservice-usa@elsevier.com

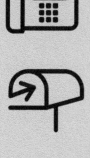

800-654-2452 (subscribers in the U.S. & Canada)
314-447-8871 (subscribers outside of the U.S. & Canada)

Fax number: 314-447-8029

Elsevier Health Sciences Division
Subscription Customer Service
3251 Riverport Lane
Maryland Heights, MO 63043

*To ensure uninterrupted delivery of your subscription, please notify us at least 4 weeks in advance of move.

Printed and bound by CPI Group (UK) Ltd, Croydon, CR0 4YY

07/10/2024

01040503-0001